The Journal of Mind and Behavior

Editorial Board

MW00906393

CONTENTS OF BACK ISSUES

The Poverty of Paradigmaticism: A Symptom of the Crisis in Sociological Explanation. *Gerard A. Postiglione, University of Hong Kong, and Joseph A. Scimecca, George Mason University.*
Social Change Versus Perceived Villainy. *Albert Lauterbach, Sarah Lawrence College.*
Left and Right in Personality and Ideology: An Attempt at Clarification. *William F. Stone, University of Maine.*
Benefic Autonomy: Thomas More as Exemplar. *Steven E. Salmony, The John Umstead Hospital, and Richard Smoke, Peace and Common Security.*
Toward a Science of Experience. *A. Kukla, University of Toronto.*
Retrospective Phenomenological Assessment: Mapping Consciousness in Reference to Specific Stimulus Conditions. *Ronald J. Pekala, Coatesville V.A. Medical Center, and Cathrine F. Wenger, City College of Detroit.*
Toward Pepitone's Vision of a Normative Social Psychology: What is a Social Norm? *Leigh S. Shaffer, West Chester State College.*

Volume 4, Number 3, Summer 1983

Von Osten's Horse, Hamlet's Question, and the Mechanistic View of Causality: Implications for a Post-Crisis Social Psychology. *Ralph L. Rosnow, Temple University.*
Functionalism and the Definition of Theoretical Terms. *Austen Clark, University of Tulsa.*
The Theory of "Formative Causation" and its Implications for Archetypes, Parallel Inventions, and the "Hundredth Monkey Phenomenon." *Carolin S. Keutzer, University of Oregon.*
Synthesizing the Everyday World. *Andrew R. Fuller, The College of Staten Island, C.U.N.Y.*
On the Nature of Relationships Involving the Observer and the Observed Phenomenon in Psychology and Physics. *Douglas M. Snyder, The Professional School.*
Homeopathy and Psychiatry. *Daphna Slonim, UCLA-Sepulveda, V.A. Medical Center, and Kerrin White, McLean Hospital.*

Volume 4, Number 4, Autumn 1983

The Opening of the Black Box: Is Psychology Prepared? *Uriel G. Foa and David L. Margules, Temple University.*
The Experience of a Conscious Self. *Thomas Natsoulas, University of California, Davis.*
Causal Attributions: Phenomenological and Dialectical Aspects. *Robert E. Lana and Marianthi Georgoudi, Temple University.*
The Implications of Langer's Philosophy of Mind for a Science of Psychology. *Joseph R. Royce, University of Alberta.*
General Contextualism, Ecological Science and Cognitive Research. *Robert R. Hoffman, Adelphi University, and James M. Nead, University of Minnesota.*

Volume 5, Number 1, Winter 1984

Desires Don't Cause Actions. *J. Michael Russell, California State University, Fullerton.*
Natural Science and Human Science Approaches to the Study of Human Freedom. *Malcolm R. Westcott, York University.*
Empirical Structures of Mind: Cognition, Linguistics, and Transformation. *Robert Haskell, University of New England.*
The Pleasures of Thought: A Theory of Cognitive Hedonics. *Colin Martindale, University of Maine, Orono.*
Lucid Dreaming: A Review and Experiential Study of Waking Intrusions during Stage REM Sleep. *Edward Covello, Pacific-Sierra Research Corporation.*
A Critical Look at Castaneda's Critics. *Anton F. Kootte, University of North Florida.*

Volume 5, Number 2, Spring 1984

The Principle of Parsimony and Some Applications in Psychology. *Robert Epstein, Northeastern University and Cambridge Center for Behavioral Studies.*
Affection as a Cognitive Judgmental Process: A Theoretical Assumption Put to Test Through Brain-Lateralization Methodology. *Joseph F. Rychlak, Loyola University of Chicago, and Brent D. Slife, University of Santa Clara.*
A Psycho-Neuro-Endocrine Framework for Depression: A Clinically Eclectic Approach. *Elliot M. Frohman, University of California at San Diego and The Winfield Foundation.*

A Biofunctional Model of Distributed Mental Content, Mental Structures, Awareness, and Attention. *Asghar Iran-Nejad and Andrew Ortony, University of Illinois at Urbana-Champaign.*
The Double Bind and Koan Zen. *Patrick Jichaku, George Y. Fujita, and S.I. Shapiro, University of Hawaii.*
Occultism is not Science: A Reply to Kootte. *Richard de Mille, Santa Barbara, California.*

Volume 5, Number 3, Summer 1984

The Classification of Psychology among the Sciences from Francis Bacon to Boniface Kedrov. *Claude M.J. Braun, University of Quebec at Montreal, and Jacinthe M.C. Baribeau, Concordia University, Montreal.*
What is a Perceptual Mistake? *Aaron Ben-Zeev, University of Haifa.*
Affect: A Functional Perspective. *Asghar Iran-Nejad, Gerald L. Clore, and Richard J. Vondruska, University of Illinois at Urbana-Champaign.*
The Subjective Organization of Personal Consciousness: A Concept of Conscious Personality. *Thomas Natsoulas, University of California, Davis.*
The Effects of Sensation Seeking and Misattribution of Arousal on Dyadic Interactions Between Similar or Dissimilar Strangers. *Sarah Williams and Richard M. Ryckman, University of Maine at Orono.*
Fatalism as an Animistic Attribution Process. *Leigh S. Shaffer, West Chester University.* .

Volume 5, Number 4, Autumn 1984

Logical Learning Theory: Kuhnian Anomaly or Medievalism Revisited? *Joseph F. Rychlak, Loyola University of Chicago.*
Mental Activity and Physical Reality. *Douglas M. Snyder, Berkeley, California.*
Unity and Multiplicity in Hypnosis, Commissurotomy, and Multiple Personality Disorder. *David G. Benner, Wheaton College, and C. Stephen Evans, St. Olaf College.*
A Comparison of Three Ways of Knowing: Categorical, Structural, and Affirmative. *Viki McCabe, University of California, Los Angeles.*
Two Alternative Epistemological Frameworks in Psychology: The Typological and Variational Modes of Thinking. *Jaan Valsiner, University of North Carolina at Chapel Hill.*
Background and Change in B.F. Skinner's Metatheory from 1930 to 1938. *S.R. Coleman, Cleveland State University.*
A Critical Look at "A Critical Look": Castaneda Recrudescent. *Jordan Paper, York University.*
Logic is not Occultism. *Anton F. Kootte, University of North Florida.*

Volume 6, Numbers 1 and 2, Winter and Spring, 1985 (Special Issue)

The Sexual Body: An Interdisciplinary Perspective by Arthur Efron, SUNY-Buffalo.
Chapter One: *Introduction: The Perspective of the Sexual Body.*
Chapter Two: *Psychoanalysis as the Key Discipline.*
Chapter Three: *Analogues of Original Sin: The Postulate of Innate Destructive Aggression.*
Chapter Four: *The Reichian Tradition: A View of the Sexual Body.*
Chapter Five: *Challenges to Psychoanalytic Theory: Recent Developments.*
Chapter Six: *Reinventing the Asexual Infant: On the Recent "Explosion" in Infant Research.*
Chapter Seven: *The Adult Sexual Body: A Missing Theory.*
Chapter Eight: *The Sexual Body, Psychoanalysis and Science: Bowlby, Peterfreund, and Kohut.*
Chapter Nine: *Lichtenstein, Holland, and Lacan: Ambivalence Toward the Sexual Body, Cooptation, and Defiance.*
Chapter Ten: *World Hypotheses and Interdisciplinary Sciences in Intimate Relation.*

Volume 6, Number 3, Summer 1985

The Ethical Ramifications of Mediation Theory. *Paul G. Muscari, State University College of New York at Glens Falls.*
Logical Behaviorism and the Simulation of Mental Episodes. *Dale Jacquette, University of Nebraska at Lincoln.*
An Introduction to the Perceptual Kind of Conception of Direct (Reflective) Consciousness. *Thomas Natsoulas, University of California, Davis.*
The Fallacious Origin of the Mind-Body Problem: A Reconsideration of Descartes' Method and Results. *Jerry L. Jennings, University of Pennsylvania.*

Consciousness, Naturalism, and Nagel. *Owen Flanagan, Duke University and Wellesley College.*
The Transpersonal Psychology of Patañjali's *Yoga Sútra* (Book I: *Samádhi*): A Translation and Interpretation. *Richard J. Castillo, University of Hawaii.*
The Effects of Oppositional Meaning in Incidental Learning: An Empirical Demonstration of the Dialectic. *Richard N. Williams and John Paul Lilly, Brigham Young University.*

Volume 6, Number 4, Autumn 1985

Retarded Development: The Evolutionary Mechanism Underlying the Emergence of the Human Capacity for Language. *Sonia Ragir, College of Staten Island.*
Awareness I: The Natural Ecology of Subjective Experience and the Mind-Brain Problem Revisited. *Mark W. Ketterer, Oklahoma College of Osteopathic Medicine and Surgery.*
Preserved and Impaired Information Processing Systems in Human Bitemporal Amnesiacs and Their Infrahuman Analogues: Role of Hippocampectomy. *Paulette Donovan Gage, University of Maine at Orono.*
A Critique of Three Conceptions of Mental Illness. *W. Miller Brown, Trinity College.*
The Subjective Character of Experience. *Paul G. Muscari, State University College of New York at Glens Falls.*

Volume 7, Number 1, Winter 1986

Formalism and Psychological Explanation. *John Heil, Virginia Commonwealth University.*
Biological Theories, Drug Treatments, and Schizophrenia: A Critical Assessment. *David Cohen, University of California, Berkeley, and Henri Cohen, Université du Quèbec á Montrèal.*
Understanding Surprise-Ending Stories: Long-Term Memory Schemas Versus Schema-Independent Content Elements. *Asghar Iran-Nejad, The University of Michigan.*
Mechanist and Organicist Parallels Between Theories of Memory and Science. *Robert F. Belli, University of New Hampshire.*
On the Radical Behaviorist Conception of Consciousness. *Thomas Natsoulas, University of California, Davis.*

Volume 7, Numbers 2 and 3, Spring and Summer 1986

Cognition and Dream Research by Robert E. Haskell (Ed.), University of New England.

Cognitive Psychology and Dream Research: Historical, Conceptual, and Epistemological Considerations. *Robert E. Haskell, University of New England.*
An Empirical Foundation for a Self Psychology of Dreaming. *Harry Fiss, University of Connecticut.*
Dreaming: Cortical Activation and Perceptual Thresholds. *John S. Antrobus, The City College of New York.*
Some Relations Between the Cognitive Psychology of Dreams and Dream Phenomenology. *Harry Hunt, Brock University.*
REM Sleep and Neural Nets. *Francis Crick, The Salk Institute, and Graeme Mitchison, Kenneth Craik Laboratory.*
Lucid Dreaming: Physiological Correlates of Consciousness During REM Sleep. *Stephen LaBerge, Lynne Levitan, and William C. Dement, Stanford University.*
Effects of Environmental Context and Cortical Activation on Thought. *Ruth Reinsel, Miriam Wollman, and John S. Antrobus, The City College of New York.*
Lucid Dreaming Frequency in Relation to Vestibular Sensitivity as Measured by Caloric Stimulation. *Jayne Gackenbach, University of Northern Iowa, Thomas J. Snyder, Iowa Area Education Agency 6, LeAnn M. Rokes, University of Northern Iowa, and Daniel Sachau, University of Utah.*
The Dream-Scriptor and the Freudian Ego: "Pragmatic Competence" and the Superordinate and Subordinate Cognitive Systems in Sleep. *Frank Heynick, Eindhoven University of Technology.*
Structural Anthropology and the Psychology of Dreams. *Adam Kuper, Brunel University.*
Logical Structure and the Cognitive Psychology of Dreaming. *Robert E. Haskell, University of New England.*
Subliminal Perception and Dreaming. *Howard Shevrin, University of Michigan Medical Center.*
Evaluating Dream Function: Emphasizing the Study of Patients with Organic Disease. *Robert C. Smith, Michigan State University.*

The Insufficiency of Mechanism and Importance of Teleology. *Brent D. Slife, Baylor University.*
On Ersatz Teleologists and the Temptations of Rationalism: Some Reactions to Some of the Reactions. *James T. Lamiell, Georgetown University.*
Are We All Clear On What a Mediational Model of Behavior Is? *Joseph F. Rychlak, Loyola University of Chicago.*

Volume 8, Number 3, Summer 1987

Emerging Views of Health: A Challenge to Rationalist Doctrines of Medical Thought. *William J. Lyddon, University of California, Santa Barbara.*
Information, Communication and Organisation: A Post-Structural Revision. *Robert Cooper, University of Lancaster, England.*
How Thoughts Affect the Body: A Metatheoretical Framework. *Irving Kirsch, University of Connecticut, and Michael E. Hyland, Plymouth Polytechnic.*
Consciousness and Commissurotomy: I. Spheres and Streams of Consciousness. *Thomas Natsoulas, University of California, Davis.*

Volume 8, Number 4, Autumn 1987

Inhibition in the Brain by Charles E. Ribak (Ed.), University of California, Irvine.
Biochemistry of Glycinergic Neurons. *Edward C. Daly, Roudebush VA Medical Center.*
Immunocytochemical Characterization of Glycine and Glycine Receptors. *R.J. Wenthold, National Institutes of Health, and R.A. Altschuler, University of Michigan.*
Distribution of Inhibitory Amino Acid Neurons in the Cerebellum With Some Observations on the Spinal Cord: An Immunocytochemical Study With Antisera Against Fixed GABA, Glycine, Taurine, and β-Alanine. *Ole P. Ottersen and Jon Storm-Mathisen, University of Oslo.*
GABA-Peptide Neurons of the Primate Cerebral Cortex. *Edward G. Jones, University of California, Irvine.*
GABAergic Inhibition in the Neocortex. *K. Krnjević, McGill University.*
Physiology of GABA Inhibition in the Hippocampus. *R.C. Malenka, R. Andrade and R.A. Nicoll, University of California, San Francisco.*
Inhibitory Processes in the Thalamus. *M. Steriade and M. Deschênes, Université Laval.*
Neurotransmitter Modulation of Thalamic Neuronal Firing Pattern. *David A. McCormick and David A. Prince, Stanford University School of Medicine.*
What Do GABA Neurons Really Do? They Make Possible Variability Generation in Relation to Demand. *Eugene Roberts, Beckman Research Institute of the City of Hope.*
GABAergic Abnormalities Occur in Experimental Models of Focal and Genetic Epilepsy. *Charles E. Ribak, University of California, Irvine.*
Inhibition, Local Excitatory Interactions and Synchronization of Epileptiform Activity in Hippocampal Slices. *F. Edward Dudek, Tulane University School of Medicine, and Edward P. Christian, University of Maryland School of Medicine.*
Inhibition in Huntington's Disease. *M. Flint Beal, David W. Ellison and Joseph B. Martin, Massachusetts General Hospital.*

Volume 9, Number 1, Winter 1988

On Complementarity and Causal Isomorphism. *Douglas M. Snyder, Berkeley, California.*
Methodological Complementarity: With and Without Reductionism. *Michael E. Hyland, Plymouth Polytechnic, and Irving Kirsch, University of Connecticut.*
On Human Nature: A Look at the Subject from Karol Wojtyla's Work *The Acting Person.* *Paul G. Muscari, State University College of New York at Glens Falls.*
On the Radical Behaviorist Conception of Pain Experience. *Thomas Natsoulas, University of California, Davis*
From Philology to Existential Psychology: The Significance of Nietzsche's Early Work. *Jerry L. Jennings, University of Pennsylvania.*

Volume 9, Number 2, Spring 1988

Are "Dialogic" Data Positive? *Salomon Rettig, Hunter College.*
Relativity, Complementarity, Indeterminacy, and Psychological Theory. *Mark Garrison, Kentucky State University.*

Information-Processing and Constructivist Models of Cognitive Therapy: A Philosophical Divergence. *William J. Lyddon, University of California, Santa Barbara.*

Is Any State of Consciousness Self-Intimating? *Thomas Natsoulas, University of California, Davis.*

Volume 9, Number 3, Summer 1988

Neuroradiology: Applications in Neurology and Neurosurgery by Stanley van den Noort and Elliot M. Frohman (Editors), California College of Medicine, Irvine.

Imaging for Neurological Disease: Current Status and New Developments. *Stanley van den Noort, Elliot Frohman and Teresa Frohman, University of California, Irvine.*

The Radiological Diagnosis of Primary Brain Tumours. *Henry F.W. Pribram, University of California, Irvine.*

Principles and Applications of Magnetic Resonance Imaging (MRI) in Neurology and Neurosurgery. *T.M. Peters, Montreal Neurological Institute.*

Functional Stereotactic Neurosurgery With Magnetic Resonance Imaging Guidance. *Ronald F. Young, University of California, Irvine.*

Magnetic Resonance Imaging in Neuro-ophthalmology. *Edward K. Wong, Jr. and Bradley P. Gardner, University of California, Irvine.*

Use of Intraoperative Angiography in Neurosurgery. *Leslie D. Cahan, California College of Medicine, Grant B. Hieshima, Randall T. Higashida and Van V. Halbach, San Francisco School of Medicine.*

Anatomical Definition in PET Using Superimposed MR Images. *Ranjan Duara, Anthony Apicella, David W. Smith, Jen Yueh Chang, William Barker and Fumihito Yoshii, Mount Sinai Medical Center.*

Neuroimaging of Head Injury. *Maria Luisa Pasut and Sergio Turazzi, University Hospital, Verona, Italy.*

Alzheimer's Disease, Dementia and Down Syndrome: An Evaluation Using Positron Emission Tomography (PET). *Neal R. Cutler, Center for Aging and Alzheimer's, and Prem K. Narang, Adria Labs, Columbus.*

Neurotransmitter Receptor Imaging in Living Human Brain with Positron Emission Tomography. *Stephen M. Stahl, Rosario Moratalla and Norman G. Bowery, Merck Sharp and Dohme Research Laboratories.*

SPECT Imaging in Alzheimer's Disease. *B. Leonard Holman, Brigham and Women's Hospital, Keith A. Johnson, Massachusetts General Hospital, and Thomas C. Hill, New England Deaconness Hospital.*

Digital Subtraction Angiography. *John R. Hesselink and Steven M. Weindling, University of California Medical Center, San Diego.*

Volume 9, Number 4, Autumn 1988

Kuhn's *Structure of Scientific Revolutions* in the Psychological Journal Liturature, 1969–1983: A Descriptive Study. *S.R. Coleman and Rebecca Salamon, Cleveland State University.*

Existence and the Brain. *Gordon G. Globus, University of California, Irvine.*

Test of a Field Model of Consciousness and Social Change: The Transcendental Meditation and TM-Sidhi Program and Decreased Urban Crime. *Michael C. Dillbeck, Maharishi International University, Carole Bandy Banus, George Washington University, Craig Polanzi, Southern Illinois University, and Garland S. Landrith, III, Maharishi International University.*

The Schema Paradigm in Perception. *Aaron Ben-Zeev, Univeristy of Haifa.*

Consciousness and Commissurotomy: II. Some Pertinencies for Intact Functioning. *Thomas Natsoulas, University of California, Davis.*

The Intentionality of Retrowareness. *Thomas Natsoulas, University of California, Davis.*

Volume 10, Number 1, Winter 1989

Consciousness and the Incompleteness of the Physical Explanation of Behavior. *Avshalom C. Elitzur, Weizmann Institute of Science.*

Experimental Semantics: The Lexical Definitions of "Prejudice" and "Alcoholic." *William T. O'Donohue, University of Maine.*

The Distinction Between Visual Perceiving and Visual Perceptual Experience. *Thomas Natsoulas, University of California, Davis.*

An Examination of Four Objections to Self-Intimating States of Consciousness. *Thomas Natsoulas, University of California, Davis.*

Casual Isomorphism: A Concept in Search of a Meaning: Complementarity and Psychology. *Douglas M. Snyder, Berkeley, California.*

Circulation Department
THE JOURNAL OF MIND AND BEHAVIOR
P.O. Box 522, Village Station
New York City, N.Y. 10014

	Students*	Individuals	Institutions
1 year	☐ $25.00	☐ $35.00	☐ $ 55.00
2 years	☐ $40.00	☐ $64.00	☐ $100.00
3 years	☐ $55.00	☐ $93.00	☐ $150.00

Name _____

Street _____

City and State _____

Country _____

Please enclose prepayment or purchase order. We accept checks drawn on US accounts only. (Exception: checks drawn on Canadian banks in US-Dollars, add $3.50 service charge.)   *with photocopy of student I.D.

Challenging the Therapeutic State:
Critical Perspectives on Psychiatry and the Mental Health System

Edited by

David Cohen, Ph.D.
Université de Montréal

The
Journal of
Mind and Behavior

SPECIAL ISSUE
Volume 11, Numbers 3 and 4
Summer and Autumn, 1990

Library of Congress Cataloging in Publication Data

The Journal of mind and behavior. – Vol. 1, no. 1 (spring 1980)–
    – ₍New York, N.Y.: Journal of Mind and Behavior, Inc.₎
    c1980–

    1. Psychology–Periodicals. 2. Social psychology–Periodicals 3. Philosophy–Periodi-
cals. I. Institute of Mind and Behavior
BF1.J6575   150′.5   82-642121
ISSN 0271-0137   AACR 2 MARC–S

The Journal of Mind and Behavior

Summer/Autumn 1990   an interdisciplinary journal   Vol. 11 Nos. 3 and 4
Special Issue: Challenging the Therapeutic State:
Critical Perspectives on Psychiatry and the Mental Health System

CONTENTS

continued next page

ISBN 0-930195-05-1   ISSN 0271-0137

Preface

"Although we may not know it, we have, in our day, witnessed the birth of the Therapeutic State." Thus did Thomas Szasz, discussing the "therapeutic approach to justice," first note in 1963 the setting up of the state as a therapeutic instrument. Today, the therapeutic state is full-grown, and its approach to justice is merely one facet of a much larger, diffuse enterprise: the medicalization of life.

The primary manifestation of the therapeutic state is the mental health system. This system includes a vast array of connected ideas and theories, legal codifications and moral justifications, therapeutic practices and helping professions, institutional locii, supporters and opponents. The system does not seek merely to eliminate or control "mental illness," but to manage all aspects of social life with the aim of producing or maintaining "mentally healthy" citizens. It constitutes one of the most encompassing projects in socio-political history, and its ideology — the medical model — now reigns supreme in the post-industrial world, explaining the innermost thoughts of individuals and shaping the social policies of nations.

Psychiatry is the profession most closely linked with the rise of the therapeutic state and the mental health system. Psychiatry in the United States and Canada is in a period of normal science, proposing ever-expanding nosologies and uncovering tens of millions of people with "diagnosable mental disorders." Caught in a current of biological theorizing and psychotechnological manipulations supported by powerful economic and political interests, the profession and its allies seem unable or unwilling to realize how the human and monetary costs of the therapeutic state have only grown with its success.

The authors in this collection, representing more than ten different disciplines, do not share a single perspective on madness, deviance, psychiatry, or social control. However, they express the view that the systematic application of the medical model and its technologies in contemporary life has produced and continues to produce intellectual confusion, iatrogenic disorders, social enfeeblement and other difficulties. I hope these essays help to chart courses toward a more humanistic, pluralistic, and non-coercive system of "helping" those we call the "mentally ill" — usually troubled, unhappy, and poor people who break our rules, annoy us, or threaten our values and peace of mind.

I wish here to pay tribute to the memory of R.D. Laing, who died August 23, 1989, after he had begun work on his contribution to this special issue. The volume would not have seen the light of day without the good will and efforts of Ray Russ; nor could I have devoted the necessary energies without support from the School of Social Service of Université de Montréal.

Montréal
November 1990

David Cohen, Ph.D.
Université de Montréal

©1990 The Institute of Mind and Behavior, Inc.
The Journal of Mind and Behavior
Summer and Autumn 1990, Volume 11, Numbers 3 and 4
Pages 247 [1] – 258 [12]
ISSN 0271–0137
ISBN 0-930195-05-1

Introduction:
The Medical Model as the Ideology
of the Therapeutic State

Ronald Leifer

Ithaca, New York

The modern, therapeutic state came into existence as a result of the political transformation from Rule of Man to Rule of Law. This transformation carries with it an internal contradiction: while people value individual freedom under Rule of Law, they wish for a greater degree of social control than is provided by law. Under the ideology of the medical model, psychiatry provides this extra-legal social control. Politically, this model justifies the involuntary incarceration of those people not found guilty of crimes but regarded as strange, threatening or dangerous. This justification rests on switching from the moral model of behavior, which implies choice and responsibility, to a causal-determinist model which implies no choice and non-responsibility. This socially useful deception blinds us to ourselves and to the nature of our personal and public problems, while rendering us less capable of intelligently discussing and dealing with these problems.

Modern psychiatry can be adequately understood only from the broad perspective of history, political sociology, and the dynamics of the human mind. Indeed, there is an intrinsic connection between modern psychiatry and the democratic revolutions now erupting in the communist societies of eastern Europe and elsewhere. These contemporary revolutions have their roots in the French Revolution and in the rise of the modern state, and before that in the relative pluralism of the Athenian aristocracy, and prior to both in the profound and ambivalent wish for freedom of every human heart.

The growing protests of survivors of involuntary psychiatric confinement and treatment are also a contemporary expression of the spirit of freedom and the desire for democratic change. These survivors are rising against their opressors with no less vigor of spirit and no less moral and political justifica-

Requests for reprints should be sent to Ronald Leifer, M.D., 115 DeWitt Park Apartments, Ithaca, New York 14850.

tion than the oppressed citizens of modern totalitarian states. There are strong similarities in the political context of the inmates of Pinel's lunatic asylum, the Russian dissidents who are diagnosed as "sluggish schizophrenic" and incarcerated in a Gulag, and the involuntary patient in the modern American psychiatric hospital.

These three seemingly disparate historical situations are all manifestations of the Therapeutic State. The term "therapeutic state" may be misleading if we infer that anything called "therapeutic" must be beneficial. On the contrary, the term is a political euphemism used to frame certain motives and actions of the state as benevolent, in the image of the medical model. The medical model is the official ideology of the therapeutic state. To understand the therapeutic state and the political function of the medical model, it is helpful to sketch a broad outline of political history.

Psychiatry and the Rise of the Therapeutic State

Two general forms of human government existed prior to the birth of the modern state. Original, primitive human "communities" consisted mainly of coalitions of families and clans into small groups in which every member had a face to face interaction with every other member. At the head of each clan stood a respected elder or cluster of elders whose knowledge, wisdom and status were perceived as essential for the survival of the group. Authority was hierarchical, as in the family. The elders and the priests guided the group, with the cooperation and participation of more ordinary members. All social functions — birth, child-rearing, social control, food-gathering and distribution, marriages, funerals, justice, etc. — were performed by the community under the aegis of the community's religion.

Over time, as the human population grew and communities came into contact and commerce with one another, large settlements developed along the banks of fertile rivers and the crossroads of trade routes. These settlements amalgamated into cities and civilizations. Early societies governed themselves by means of competing clans ceding authority to a superordinate king in whose persona was vested the power to rule the merged populations. Although pockets of democracy have existed throughout history, in most regions of the world a sovereign king ruled with supreme authority or by Divine Right. Laws were issued by royal decree, and enforced by armed militia. For obvious reasons, this form of government is known as Rule of Man.

The eighteenth century democratic revolutions in Europe and America replaced Rule of Man by Rule of Law. (Today, the democratic revolutions in Communist countries, as the earlier democratic revolutions against absolute monarchy, also involve a political transformation to Rule of Law.) This transformation carries with it social and political contradictions which are projections of a profound ambivalence inherent in the ordinary human mind, an ambivalence whose understanding is essential to appreciate the major social function of modern psychiatry.

The fundamental ambivalence is that people love and desire both freedom and social order. These are mutually limiting, however. When freedom increases in society, so does turbulence. On the other hand, a stable, tranquil, virtuous social order requires the restriction of civil liberties and rights. Rule of Man provides a greater degree of (overt) social control than Rule of Law. Indeed, the function and justification for tyranny has always been the call for social order. The absolute monarch could enforce public order and obedience through arbitrary arrest and detention of any citizens and seizure of their property. The democratic revolutions of the past two centuries, which instituted Rule of Law, ended this totalitarian system of social and political control by limiting the power of the state. Rule of Law provides that an individual cannot be deprived of life, liberty or property unless convicted of violating the law by a jury of peers on the basis of evidence presented according to strict rules of procedure. These rules severely limit the state's power to control and regulate its citizens.

The transformation to Rule of Law created the problem that while people value freedom under Law, they also demand a greater degree of social control and order than is provided by Rule of Law. Therein lies the historical mission of public psychiatry. *The main social function of public psychiatry is to provide a mechanism for covert, extra-legal social control without violating the principle of Rule of Law.* This is accomplished by redefining deviant and undesirable conduct as mental illness.

This semantic and ideological revision occurred during what official psychiatric history calls The First Psychiatric Revolution. According to this version of history, Philippe Pinel introduced democracy and science — the twin hallmarks of the French Revolution — into the asylums of Paris. He introduced democracy by liberating *some* of the inmates of the Salpêtrière and Bicêtre. He allegedly introduced science by classifying the inmates according to the prevailing psychiatric diagnoses of the times.

This version of history is an ideological apology for the political function of psychiatry as an instrument of covert social control. By focusing on the few — celebrated inmates liberated by Pinel rather than the many detained by him on the grounds that they were suffering from mental diseases — psychiatry is depicted as liberal and humane rather than as an institution of covert social control. Although official psychiatry describes Pinel's psychiatric classification as a scientific advance, Pinel did nothing scientific. He merely imitated the emerging scientific medicine by redefining the inmates of the asylum as ill, *by fiat* (Szasz, 1961, 1963).

The First Psychiatric Revolution marks the inauguration of the medical model of psychiatry, the chief ideological justification for psychiatry's political function of social control. The arbitrary authority to classify and control people, taken away from the absolute monarch by the democratic revolution, had now been granted to the alienist.

The Medical Model as Ideology

Redefining deviance as mental illness requires a covering ideology to justify what otherwise would be seen as the unconstitutional confinement of innocent persons. The medical model of psychiatry serves as such an ideology. The term "ideology" is used here in the classical sense as defined by Karl Mannheim (1929) to refer to a set of ideas which justifies and promotes certain prevailing interests — in this case, the public interest in an extra-legal form of social control. The medical model is well suited as ideology because it *appears* to represent the most authoritative and reliable source of knowledge, namely, science, as well as the most benevolent and compassionate branch of science, namely, medicine.

The medical model can function as an ideology because using it switches explanations of human action from the commonly used moral model to a causal-determinist (medical) model. This switch in semantics promotes a transformation of perceptions which converts the person labelled as mentally ill into the kind of object upon which psychiatrists represent themselves as qualified to act (Goffman, 1961).

There are basically two models for explaining human action (Louch, 1966). We explain "normal" behavior — our own and that of others — in moral terms, that is, in terms of the conventional purposes and meanings attached to people's actions. For example, if we were to meet a friend crossing the street and we wished to understand his actions, we might ask him where he was going and what he intended to do. If he told us he was going to the grocery to buy some milk we would be satisfied with his explanation and feel that we understand his actions. Psychologically normal behavior is behavior we can explain in terms of conventional goals and conventional means for achieving those goals.

We think of people as bad or deviant, but not necessarily abnormal, when their behavior violates social conventions. For example, if a man marries a woman for her money we might think that person is greedy and exploitative and we would judge him to be an immoral, or bad, person. If our friend whom we met crossing the street tells us he is being chased by the police, we would wonder what law (or convention) he had broken. In both cases, however, whether the actions are conventional or unconventional, they are intelligible with reference to conventional goals and means of pursuing them.

The moral model of human action (in contrast to the medical model) implies and recognizes two vital attributes of human character: freedom and responsibility. To say that behavior is purposive and conventional is to imply that it is freely chosen, that one conventional goal is valued and chosen over others. It implies also that the means of achieving those goals are valued and freely chosen. This model of human action has been compared to a game (Szasz, 1961) because human actions have goals which are achieved by following (or violating) established rules. In the game of life, if one chooses to pursue prohibited goals (such as a man having sex with his daughter) or to pursue conventional goals by prohibited means (such as stealing money instead of earning it), one is held responsible for one's actions and required to submit to the judgment of law or social convention. When the moral model is used to explain human behavior, it is assumed that the person has the capacity for free choice and is responsible and is accountable for his or her actions.

The medical model, on the other hand, is deterministic and explains human actions in terms of antecedent causes. These causes may be biochemical, social, psychological or historical. We might explain the behavior of a man getting married as the result of a hypomanic episode, social pressure, or a fixation on his mother. The desire to binge-eat can be viewed deterministically, as a consequence of depression, rather than morally, as an attempt to evade the pain of life. Similarly, a flight into religious fantasy can be interpreted as the result of dopamine deficiency instead of as a search for meaning in a world of diluted meanings. From the perspective of the medical model, the "cause" of disturbing behavior is mental illness rather than the failure or the refusal of the individual to conform to conventional goals and means for achieving them.

The medical model is used to describe people whose behavior is disturbing to the conventional social order and fits neither acceptable explanations of behavior or acceptable explanations of social conventions. The notorious case of John Hinckley is a good example. It is psychologically "normal" to attempt to assassinate a president for political reasons, but not in order to be noticed and admired by a woman. Defining a political assassination as a symptom of mental illness would invalidate the political dissent that motivated the act by defining the action as irrational, involuntary and caused rather than as rational and freely chosen. Democratic societies value dissent and, recognizing the occasional justification for political assassination, define it as crime rather than as a socially invalid act. To regard Hinckley's motivation as valid would, in effect, declare "open hunting" on all public figures whose heads might serve as personal trophies. In primitive hunting societies, displaying the head of an enemy or a totem animal would signify the power of the hunter. In modern societies, however, which are plagued by ethnic and class conflict, to sanction assassination as legitimate trophy hunting would initiate political chaos. These examples illustrate how the designations "psychological normality and abnormality" specify the acceptable and conventional boundaries within which the game of life is played. The conventional violation of conventional rules is regarded as sane and draws penalties. The unconventional violation of conventional rules is labelled insane and results in being thrown out of the game.

Another example can be drawn from the religious sphere. It is well known that "schizophrenic" symptomatology often takes religious form. But what is sane religion and what is insane? It is considered sane to pray to an invisible God whose existence cannot be objectively demonstrated. If that God answers back, however, it is a symptom of mental illness. Praying is socially safe. The claim to have heard God's voice is a threat to society, however, because it might be used to authorize socially controversial or destructive actions. Society cannot tolerate such usurpation of its authority and, thus, designates hearing God's voice as a symptom of mental illness rather than an authentic event.

Therein lies the distinction between sanity and madness. Sane behavior is socially meaningful and is described with the moral model. Insane behavior is drained of its social meaning by describing it in the causal-deterministic language of the medical model. In sum, people whose behavior places them outside the boundaries of conventional good and evil are diagnosed as mentally ill. Their behavior is explained in terms of causes which shape it rather than in terms of their extraordinary purposes and their strange manners of pursuing them.

The use of the causal-deterministic model to explain human action is a political decision because any human behavior can be viewed and explained either as caused or as freely chosen. Most modern psychology explains normal *and* abnormal human behavior with some version of the causal-deterministic model, while classical social science used primarily the moral-purposive model. From the perspective of the moral model, so-called mentally ill people are likely to pursue unconventional goals through conventional means, to pursue conventional goals through unconventional means, or both.

The medical model of human behavior blurs the distinction between body and mind, and between happenings and doings. Happenings occur independently of human will, as physical illness does. Doings are motivated actions. The medical model views the mind as a part of the body, as a happening, and views moral actions invested with moral meanings by the subject or others as morally neutral events. This characteristic of the medical model makes it particularly useful as an ideology for covert social control, for the model makes it appear not only that the individual is not acting freely and intelligibly by holding certain values and pursuing certain goals, but that the individual may be actually *incapable* of free and responsible action. This belief is then used to justify depriving people of their rights and confining them against their will. Thus, the medical model serves as an ideology for the historic psychiatric function of providing a covert, extra-legal form of social control in societies governed by Rule of Law.

The Medical Model and Psychiatric Identity

Sigmund Freud changed the history of psychiatry in many ways, among others by inventing psychotherapy and instituting the private practice of psychiatry between consenting adults. Psychotherapy serves a different social function than the control of deviance. Psychotherapy evolved from the religious function of spiritual guidance, or "the cure of souls" (Nelson, 1965; Rank, 1941). With the decline of religion, the cure of souls evolved into ethical and moral guidance and, with the rise of modern psychology in the late nineteenth century, into psychological guidance.

In its ideal form, psychotherapy does not serve the function of social control and so has no need for the medical model. Nevertheless, Freud wanted to be viewed as a scientist and he often adopted the frameworks of the physical and biological sciences to understand the "symptoms" of his private patients. As a result, he struggled with the medical model, complaining that his case histories — which he wished would appear as scientific as medical case histories — often sounded like novels. Freud remained ambivalent about the proper classification of psychotherapy as medicine or secular pastoral work (Freud, 1927).

Eventually, the introduction of psychoanalysis, depth psychology, and humanistic psychology led to a profound split between those who served the function of social control and those who served the function of spiritual guidance. This split became most profound in the early 1960s. On one hand, psychiatrists working in the state mental hospitals began to use recently discovered drugs to control and manage psychiatric inmates. These chemical tools for controlling behavior spurred hopes that scientific research in brain physiology would result in new insights into the biological causes and the medical cures of mental illness. On the other hand, psychoanalytically oriented psychotherapists were turning to the humanities and social sciences for new understandings of mental and emotional problems. Increasing numbers of non-medical psychotherapists, particularly social workers and psychologists, were entering private practice and transforming psychotherapy into a non-medical enterprise that more closely resembled education and the New Age religion than classical medical treatment.

This split in the social practices and theoretical orientations of psychiatry generated a crisis in psychiatric identity. Psychiatrists — long sensitive to being regarded as second class citizens by their medical colleagues — began to resent and resist the increasing tide of non-medical competitors and their non-medical ideas. Heated arguments ensued in professional psychiatric circles about the contradiction in psychiatric identity. Is psychiatry a medical science which uses the medical model to understand the causes and treatments of mental disease? Or is it a social art which employs the insights of sociology, anthropology, psychology, political science, etc., to understand and help clients deal with problems in living? This question had urgent practical consequences. Aside from competition between medical and non-medical practitioners, academic psychiatrists in medical schools feared that if their programs slanted too strongly toward the humanities and social sciences, they would lose credibility as well as funding from government agencies for psychiatric research and training.

At the department of psychiatry of the State University of New York, Syracuse, this crisis of psychiatric identity reached explosive proportions. In 1961, Thomas Szasz had just published his now classic book, *The Myth of Mental Illness*. Szasz also openly criticized coercive psychiatric practices, particularly involuntary psychiatric confinement. Ernest Becker, an anthropologist hired by this psychoanalytically oriented department to teach social science to psychiatric residents, was working on new, non-medical understandings of depression and schizophrenia (Becker, 1962, 1963, 1964, 1969, 1973). I was a junior, non-tenured member of that department at the time, working on my own contribution to the "new psychiatry" (Liefer, 1969).

To fight the threat to the medical model posed by this group of critics and innovators, Paul Hoch, Director of the New York State Department of Mental Hygiene and representing the state psychiatrists, ordered Marc Hollander, who was both Director of the Syracuse State Psychiatric Hospital *and* Chairman of the Department of Psychiatry at Upstate Medical Center, to forbid Szasz to teach or lecture at the State hospital (which was the seat of the academic department of psychiatry). Becker and I and a few others protested. Hollander fired Becker for criticizing him. Because of his association with Szasz and his own assault on the medical model, Becker was blackballed from academic psychiatry and, after a long, peripatetic career, found an appointment at the University of Vancouver; he died prematurely in 1974, two months before receiving the Pulitzer Prize for *The Denial of Death* (see Leifer, 1986). Szasz, who was tenured, successfully fought Hollander's attempts to suppress him. As a result, Hollander resigned. His successor, David Robinson, refused to renew my appointment on the grounds that my forthcoming book, *In the Name of Mental Health*, would give the impression that Syracuse was an "anti-psychiatry" center and that the National Institute of Mental Health would refuse to grant funds for research and training. These acts of repression and punishment for those who deviated from the official line and criticized coercive psychiatry, represent only some of psychiatry's continual efforts to reassert its medical identity and reaffirm the medical model as an ideology for the extra-legal control of behavior.

The direction psychiatry has taken from this conflict is clear. Psychiatry has made every effort to affirm its medical identity. In all the public media and in professional writings and talks, psychiatrists assert repeatedly, as if it were a scientific fact, that "mental illness is like any other illness." Organized psychiatry has engaged in a massive campaign to convince the public that advances in medical science have discovered the physiological causes of such "real" diseases as mania, depression, schizophrenia, panic, and even obsessive compulsive disorders. This campaign has been so successful that most people do indeed believe that mental illnesses are biological entities which exist independently of human perceptions and labelling strategies.

We must, however, continue to insist on pressing a number of difficult questions to the intellectual community about the scientific validity of the medical model and the legitimacy of the political functions of psychiatry. Regarding the mind as a part of the body and explaining human behavior in terms of genetics and brain physiology raises serious logical, ethical and political problems (Leifer, 1989; Ryle, 1949). Law, the dramatic arts and our ordinary understanding of human situations depend on the use of the moral model of human behavior. If behavior were always described with the causal-determinist model, choice and responsibility would become meaningless terms. No one could be held accountable for his or her actions, and the drama of our lives would lose significance. This problem is not sufficiently discussed, in my opinion, because open dialogue on this issue would undermine the medical identity of psychiatrists and would call into question the morality of using the medical model as an ideology to justify social control.

Moreover, how can we respect an allegedly scientific medical model when it is used to justify extra-legal confinement and involuntary pharmacological assault? How can we respect the objectivity of psychiatry when the primary conceptual model of psychiatrists serves their interests to be viewed as physicians (who have a monopoly, or at least a substantial advantage, in the billion dollar mental health field)? There are conflicts of interest here, as surely as if a racist were asserting as scientific fact the superiority of his or her race. Psychiatrists have a prejudicial interest in the medical model. Their very identity as medical doctors depends upon it. Society, as I have argued, also has a vested interest in the medical model.

The pharmaceutical industry also benefits enormously from the claim that mental illnesses have biological causes and can be treated with drugs. The medical model converts "drugs" into "medicines." Psychiatrists and drug companies both benefit from their intercourse — the first because the image of doctors prescribing medicines to treat mental illnesses bolsters the medical model, the second because their "medicines" sell. Is it proper for pharmaceutical companies to finance academic research, to advertise in psychiatric journals, to sponsor allegedly scientific conferences, and to advertise the medical model along with their products? Is it proper for psychiatrists to promote the use of drugs made by companies which, in turn, reinforce the medical model of psychiatry? Undoubtedly, drugs may positively or negatively influence mental states and behavior. This, however, does not imply that "abnormal" mental states are caused by physiological factors. I question the propriety of the relationship between academic, allegedly scientific, psychiatry and the pharmaceutical companies which profit from the medical model which they subsidize.

The Costs of the Medical Model of Psychiatry

We pay a high price for the social and political advantages of the medical model. We deceive ourselves about the social, political, moral and psychological nature of the problems we define as medical-psychiatric. This self-deception cripples our intelligence and renders us less capable of understanding and implementing effective measures to deal with these problems.

Psychotherapy is a good example of how the medical model may handicap. If the psychotherapy patient is viewed as medically sick, his or her symptoms or problems are seen as caused by some agency external to his or her will — unfortunate genes, errant biochemistry, a malfunctioning family, a malevolent mother, and so on. How can these factors then be changed by the patient's own efforts? If psychotherapy is to be effective, individuals must take their lives into their own hands, take responsibility for becoming aware and changing themselves — for accepting reality, for exercising self-discipline and restraint, for choosing constructive rather than destructive attitudes and actions. The medical model interferes with this task, and hence interferes with psychotherapy. It blinds us to ourselves and the nature of our suffering, and promotes a distorted, irresponsible attitude toward life.

The problem of drug addiction also highlights the confusion surrounding the medical model. Viewed through this model, addiction is a disease, the cause of which is variously attributed to the drug-pusher, the drug itself, genetic predisposition, psychological stress, social conditions, and so on. When the addict undergoes treatment, however, the model reverts to a strong version of the moral model: the addict is held strictly responsible for his or her habits, attitudes, actions and life-style. Arguably, the function of the medical model is to excuse the addict from responsibility and provide a social alternative to the harsh and futile criminalization of the addict. If drugs were decriminalized, the medical model of addiction would be not only unnecessary but also counterproductive.

Another situation in which the medical model solves certain social problems at the price of blinding and crippling us lies in the control of unruly children. If a child falls outside of the conventions established by the school as normal, the child is likely to be diagnosed as mentally ill. Hyperactivity, now called ADD or Attention Deficit Disorder, is a good illustration. A "normal" child is expected to sit in the classroom quietly and attentively for eight hours a day without creating a disturbance. Some children are not interested in what or how the schools teach, or they are bored with their teachers, or preoccupied by erotic or aggressive feelings, or by problems at home. If a child is distracted, or temperamentally active and inclined to engage in physical activity, he or she is vulnerable to being diagnosed as "having ADD" and assigned to a "special" class with other "special" children, and to receive medication. In other historical societies, a hyperactive child could be a champion hunter and hero to the people. In the modern school, such a child is an anachronism. Rather than view the situation as one in which the school is too rigid to adapt itself to the needs of the child, the medical model sees the child as unable to adapt to the needs of the school. This facilitates the management of students while leaving the school immune to criticism.

The medical model also serves as an ideology for the control and management of the elderly. When old people are confined to nursing homes which do not provide adequate care, companionship or activities, they usually become depressed and disoriented. They are then seen as suffering from mental illnesses and subsequently medicated. Rather than viewing the problem in terms of the economics and other inadequacies of nursing care for the elderly, the problem is defined in terms of psychiatric problems of the institutionalized aged.

Another example of the use of the medical model to solve a social problem concerns the control of inmates in overcrowded prisons using psychiatric drugs. The director of the New York State prison system recently announced that, due to overcrowding, prison inmates will be double bunked ("New York," 1990). At the same time, the Supreme Court ruled that prison inmates may be given psychiatric drugs without their consent ("Court Upholds," 1990). Ironically, people convicted and imprisoned for selling illegal drugs in an essentially voluntary transaction may now have psychiatric drugs forced on them by the state.

In sum, while the medical model is politically useful as an ideology to disguise social control as benevolent caring, we pay the price of blinding ourselves to ourselves. To the extent that we view humanity through the lenses of "scientific" psychiatry, we shall see ourselves as objects whose structure, character and functions are slavishly determined by laws of cause and effect. It follows then, that our fate is in the hands of experts who justify their power as both scientific and benevolent. This point of view, working hand in hand with the powerful, bureaucratic "therapeutic" state, can lead us down the dangerous path.

Far from representing the finest human thinking, the medical model actually represses creative ways of understanding and taking responsibility for ourselves and our lives. The medical model stands for constricted consciousness and the standardization of behavior. Here is the question I would like to see addressed in public debates: Is an extra degree of social control, one that often hurts and humiliates people, worth the price of endarkenment and enfeeblement? At a time when the human species is threatened with self-extinction, can we afford to blind and cripple ourselves with a politically convenient deception?

References

Becker, E. (1962). *The birth and death of meaning.* New York: The Free Press.

Becker, E. (1963). Social science and psychiatry: The coming challenge. *Antioch Review, 23,* 353–366.

Becker, E. (1964). *Revolution in psychiatry.* New York: The Free Press.

Becker, E. (1969). *Angel in armor: A post-Freudian perspective on the nature of man.* New York: George Braziller.

Becker, E. (1973). *The denial of death.* New York: The Free Press.

Court upholds forced treatment of mentally ill by prison officials. (1990, February 28). *The New York Times,* p. 1.

Freud, S. (1927). Postscript to the question of lay analysis. In *The standard edition of the complete psychological works of Sigmund Freud* (Volume 20, pp. 252–256). London: The Hogarth Press.

Goffman, E. (1961). *Asylums: Essays on the social situation of mental patients and other inmates.* New York: Doubleday.

Leifer, R. (1966). Avoidance and mastery: An interactional view of phobias. *Journal of Individual Psychology, 22,* 80–93.

Leifer, R. (1969). *In the name of mental health: The social functions of psychiatry.* New York: Science House.

Leifer, R. (1986). The legacy of Ernest Becker. *Kairos, 2,* 8–21.

Leifer, R. (1989). The deconstruction of self. *Journal of Contemplative Psychology, 4,* 153–171.

Louch, A.R. (1966). *Explanation and human action.* Berkeley: University of California Press.

Mannheim, K. (1929). *Ideology and utopia.* New York: Harcourt, Brace and World.

Nelson, B. (1965). Self image and systems of spiritual direction in the history of European civilization. In S.Z. Kalusner (Ed.), *The quest for self-control: Classical philosophies and scientific research* (pp. 49–103). New York: The Free Press.

New York plans to double bunk inmates in 10 of its state prisons. (1990, March). *The New York Times,* p. 1.

Rank, O. (1941). *Beyond psychology.* Camden, New Jersey: Hadden-Craftsmen.

Ryle, G. (1949). *The concept of mind.* New York: Barnes and Noble.

Szasz, T. (1961). *The myth of mental illness.* New York: Hoeber-Harper.

Szasz, T. (1963). *Law, liberty and psychiatry.* New York: Macmillan.

©1990 The Institute of Mind and Behavior, Inc.
The Journal of Mind and Behavior
Summer and Autumn 1990, Volume 11, Numbers 3 and 4
Pages 259 [13] – 284 [38]
ISSN 0271-0137
ISBN 0-930195-05-1

Toward the Obsolescence of the Schizophrenia Hypothesis

Theodore R. Sarbin

University of California, Santa Cruz

The disease construction of schizophrenia is no longer tenable. That construction originated during a period of rapid growth of biological science based on mechanistic principles. Crude diagnostic measures failed to differentiate absurd, unwanted conduct due to biological conditions from atypical conduct directed to solving existential or identity problems. The construction was communicated — in the absence of solid evidence — by medical practitioners by means of symbolic, rhetorical, and organizational acts. The patient came to be regarded as an object without agency or goals. In spite of enormous research funding, no biological or psychological marker has been discovered that would differentiate diagnosed schizophrenics from normals without creating unacceptable proportions of false positives and false negatives. Employing a moral category, "unwanted conduct," as a criterion, and tacitly transforming moral judgments to the medical category, schizophrenia, leads to the use of schizophrenia/nonschizophrenia as the independent variable in research designs. The failure of eight decades of research to produce a reliable marker leads to the conclusion that schizophrenia is an obsolescent hypothesis and should be abandoned.

Any effort to criticize or clarify the concept of schizophrenia must begin from the position that "schizophrenia" is a hypothetical construct. Notwithstanding the use of the term to denote a firm diagnostic entity by most textbook writers and clinical practitioners, investigators by the hundreds are still trying to establish the empirical validity of the construct. The output of published and unpublished research directed toward establishing empirical validity has been enormous, yet schizophrenia remains an unconfirmed hypothesis. A great deal of the research is directed to the task of breaking out of the circular reasoning in which "schizophrenia" appears on both sides

This essay borrows from a more extended set of arguments prepared for an international conference on schizophrenia at Clark University, Worcester, Massachusetts, June 10-11, 1990. The conference paper will be included in a book recording the proceedings. I am grateful to a number of friends and colleagues who offered suggestions to improve the essay, among them, Mary Boyle, Ralph M. Carney, David Cohen, Philip Cowan, Daniel B. Goldstine, Norman S. Greenfield, James C. Mancuso, and Frederick J. Ziegler. Requests for reprints should be sent to Theodore R. Sarbin, Ph.D., Adlai E. Stevenson College, University of California, Santa Cruz, California 95064.

of a causality equation: unwanted behaviors are taken to be symptoms of schizophrenia; schizophrenia is the cause of unwanted behaviors.

Historical accounts of psychiatry and psychology make clear that the core hypothesis — schizophrenia as a disease entity — continues to serve as an implicit guide to the construction of current versions of the schizophrenia concept. The schizophrenia construction continues to be employed in spite of the well-documented fact that it has been submitted to repeated empirical tests and has been found wanting. My thesis is that decades of research have not provided determinate findings that justify continuing the use of schizophrenia-nonschizophrenia as an independent variable. Having voiced this claim, I quickly add that my judgment of the failure of the schizophrenia hypothesis is in no way a disclaimer to the observation that some people, under some conditions, engage in conduct that others might identify as mad, insane, bizarre, foolish, irrational, psychotic, deluded, inept, unwanted, absurd, or plain crazy.

The focus of my paper is that schizophrenia is a construction put forth by nineteenth century physicians and elaborated within an epistemological context that supported the notion that unwanted conduct was caused by disease processes. Historical forces in the nineteenth century influenced doctors to regard perplexing conduct as the outcome of a subtle brain disease. The opacity of the term "schizophrenia" directed scientists and practitioners to employ a prototype when writing their own definitions or when labelling putative patients. The contemporary construction of schizophrenia is consistent with the prototype of a person with an infectious brain disease. The crude diagnostic efforts of the late nineteenth and early twentieth centuries failed to differentiate patients with organic brain disease from patients employing atypical conduct to solve their identity and extistential problems. Because so many diagnosed schizophrenics did not fit the specifications of the prototype, some authorities, notably Eugen Bleuler, suggested the employment of the plural, "the schizophrenias." This stratagem has not been productive, but has preserved schizophrenia as a sacred emblem of psychiatry when experiments have yielded indeterminate results. "The schizophrenias" and its modern equivalent "schizophrenia spectrum disorders" have also been employed to increase the size of an experimental sample in order to achieve statistical significance. Such miscellaneous categories do little more than supply Greek or Latin labels to formalize the lay concept that "people can be crazy in different ways and for different causes or reasons."

Nearly 50 years ago, when I had my first encounters with hospitalized patients, I was confronted with the official lore that schizophrenia was a disease. I did not accept, however, the official lore without reservation. Day to day interactions with inmates of a mental hospital influenced me to be tentative about adopting the prevailing doctrine. In the course of working with men and women who had been diagnosed as schizophrenic by appropriately-qualified psychiatrists, I became aware of the multifarious actions that were interpreted as "presenting symptoms" — actions that family members or employers could not readily assimilate into their constructions of acceptable conduct.

My first patient was a middle-aged women who held the belief that agents of a foreign power were conspiring to kidnap her; the second was a man who believed that his neighbor was directing magnetic rays to the nails in his shoes so that walking was a great effort; a third was a 40 year-old man who argued with an absent opponent about metaphysical propositions; a fourth inmate behaved as if he had lost all power of speech; a fifth would not leave his room, even for meals, afraid that he would be the object of massive microbial invasions; a sixth, a seminary student, claimed to be a saint of the thirteenth century; a seventh, a retired baker, held friendly conversations in the privacy of his room with two long-dead religious figures.

Along the way, I worked with other schizophrenics whose "presenting symptoms" added to the heterogeneous array of actions, the meaning of which could only be constructed from detailed knowledge of their self-narratives. One of these cases was a young man who, for reasons that he initially kept secret, refused to eat, although he acknowledged that no one was trying to poison him nor was he bent on suicide. I spent hours with a college student who held the belief that the disembodied spirit of a convicted mass-murderer had entered his body. Another clinical experience involved trying to understand the reasons that a 20 year-old woman claimed that her recently-deceased brother was alive and visited her frequently.

In most cases, these actions were so specific to the individual's life story that it was difficult for me to accept the explanation that some brain anomaly could account for the heterogeneity. The notion of a common cause for such an assortment of human actions can be entertained only if, in Procrustean fashion, we reduce the interesting array of polymorphous actions to a small number of categories, for example, delusions, flattened affect, and hallucinations, and further, if we arbitrarily redefine the categories as "symptoms" of a still-to-be-discovered disease entity. Such a redefinition obliterates the specificity, the individuality, and the problem-solving features of each person's conduct. Further, the acceptance of the redefinition renders irrelevant the search for intentions and meanings behind perplexing interpersonal acts.

Search Strategies

In the early 1960s, I undertook seriously to question the lore that had grown up around the schizophrenia concept. I followed two strategies: the first was to determine the epistemic and social pathways from particular actions of putative patients to diagnostic judgments by mental health professionals; the second was to determine from a search of the published experimental literature whether a stable set of referents had been discovered that would give body to the schizophrenia hypothesis.

The Search for Unique Symptoms

To implement the first strategy, I chose to delimit my search to behavior that is regarded as a "symptom" of schizophrenia by knowledgeable specialists. In an informal survey, I presented to 15 colleagues (psychiatrists, clinical psychologists, psychoanalysts) the following question: Of the many behaviors that are supposed to point to a diagnosis of schizophrenia, which would you regard as the single most significant item of behavior in establishing a diagnosis of schizophrenia? All but three of the respondents listed "hallucinations," and many added that the presence of hallucinations reflected an underlying thought disorder. The results of this informal survey were similar to those reported by Willis and Bannister (1965) who surveyed the opinions of 346 English psychiatrists. This more extensive survey made clear that "thought disorder" was considered the most important characteristic of schizophrenia.

For the next few years, I studied "hallucinations" in the laboratory, in the clinic, and in the library (Sarbin, 1967, 1972a; Sarbin and Juhasz, 1967, 1970, 1975, 1978, 1982). I was interested in the judgmental processes of diagnosticians who would classify a person's reported imaginings as "hallucination." But before addressing the diagnostic process, it was important to determine whether "hallucination" was a property exclusively of persons who were candidates for psychiatric diagnosis, persons who, in the professional vernacular, had sick minds or damaged brains. In tracing the history of the term "hallucination" from the sixteenth century to the present, it became clear that the conduct upon which the attribution "hallucination" is made is no more than the self-report of imaginings. It is important to note that imaginings (no matter how wild) that are not reported through word or deed do not become candidates for the label "hallucination."

The word "hallucination" belongs, in behavioral terms, to a family of words that includes day-dreaming, imagining, fantasy, fancy, fictions, inventions, and fabrications. Common examples of imagining include childhood imaginary companions, adult dreams of glory, imaginary interactions with celebrity figures, "the voice of conscience," and playful or romantic fantasies. The imaginings that are constructed by so-called normals appear to cover the same range of topics as the imaginings of psychiatric patients. The claim of "reality" for the imagining is not exclusive to persons identified as schizophrenic. In one experiment, for example, volunteer college students were induced to imagine tasting salt solutions and subsequently were willing to testify in a court of law that they had tasted salt. They had only tasted distilled water (Juhasz and Sarbin, 1966).

Besides membership in a readily-understood class of behaviors, the word "hallucination" belongs to another class, the defining property of which is a pejorative value judgment. The value judgment, of course, is rendered not by the putative patient, but by another, usually a person with greater social power than the "hallucinator." To employ the concept of hallucination, then, involves two actors, the person reporting his or her imaginings and the person who is empowered to pass judgment upon such imaginings.

Since the turn of the century, psychologists have been exploring the proposal that "hallucinations" are not uncommon among the general population. That is to say, people have experiences in which they assign a high degree of credibility to imaginings, in some cases they assign the same degree of credibility as to veridical perceptions. Ethnographic studies of subcultural pockets in the United States make clear that reported imaginings (e.g., "I could feel the Holy Ghost enter my body") are not identified as hallucinations by fellow participants in the culture. In fact, such a report sometimes leads to the person being assigned honorific status in the subculture. The same imagining reported to a conventional diagnostician in a forensic or clinical context could be evaluated as meeting the official criteria for hallucination and could lead to the diagnosis of schizophrenia. Whether or not the "hallucinator" would be classified as schizophrenic would depend upon other moral judgments. If, in the eyes of the diagnostician, the person had already suffered a degradation of identity, then the reported imagining could be employed to support the schizophrenia diagnosis. Social status considerations may insidiously insert themselves into the clinician's diagnostic matrix. The frequency of schizophrenia diagnoses among persons who are poor and black supports the claim that social structural features of the diagnostic setting supply a readiness for professionals to employ pejorative interpretations of atypical conduct. For a person whose identity has not been previously degraded, the reported imagining can be assigned to other classes, such as creative imaginings, poetic language, mystical experience, even metaphor.

Social status appears to play a part in diagnosticians' categorizing of perplexing behaviors, among them, admissions of atypical beliefs. Such beliefs of a socially degraded person, sometimes shared as in popular superstitions, are more likely to be regarded as "delusions" and thus symptomatic of schizophrenia. The superstitions of persons whose social identities have not been devalued are likely to be interpreted as quaint, or accepted as harmless, empirically-empty beliefs. Whether or not a particular belief is identified as delusional has nothing to do with "truth." One can point to beliefs held by previous generations of scientists that were declared erroneous by later scientists. Delusion would not be employed as a term to mark the false beliefs of respected scientists.

The conclusion to my efforts to understand hallucination and delusion was that the process of constructing imaginings and beliefs was the same for so-called schizophrenics and so-called normals. The technical and pejorative terms, hallucination and delusion, were selectively assigned by clinicians to devalued or degraded persons as symptoms of disease. In most instances, those who employed these terms were unconcerned with fathoming the meanings of such behaviors or the part such behaviors played in the patient's life story. Among the exceptions to this generalization is a study reported by Benjamin (1989). In a carefully crafted investigation she demonstrated that the auditory hallucinations of psychiatric patients were meaningful and reflected widely observed interpersonal themes. Further, the "voices" appeared to have an important adaptive function for the patients.

The Search for Research Support

The second strategy in my search was to determine to what extent, if any, the published research could be used to support the schizophrenia hypothesis. It was not unreasonable to suppose that the schizophrenia hypothesis must have some validity because so much journal space was devoted to experimental studies. In the early 1970s, I made some casual forays into the experimental literature, looking for support for the then-popular theories of schizophrenia (Sarbin, 1972b). My preliminary analysis made clear that most of the theories of schizophrenia had been initially supported on the basis of one or two experiments. When replicated by other investigators, the results of the experiments proved to be artifacts. Each theory had a short period of enthusiastic support and then a marked decline. The rise and fall of theories of schizophrenia led me to conclude that such theories have a half-life of about five years. The conclusion applied to somatic theories and psychological theories alike (Sarbin, 1972a). Cutting (1985) arrived at a similar conclusion and added: ". . . of all the proposed causes of schizophrenia, biochemical ones have the shortest life-span" (p. 138).

My preliminary excursions called for a more systematic analysis of the published literature. Professor James Mancuso joined me in a project to review every research article on schizophrenia published in the *Journal of Abnormal Psychology* for the 20-year period beginning in 1959[1] (Sarbin and Mancuso, 1980). We selected this journal because of its high standards, the average manuscript rejection rate being about 80 percent. (To avoid the criticism that

---

[1]Until 1964, *Journal of Abnormal and Social Psychology.*

we had introduced a bias in selecting a psychological journal, we appended to our analysis a review of selected articles from psychiatric journals.) We found 374 reports of experiments designed to illuminate the concept of schizophrenia. By any standard, the published research on schizophrenia during the 20-year period represented a prodigious effort. It is abundantly clear that in the period under review, students of deviant conduct focused on the central problem: to identify a reliable diagnostic marker, psychological or somatic, that would replace subjective (and fallible) diagnosis. The discovery of such a marker would establish the long sought-for validity for the postulated entity, schizophrenia.

In nearly all the studies, schizophrenia/nonschizophrenia was the independent variable. To accomplish their mission, investigators compared the *average* responses of "schizophrenics" on experimental tasks with the *average* responses of persons who were not so diagnosed. It is no exaggeration to say that the experimental tasks devised by creative investigators numbered in the hundreds. All were constructed for the purpose of rigorously testing miniature hypotheses, the origins of which were linked to the postulate that schizophrenia was an identifiable mental disease or disorder. The choice of these variables was influenced by the lore of schizophrenia, beliefs that could be traced to Kraepelin's and Bleuler's claims that schizophrenics were cognitively or linguistically flawed; perceptually inefficient; affectively dysfunctional; and psychophysiologically impaired. The experimental hypotheses were formulated from the expectation that whatever the task, the schizophrenics would perform poorly when compared with the performance of a control group. The range and variety of the experimental tasks suggests that the formulators of these experimental hypotheses shared the conviction that "schizophrenics" were persons who were basically flawed, that the putative disease affected all somatic and psychological systems.

Mancuso and I analyzed 374 studies on several dimensions. We drew a number of conclusions, among them, that the criteria for selecting subjects were less than satisfactory. The unreliability for psychiatric diagnosis notwithstanding, the experimenters were satisfied to accept diagnoses made by "two staff psychiatrists," "by a psychiatrist and a psychologist," "by consensus in diagnostic staff conference," etc. It is unknown to what extent the diagnosticians employed the *Diagnostic and Statistical Manual-II*, although it is likely that the lore contained in the *Manual* provided the diagnostic criteria.[2] The

---

[2] The constantly changing criteria for schizophrenia in the various editions of the *Diagnostic and Statistical Manual* render it well-nigh impossible to aggregate the results of research studies. Blum (1978) compared diagnostic practices in 1954, 1964, and 1974 in the same hospital. About one-third of persons diagnosed as schizophrenic in 1954 would acquire a different diagnosis 20 years later. DSM-III, DSM-III-R, and other diagnosis handbooks, each with a different set of criteria, contribute to the problem.

dependent variables were assessed with great precision, sometimes to two decimal places. In contrast, the independent variable, schizophrenia/non-schizophrenia, was assessed either by the subjective and fallible judgments of clinicians, or by a vote taken in a diagnostic staff conference.

To bring our analysis up to date, we performed the same analysis on the reports published in the *Journal of Abnormal Psychology* for the ten-year period, 1979–1988. It was in this period that DSM-III and DSM-III-R came into use, and that structured interviews were refined to increase the reliability of diagnosis. Because validity is dependent upon reliable assessments, scientists expected that these systematic aids to diagnosis would facilitate the discovery of valid markers for schizophrenia. Members of the profession were optimistic that these improvements would firmly establish the ontological status of schizophrenia. Our preliminary examination of the reports shows that the experiments reported during the period 1979–1988 followed the same pattern that we had discerned in the earlier analysis. Underlying the research hypotheses is the Kraepelinian premise that schizophrenics are basically flawed organisms (Sarbin, Mancuso, and Podczerwinski, in preparation).

About 80 percent of the studies reported that schizophrenics performed poorly when compared to control subjects. Variability in performance was the rule. Although the published studies reported mean differences between groups as statistically significant, the differences were small. In those studies where it was possible to reconstruct distributions, it was immediately clear that the performances of the schizophrenic samples and the normal samples overlapped considerably. An examination of a number of such distributions points to an unmistakable conclusion: that most schizophrenics cannot be differentiated from most normals on a wide variety of experimental tasks. If one were to employ the dependent variable as a marker for schizophrenia in a new sample, the increase in diagnostic accuracy would be infinitesimal.

That so many studies showed small mean differences has been taken to mean that the schizophrenia hypothesis has earned a modicum of credibility. The degree of credibility dissolves when we consider a number of hidden variables that could account for the observed differences. A large number of reports noted that the schizophrenic subjects were on neuroleptic medication. It is appropriate to ask whether the small mean differences could be accounted for by the drugged status of the experimental subjects and the non-drugged status of the controls. Other hidden variables are socioeconomic status and education. At least since 1855, it has been noted that the diagnosis of insanity (later dementia praecox and schizophrenia) has been employed primarily as a diagnosis for poor people (Dohrenwend, 1990). Many of the experimental tasks called for cognitive skills. The mean difference in performance on such tasks could well be related to cognitive skills, a correlate of education and socioeconomic status. Some experimenters noted the difficulty in recruiting control subjects whose educational level matched the low levels of schizophrenic samples, in many instances, about tenth grade.

Not assessed in these studies were the effects of patienthood. At the time the hospitalized patients were recruited to be subjects, they had been the objects of legal, medical, nursing, and in some cases, police procedures, not to mention mental hospital routines and their effects on personal identity. As mentioned before, only cooperative, i.e., docile, patients were recruited. It would be instructive to investigate to what degree docility influences the subjects' approach to experimental tasks.

Any of the hidden variables could account for the small mean differences observed in experimental studies. One conclusion is paramount: the 30 years of psychological research covered in our analyses has produced no marker that would establish the validity of the schizophrenia disorder. The argument could be made that psychological variables are too crude to identify the disease process. Biochemical, neurological, and anatomical studies, some would argue (e.g., Meehl, 1989), are more likely to reveal the ultimate marker for schizophrenia. However, reported findings employing somatic dependent variables follow the same pattern as for psychological studies. Variation is the rule. For example, one variable of interest for those who would locate the seat of schizophrenia in the brain is the size of the hemispheric ventricles. Several studies employed computer tomography to measure the size of the ventricles. Homogenizing the results of measurement, they found that the schizophrenic group had larger ventricles than the controls. The degree of variation, however, was such as to preclude using the ventricular size as a diagnostic instrument (Nasrallah, Jacoby, McCalley-Whitters, and Kuperman, 1982; Weinberger, Torrey, Neophytides, and Wyatt, 1979). Another set of investigators, presumably employing a more refined method for measuring the scans, reported no differences between schizophrenics and controls (Jernigan, Zatz, Moses, and Berger, 1982a, 1982b). Another hypothesis, disarray of pyramidal cells in the hippocampus, was advanced by several researchers as a potential marker for schizophrenia. Christison, Casanova, Weinberger, Rawlings, and Kleinman (1989) conducted precise measurements on brains stored in the Yakovlev collection. They found no differences in hippocampal measurements when the brains of schizophrenics were compared to the brains of controls.

It is important to note the high degree of variability in biomedical and psychological measurements. To isolate the elusive marker, investigators must discover indicators that cluster near the mean for the experimental sample and at the same time do not overlap with the control sample or with other presumed diagnostic entities. None of the studies we reviewed met this requirement.

Schizophrenia as Disease: A Social Construction

The prevailing mechanistic framework directs practitioners to perceive crazy behavior as caused ultimately by anatomical or biochemical anomalies. An alternative framework is available, one not dependent on the notion that human beings are passive objects at the mercy of biochemical forces. The starting point in this framework is the observation that candidates for the diagnosis of schizophrenia are seldom people who seek out doctors for the relief of pain or discomfort. Rather, they are persons who undergo a pre-diagnostic phase in which moral judgments are made on their nonconforming or perplexing actions by family members, employers, police officers, or neighbors. In the absence of reliable tests to demonstrate that the unwanted conduct is caused by anatomical or biochemical distortions, diagnosticians unwittingly join in the moral enterprise. They confirm the initial pre-diagnostic judgment that the deviant behavior belongs to a class of behaviors that are unwanted. After appropriate rituals, diagnosticians can confirm the moral verdict and encode it with a proper medical term, schizophrenia.

The foregoing remarks are preliminary to my argument that schizophrenia is a social construction initially put forth as a hypothesis by medical scientists and practitioners. A social construction is an organized set of beliefs that has the potential to guide action. The construction is communicated and elaborated by means of linguistic and rhetorical symbols. The categories are vicariously received, passed on from generation to generation through symbolic action. Like any construction, the schizophrenia hypothesis serves certain purposes and not others. A pivotal purpose for schizophrenia is diagnosis — professional practice requires diagnosis before treatment can be rationally prescribed. It is important to remind ourselves that any social construction can be abandoned when alternate constructions are put forth that receive symbolic and rhetorical support from scientific and political communities.

To find the origin of the schizophrenia construction, one must refer to historical sources. Because of space limitations, a full historical account is not possible. Instead I point to some pertinent observations. Ellard (1987), an Australian psychiatrist, has contributed a provocative argument under the title "Did Schizophrenia Exist Before the Eighteenth Century?" Ellard's historical analysis begins from a skeptical posture, namely, to "reflect on the question whether or not there has ever been an entity of any kind at all that stands behind the word, 'schizophrenia', and if so, what its true nature might be" (p. 306). Citing well-known authorities, Ellard points to significant changes in the description of schizophrenia over the past 50 or 60 years. He cites the common observation that contemporary clinicians seldom encounter patients who fit the prototype advanced by Kraepelin and Bleuler. If the nosological criteria for schizophrenia changed so radically in a half-century, is it not conceivable that the criteria changed significantly in the half-century before Kraepelin and Bleuler? – and in the half-century before that?[3] Ellard makes clear that schizophrenia is a construction of medical scientists that is historically-bound.

As a point of departure, Ellard takes the construction and eventual abandonment of the nineteenth century diagnosis, masturbatory psychosis. Medical orthodoxy posited a psychosis characterized by restlessness, silliness, intellectual deterioration, and inappropriate affect. The entrenched belief in the association between biological activities and crazy behavior nurtured the idea of masturbatory insanity well into the twentieth century. Although at one time professionally acceptable, it was ultimately abandoned as an empty if not counterproductive hypothesis.

Employing the vaguely-defined "thought disorder" as the criterion of schizophrenia, Ellard searched the literature for evidence of cases noted by physicians and historians. His reading of case histories and medical records led to the conclusion that insanities involving "thought disorders" were identified in the eighteenth and nineteenth centuries, but such cases were exceedingly rare in the seventeenth century. It remains for future historians to identify the social, political, and professional conditions that brought about the creation of a diagnosis centered on ambiguously-defined "thought disorder."[4]

Ellard's observation about the changing criteria for schizophrenia receives strong support from a historical analysis prepared by Boyle (in press) in which she advanced a convincing explanation for the changing symptom picture.

---

[3]It appears that the rate of change in the criteria for schizophrenia is accelerating. In less than a decade, two revisions of the *Diagnostic and Statistical Manual* appeared. DSM-III was published in 1980 and DSM-III-R in 1987. A new revision, DSM-IV, is in the offing. These *Manuals* are products of consensual judgments by psychiatric experts nominated by Task Forces of the American Psychiatric Association. In the 1970s, the Present State Examination (PSE) was developed in England and implemented by a computer system for making diagnoses (Wing, Cooper, and Sartorius, 1974). The criteria in the PSE were taken from Schneider (1959) who, for example, regarded certain "hallucinations" as "first rank" symptoms. The earlier editions of the American Manual had adapted Bleuler's four "A's" as criteria (anhedonia, associations, ambivalence, and autism) and looked upon "hallucinations" as accessory, not central, phenomena. More recent editions are neo-Kraepelinian – hallucinations and delusions are categorized as psychotic phenomena. The overlap between the two systems is far from perfect, each selects different candidates for what appear to be the same diagnostic categories. The two systems were compared on an outpatient psychiatric population by van den Brink, Koeter, Ormel, Dijkstra, Giel, Sloof, and Woolfarth (1989). The two systems converged on 115 of 175 patients, yielding a kappa coefficient of .32.

[4]The origins of the antecedents to the schizophrenia diagnosis occurred about the same time as the construction of the notion of the modern nuclear family (Gubrium and Holstein, 1990). The most frequent path to the mental hospital is the complaints of family members. These observations might lead a historical researcher to take a fresh look at family communications hypotheses such as those advanced by Bateson, Jackson, Haley, and Weakland (1956), Singer and Wynne (1963), and others.

Like Ellard, Boyle cites the well-documented observation that the kind of deteriorated cases described by Kraepelin and Bleuler are rarely, if ever, seen in modern times. Kraepelin recorded somatic signs and symptoms of some of his dementia praecox patients that were consistent with his gloomy prognosis of outcome: "marked peculiarities of gait. . ., excess production of saliva, and urine; dramatic weight fluctuations; tremor; cyanosis of the hands and feet; constraint of movement and the inability, in spite of effort, to complete 'willed' acts" (cited in Boyle, in press). Kraepelin also reported brain damage as revealed microscopically at post-mortem. Bleuler noted similar phenomena, for example, he claimed to be able to diagnose a schizophrenic by his or her gait.

When Kraepelin and Bleuler were establishing the diagnoses of dementia praecox and schizophrenia, they had no way of knowing that their patient populations might have included a sizable number of persons suffering from post-encephalitic parkinsonism. It was not until 1917 that the Austrian neurologist, von Economo, identified encephalitis lethargica, popularly known as sleeping sickness. The sequelae to the infection included post-encephalitic parkinsonism, signs and symptoms very much like the signs and symptoms that Kraepelin had noted for dementia praecox. A number of encephalitis epidemics had swept through Europe culminating in the epidemic of 1916–1927. Before von Economo's identification of encephalitis lethargica, persons presenting themselves to clinics and hospitals with the symptoms of post-encephalitic parkinsonism could be tagged with any number of diagnoses, including dementia praecox. Modern-day psychiatrists and neurologists do not see crazy patients who fit Kraepelin's and Bleuler's descriptions, patients who display the features of post-encephalitic parkinsonism. The change in symptom-picture over the past 50 or 75 years, then, is the result of not including encephalitic patients in the pool of patients who come to the attention of mental health professionals.

Boyle's historical account lends credibility to the thesis that post-encephalitic parkinsonism was unwittingly employed as the prototype for dementia praecox and schizophrenia. Thus the social construction of schizophrenia as a form of disease was facilitated by erroneously sorting into a single class two types of persons: undiagnosed post-encephalitic (or other organic) patients, and persons who had engaged in various kinds of unwanted conduct to solve life problems. The latter, who presented conduct only superficially similar to brain-damaged individuals, were assimilated to the former.[5]

---

[5]In addition to the confounding of diagnoses, Kraepelin's construction of dementia praecox was in part developed during his tenure at the University of Dorpat (now Tartu in Estonia). The nature of his contacts with non-German speaking clinic patients influenced the development of his "degeneration" theory. He made his diagnostic judgments second-hand, so to speak. An interpreter had to translate into German patients' stories which were told in a non-literary and less inflexional form of Estonian (Berrios and Hauser, 1988).

Sustaining the Social Construction of Schizophrenia as a Disease

Two features sustain the validity of any social construction: (1) its utility in solving certain societal problems, and (2) the support it receives from authoritative sources and from the forces of concurrent ideological commitments.

The Medicalization of Deviant Conduct

The social construction of schizophrenia was elaborated in the context of the asylum movement. The history of the nineteenth century asylum movement makes clear how madness was medicalized (Sarbin, 1990). In the ferment produced by rapid strides in all branches of science and technology, madness became a fit subject for scientific work. It was in the nineteenth century that medical practitioners introduced a host of new diagnoses (Rosenberg, 1989). When called upon to deal with crazy people, in the spirit of the rapidly-advancing medical science, these practitioners formulated new diagnoses, among them, dementia praecox.

The context for this new medical activity was the asylum, soon to be renamed mental hospital. The mental hospital filled a number of societal needs, the most salient of which was social control − the maintenance of order. A cursory glance at the treatments introduced over the past 150 years demonstrates clearly the operation of a mechanistic and medical ideology to solve the control problem. Locked wards and physical restraints were supplemented with treatments that were manifestly medical. Bloodletting and emetics, relics of Galenic theory, were widely practiced and ultimately abandoned. Treatments that were consistent with the developing medical theories were invented, among them, unlimited surgery to rid the patient's body of focal infections. Scull (1987) has written a Gothic horror tale of the focal infection theory and the unwarranted surgery practiced by dentists and surgeons in their efforts to control unwanted behavior. Enthusiasm for such treatments went unchecked until it became public knowledge that the high mortality rates ensuing from treatments could not justify the small number of patients whose behavior was brought under control. The more recent history of insulin, metrazol, and electric shock therapies provide additional support to the claim that social control was the object of the therapies. Frontal lobotomy as a means of behavior control was another treatment based on the entrenched belief that unwanted conduct was somehow caused by malfunctioning frontal lobes (Valenstein, 1986). Just a short time ago, biologically-oriented psychiatrists, influenced by the same ideology, employed hemodialysis in an effort to rid patients of the presumed schizotoxin.

The most recent application of this ideology is the attempt to control behavior through the use of neuroleptic medications, formerly called "major tranquilizers." The justification for the prescription of such medications is the dopamine hypothesis, that schizophrenic behavior is the result of an excess of dopaminergic activity. Phenothiazine medications block such activity and, in some patients, there is a diminution of unacceptable activity. It has been observed that not only unacceptable behavior is reduced, but also other activities. The behavior control brought about by the medications has its price, however. Structural and histological damage to the brain is known to follow the prolonged use of phenothiazines, among them, tardive dyskinesia which occurs in a substantial proportion of patients (Breggin, 1983; Cohen, 1989; Cohen and Cohen, 1986). Contemporary clinical practice, however, accepts the notion that dopamine blockers are the medications of choice and also the corollary notion that it would be unethical to withhold such "proven" medication from schizophrenic patients. The rationale for prescribing dopamine blockers is questioned in a recent editorial in the prestigious *New England Journal of Medicine*. "Despite a number of sugestive findings . . . there is currently no proof that either a neurotoxin or an abnormality of transmission (including a dopaminergic abnormality) is a primary feature of schizophrenia" (Mesulam, 1990, p. 843).

Clearly, the schizophrenia construction has been useful to mental health practitioners. The construction has provided a justification for diagnosis. The availablity of the diagnostic term, schizophrenia, like the availability of its superordinate, mental illness, is useful as a step in the societal process of controlling persons whose conduct is unacceptable to others. With the development of the profession of medicine and especially the discipline of psychiatry, the control of patient conduct has for the most part been accomplished by means of traditional medical procedures: surgery and medication. I have identified a few of these procedures. All had a moment in the sun and were discarded when proven to be ineffective or harmful. During the period that each of the procedures was considered professionally ethical and potentially effective, however, the sequence "first diagnosis, then treatment" gave illusory support to the construction of nonconforming conduct as a disease process. In many cases, the first step in the sequence, diagnosing, was no more than a ritual exercise because of the ignorance of the effects of available treatments and their remote outcomes.

The importance given to the development of diagnostic manuals appears to be out of proportion to their utility. The obsessive preoccupation with diagnosis is illustrated in the history of the *Diagnostic and Statistical Manual*. The *Manual* is put together by psychiatric experts guided by the need for consensus. Blashfield, Sprock, and Fuller (1990) have noted that the first *Diagnostic and Statistical Manual*, published in 1952, contained 106 categories, the second, published in 1968, contained 182, the third, published in 1980, contained 265, and the fourth, published in 1987 (DSM-III-R) contained 292. "By linear extrapolation, the DSM-IV should be expected to contain about 350 categories. . ." (p. 18). This progression raised many questions about the underlying assumptions and purposes of such diagnostic manuals.

Intrinsic and Extrinsic Support for the Disease Construction

Despite its failure when examined by empirical methods, the social construction of schizophrenia has persisted. Its persistence is a function of the support it has received. Two classes of support can be identified: support intrinsic to the biomedical model; and support extrinsic to the model in the form of social practices and unarticulated beliefs.

Biological research has served as intrinsic support for the schizophrenia construction. I need but mention the names of hypotheses that have been subjected to laboratory and clinical testing: taraxein, CPK (creatine phosphokinase), serotonin, and dopamine, among others. The composite impact of all this research activity is that an entity exists, waiting for refined methods and high technology to identify the causal morphological, neuro-transmission, or biochemical factor. As I indicated before, countless studies have not identified the disease entity. Nevertheless, the profession and the public have interpreted the sustained research activity by responsible scientists as evidence that the schizophrenia construction is a tenable one.

Guided by the mechanistic paradigm (that behavior is *caused* by antecedent physico-chemical conditions) and operating within the medical variant of that paradigm (that the causes of atypical conduct are to be found in disease entities), research scientists employed a number of broad categories as the defining criteria of schizophrenia. Such categories as cognitive slippage, anhedonia, social withdrawal, ambivalence, thought disorder, loosening of associations, delusions, inappropriate affect, and hallucinations, among others, have been employed for classifying the observed or reported conduct of persons brought to diagnosticians by concerned relatives or by forensic or social agencies. The diagnostic process involved locating the putative patient's conduct in one or more of these broad categories, and then inferring the diagnosis of schizophrenia. Thus, immediate and remote origins of the *meanings* of an individual's atypical conduct become irrelevant to the objective of the diagnosis. A scientist interested in the *person* would have little to go on from reading research reports. Readers of these reports are frustrated if they search for connections between a particular instance of unwanted conduct − the presumed basis for the diagnosis − and some dependent variable assessed after a diagnosis has been made. No causal link can be postulated to account, for example, for a schizophrenic patient's anomalous brain scan and his specific claims to having daily conversations with St. Augustine.

Typically, journal articles provide statements of statistically significant associations between such variables and *diagnoses*, not between such variables and *conduct*. Since heterogeneous acts are lumped together into homogenized diagnoses, experimental results cannot provide information that would allow inferences about the relation between the experimental variable and specific behaviors. The conventional publication style facilitates the illusory conclusion that a cause, or partial cause, of schizophrenia has been discovered. Because distributions of the dependent variable are not usually published, the reader cannot calculate the proportions of false positives and false negatives that would be generated if the dependent variable were to be used as a diagnostic instrument. Not reporting the proportion of cases contrary to the hypothesis, like the employment of diagnoses as the independent variable, facilitates the belief that some enduring property of schizophrenia has been isolated.

The traditional method of reporting scientific data helps to support the belief that some biochemical or anatomical entity corresponding to schizophrenia exists. The common practice is to report the differences between the means of the experimental subjects and the means of the controls. If the differences between the means are statistically significant, then it is assumed that the variable under consideration is related to the dichotomy: schizophrenia-nonschizophrenia. As I mentioned in connection with the analysis of 30 years of published research, the differences may be statistically significant but so small that the variable could not be employed as a diagnostic test. There is a subtle epistemological problem here: in employing group means, the experimenter homogenizes all the subjects in the experimental group and all subjects in the control group. The measurements, whether psychological, chemical, electrical, or whatever, are lumped together. They are regarded as fungible – the assessment of the cerebral ventricles of one schizophrenic is treated as if it were the same as the assessment of the ventricles of any other schizophrenic, without regard to the form, quality, and frequency of behaviors that led to the diagnosis of schizophrenia. The epistemological assumption of the significance of mean differences has proven useful in agricultural research and in insurance studies. It is hardly tenable as a basis for diagnosis.

In addition to direct biological research, the genetic transmission hypothesis has been advanced to support the construction of schizophrenia. Highly visible scientists have reported a heritability factor for schizophrenia. Wide publicity, both within the profession and outside, has been given to studies of twins and to studies of children of schizophrenics who were reared by adoptive parents (see, for example, Gottesman and Shields, 1972; Kety, Rosenthal, Wender, and Shulsinger, 1968; Kety, Rosenthal, Wender, Shulsinger, and Jacobsen, 1975). Current textbooks cite these investigations as revealed truth, but the extensive critiques of the studies are seldom noted. That the reported

studies are riddled with methodological, statistical and interpretational errors
has been repeatedly demonstrated (see especially, Abrams and Taylor, 1983;
Benjamin, 1976; Kringlen and Cramer, 1989; Lewontin, Kamin, and Rose,
1984; Lidz, 1990; Lidz and Blatt, 1983; Lidz, Blatt, and Cook, 1981; Marshall,
1986; Sarbin and Mancuso, 1980). The extent of these criticisms suggests that
establishing the validity of "schizophrenia" should have had logical priority
over the identification of its genetic features.

My aim is not to rehash the arguments pro and con of the heredity thesis,
rather to show that the wide publicity given genetic studies has served as
additional support to maintain the schizophrenia construction. My thesis
holds for genetic research as it does for psychological and biological research:
that no firm ontological basis has been established for schizophrenia. In the
absence of determinate criteria, investigators direct their efforts toward
discovering intergenerational similarities — not of identifiable behavior but
of *diagnosis*, a far cry from the subject matter of behavior genetics in which
intergenerational similarities of *behavior* are studied.[6]

In addition to intrinsic supports, it is possible to identify a number of extrinsic supports that help explain the tenacity of the schizophrenia construction. Although constructions that are congruent with the concurrent scientific paradigm may appear self-supporting, they are in great measure sustained
by forces external to the scientific enterprise.

A vast bureaucratic network at federal, state, and local levels legitimizes
biochemical conceptions of deviant conduct, including schizophrenia. Federal
agencies that control research grants advocate studies the aim of which is
the understanding and ultimately the control of "the dread disease"
schizophrenia. The National Institute of Mental Health has promoted the
schizophrenia construction in many ways, including the sponsoring of its own
professional journal, *Schizophrenia Bulletin*, now in its sixteenth year of publication. That the government is willing to spend precious tax dollars on such
an enterprise is convincing evidence to some people that "something" is there
to be studied. Some local communities have taken to the airwaves and to
the press to advocate the notion that schizophrenia and other mental illness
are like somatic illness and can be treated with appropriate medication.

In addition to bureaucratic advocacy, in recent decades the pharmaceutical
industry has been instrumental in furthering the schizophrenia doctrine.
Pharmaceutical companies support countless research enterprises in which
medications are clinically tested on patients, many of whom are diagnosed
as schizophrenic. The psychiatric journals are to a great extent subsidized

---

[6]Kety, one of the leading advocates of the genetic transmission hypothesis, wrote a critique of
Rosenhan's (1973) famous study, "Being Sane in Insane Places." In the critique, he composed
a rhetorical sentence that lends itself to a literal interpretation: "If schizophrenia is a myth, it
is a myth with a very strong genetic component" (1974, p. 961).

by pharmaceutical advertising, such advertising being directed to physicians who are legally empowered to prescribe medications.

The implicit power of bureaucracy and the commercial goals of pharmaceutical companies would be minimal if the schizophrenia messages fell on deaf ears. A readiness to believe the schizophrenia story follows from the unwitting acceptance of an ideology — a network of historically-conditioned premises.

I use the term "ideology" in the manner in which it has been employed by political scientists. "Ideology" carries the meaning that knowledge is situationally determined — the worldview and the social status of the scientist influence the content of knowledge. An examination of ideological premises illuminates how an entrenched professional organization can become so bound to a situation that its members cannot recognize facts that would dissolve its power. An ideology has a sacred quality. A challenge to a claim based on ideological premises usually invokes passionate rather than reasoned responses. Note the heated responses to the writings of Szasz, Laing, Rosenhan, and other critics of the official schizophrenia doctrine.[7]

One strand in the texture of the schizophenia ideology is the creation of the mental hospital institution. The transformation of the asylum to a mental hospital, in the context of preserving order, paved the way for regarding inmates as objects. The hospital and its medical climate were legitimated through legislative acts and judicial rulings. The courts, usually acting on the advice of physicians, granted almost unlimited power to physicians to employ their skills and their paradigms in the interest of protecting society. Because of culturally-enscripted roles for physicians and patients, once the physician made the diagnosis, the patient became a figure in an altered social narrative. The power of physicians relative to patients created a condition in which physicians could distance themselves from patients — a necessary precondition for the draconian surgical and medical treatments mentioned previously.[8]

---

[7]Hays (1984), commenting on the inclusion of a heterogeneous array of behaviors in one nosological class, addresses the matter of ideological support: "Medicine is a conservative profession. What doctors know is passed on to students. In this way they honestly associate themselves with their own body of knowledge and as responsible guarantors of its truth. It is natural for such men and women to shy away from radical formulations which threaten their hard-won data-base, introduce uncertainty, and reduce the worth of what they have learned and what they have to offer. The presentation of a conceptualization which is at variance with extant schemata may be received as an affront. . ." (p. 5).

[8]It is instructive to trace the emphasis on diagnosis to its historical roots. Craik (1959) revived the historical notion that the early Greeks recognized that different outcomes were entailed if the doctors emphasized the *disease* or the *person*. The focus on diagnosing and treating the disease is associated with a school of medical practice on the island of Cnidus. A contrary view is associated with Hippocrates of Cos. The Cosan view recognized the necessity of dealing with the whole patient, the illness in relation to biography. The doctor-patient script was a collaborative one.

The legitimate power of the physician remains as an unquestioned premise in the social construction of schizophrenia. But legitimate power is only one of the characteristics that operate as silent assumptions in physicians' enacting their roles. Physicians carry Aesculapian authority, an authority that supplements legitimate power with moral and charismatic authority (Paterson, 1966; Siegler and Osmond, 1973). Physicians are assumed to have moral power in that they are dedicated to relieving pain and curing illness. They are assumed also to have the charisma that goes with the priestly role, a derivative from the time when religious figures participated in healing activities. Aesculapian authority continues to operate as a silent premise for government bodies that allocate funds in support of research the aim of which is the control of crazy people.[9]

A parallel premise is that "certain types of people are more dangerous than other types of people" (Sarbin and Mancuso, 1980). The origins of the connection between being schizophrenic and being dangerous are obscure. Several strands in the fabric of this premise can be identified, among them, the Calvinistic equation of being poor and being damned, and the attribution "dangerous classes" to the powerless poor. "Dangerous to self or other" remains as a criterion for commitment in most jurisdictions.

The overrepresentation of poor people in the class "schizophrenics" has been repeatedly documented. In addition, Pavkov, Lewis, and Lyons (1989) have shown that being black and coming to the attention of mental health professionals is predictive of a diagnosis of schizophrenia. Recently, Landrine (1989) has concluded on the basis of research evidence that the social role of poor people is a stereotype in the epistemic structure of middle-class diagnosticians. The linguistic performances and social interactions of poor people are of the same quality as the performances of men and women diagnosed as schizophrenics, particular of the "negative type" (Andreasen, 1982), those social failures who have adopted a strategy of minimal action.

With the renewed emphasis on the Kraepelinian construction, interest in studying the relations between socio-economic status (SES) and psychiatric diagnoses has declined. This decline in interest is not due to any change in the demographics. Schizophrenia is primarily a diagnosis for poor people. The advent of neo-Kraepelinian models, especially the diathesis-stress construction, turned attention to genetics research and to the study of stress. But

---

The prevailing ideology in medicine, including psychiatry, is Cnidian. The doctor-patient script diminished the role of biography in therapy. In their research, psychologists have borrowed the Cnidian point of view. They begin the research enterprise with subjects who have been "diagnosed" as schizophrenic, thus embracing — sometimes unwittingly — the disease construction. Once the diagnosis is made, the life-narrative of the patient is irrelevant.

[9]In the interest of brevity, I have omitted a discussion of several other premises that undergird the social construction of schizophrenia. These are described in Sarbin and Mancuso (1980).

SES has not figured prominently in stress research. Dohrenwend (1990), a leading epidemiologist, has noted that ". . . relations between SES or social class and psychiatric disorders have provided the most challenging cues to the role of adversity in the development of psychiatric disorders. The problem remains what it has always been: how to unlock the riddle that low SES can be either a cause or a consequence of psychopathology" (p. 45). The adversity thesis might be illuminated through an examination of the observation that the outcome of "schizophrenia" varies with economic and social conditions (Warner, 1985). Landrine's research, cited above, adds to the puzzle another dimension: lower class stereotypes held by middle class diagnosticians.

The translation from the expression of atypical, unassimilable conduct (craziness) to being dangerous is facilitated by the myth of the "wild man within" (White, 1972). The myth grew out of beliefs held by Europeans during times when unknown lands were being discovered. Because the inhabitants of exotic places engaged in conduct that differed so markedly from western norms, Europeans looked upon such people as being unsocialized, wild savages. The continually shrinking world has unearthed no wild man of Africa, Asia, or of any other place, but the myth of the "wild man within" lingers as an unspoken basis for attributing dangerousness to crazy people. The myth found expression and *a fortiori* support in Lombroso's notion of "atavism" and Freud's concept of the impulse-ridden Id.[10]

Conclusion

To recapitulate: my thesis is that schizophrenia is a social construction, generated to deal with people whose conduct was not acceptable to more powerful others. During the heyday of nineteenth century science, the construction was guided by metaphors drawn from mechanistic biology. Physicians formulated their theories and practices from constructions that grew out of developing knowledge in anatomy, chemistry and physiology. The construction has an ideological cast − its proponents were blind to the possibilities that the absurdities[11] exhibited by mental hospital patients were efforts at sense-making. Instead proponents followed the tenets of mechanistic science: that social misconduct, like rashes, fevers, aches, pains, and other somatic conditions, was caused by disease processes. Reliable and sustained empirical evidence − a cardinal requirement of mechanistic science − has not been put forth to validate the schizophrenia hypothesis. Despite the absence of

---

[10]A pharmaceutical advertisement in one of the psychiatric journals continues the rhetorical tradition. The product, it is claimed, will *"tame the psychotic fury."*

[11]Mancuso (1989) has offered the felicitous suggestion that we employ the descriptor "absurdity" to designate disvalued conduct.

empirical support, the schizophrenia construction continues its tenacious hold on theory and practice.

My recommendation is that we banish schizophrenia to the musty historical archives where other previously-valued scientific constructions are stored, among them, phlogiston, the luminiferous ether, the geocentric view of the universe, and closer to home, monomania, neurasthenia, masturbatory insanity, lycanthropy, demon possession, and mopishness.

I emphasize that I am not recommending formulating a new descriptive term to replace schizophrenia. It is too late for that. The referents for schizophrenia are too diverse, confounded, changing, and ambiguous (Bentall, Jackson, and Pilgrim, 1988; Carpenter and Kirkpatrick, 1988). The fact that two persons (or 200) who exhibit no absurdities in common may be tagged with the same label demonstrates the emptiness of the concept.

Abandoning the schizophrenia hypothesis, however, will not solve the societal and interpersonal problems generated when persons engage in absurd, nonconforming, perplexing conduct. The first step in solving such problems calls for critical examination of the societal and political systems that support the failing biomedical paradigm. Such examination would be instrumental in replacing the mechanistic world view with a framework that would regard persons as agents trying to solve existential and identity problems.

I have already referred to the observation that the yield from the traditional approach — derived from the mechanistic metaphors — has been disappointing. This metaphysic has guided scientists and practitioners to look upon human beings as organismic objects. From this perspective, it was assumed that the behavior of organisms could be understood, predicted, and controlled through applying the root metaphor of mechanistic science — the transmittal of forces. From this belief there flowed countless hypotheses about the internal transmittal and transformation of forces. Explanations of conduct, especially deviant conduct, focused on the transmittal of forces within the brain.

The mechanistic world view is not the only metaphysical framework. An alternate framework, contextualism, leads to a totally different approach to the understanding of deviant conduct. The root metaphor of contextualism is the historical act in all its complexity. Change, novelty, variation and contingency are the categories. Unlike mechanistic constructions in which the human being is a passive object reacting to happenings within the body, the contextualist perspective directs the scientist to perceive human beings as agents, actors, performers. Within this framework, the clinician would begin his or her study by posing questions such as "what is the person trying to do or say?" "what goals is he or she trying to reach?" "what story is he or she trying to tell?" Persons are perceived as agents trying — sometimes with poorly-developed skills — to maintain their self-narratives in the face of a complex, unpredictable and confusing world. As agents, they may choose to incorporate into their sense-making the moral valuations imposed on their conduct by parents, siblings, employers, doctors or other power figures. I see the failure of modern research on absurd conduct as following from the perception of "schizophrenics" as without agency, as suffering from happenings in the brain, rather than as agents trying to solve existential and identity problems through the construction of atypical beliefs, unusual imaginings, and bizarre speech and gestural behavior. Were we to look upon such persons as agents we would become interested in how they arrive at constructions of the world that are so different from our own (Sarbin, 1969).

One implication of adopting a contextualist framework would be a reduction in the obsessive concern with diagnosis. Each person has his or her own story, and the expressed beliefs, the atypical imaginings, the instrumental acts of withdrawing from strain-producing situations are intentional acts designed to solve identity and existential problems. The actions designed to keep one's self-narrative consistent are not invariant or machine-like outcomes of postulated disease processes. Contingencies of many kinds enter into the person's adopting a deviant role and also — I hasten to add — of rejecting such a role. Invariance is not a feature of human social life.

Reconstructing the patient's self-narrative is central to psychosocial change efforts (Sarbin, 1986). We can revive the systematic case study (Fishman, 1990) which, although time-consuming, provides patients with a context for reconstructing their self-narratives. Respectful listening to patients' stories is the first step in granting them the status of agents, goal-directed beings. At the same time that they reconstruct their life-narratives, they are given the opportunity of recounting the conduct of significant others who have collaborated in forming the self-narratives.

Understanding the interpersonal or existential themes in the stories of troubled persons is hampered when we rely on the customary vocabulary of pathology: toxins, tumors, traumata, dysfunctional traits, or defective genes. Understanding is more likely to be facilitated if we follow the lead of poets, dramatists, and biographers, and focus on the language of social relationships.

References

Abrams, R., and Taylor, M.A. (1983). The genetics of schizophrenia: A reassessment using modern criteria. *American Journal of Psychiatry, 140,* 171–175.

Andreasen, N.C. (1982). Negative symptoms in schizophrenia: Definition and reliability. *Archives of General Psychiatry, 39,* 784–788.

Bateson, G., Jackson, D.D., Haley, J., and Weakland, J.H. (1956). Toward a theory of schizophrenia. *Behavioral Science, 1,* 251–264.

Benjamin, L.S. (1989). Is chronicity a function of the relationship between the person and auditory hallucination? *Schizophrenia Bulletin, 15,* 291–310.

Benjamin, L.S. (1976). A reconsideration of the Kety and Associates study of genetic factors in the transmission of schizophrenia. *American Journal of Psychiatry, 133,* 1129–1133.

Bentall, R.P., Jackson, H.F., and Pilgrim, D. (1988). Abandoning the concept of "schizophrenia": Some implications of validity arguments for psychological research into psychotic phenomena. *British Journal of Clinical Psychology*, 27, 303–324.

Berrios, G.E., and Hauser, R. (1988). The early development of Kraepelin's ideas on classification: A conceptual history. *Psychological Medicine*, 18, 813–821.

Blashfield, R.K., Sprock, J., and Fuller, A.K. (1990). Suggested guidelines for including or excluding categories in the DSM-IV. *Comprehensive Psychiatry*, 31, 15–19.

Blum, J.D. (1978). On changes in psychiatric diagnosis over time. *American Psychologist*, 33, 1017–1031.

Boyle, M. (in press). Is schizophrenia what it was? A reanalysis of Kraepelin's and Bleuler's population. *Journal of the History of the Behavioral Sciences*.

Breggin, P.R. (1983). *Psychiatric drugs: Hazards to the brain*. New York: Springer.

Carpenter, W.T., Jr., and Kirkpatrick, B. (1988). The heterogeneity of the long term course of schizophrenia. *Schizophrenia Bulletin*, 14, 645–652.

Cohen, D. (1989). Biological basis of schizophrenia: The evidence reconsidered. *Social Work*, 34, 255–257.

Cohen, D., and Cohen, H. (1986). Biological theories, drug treatments, and schizophrenia: A critical assessment. *Journal of Mind and Behavior*, 7, 11–35.

Christison, G.W., Casanova, M.F., Weinberger, D.R., Rawlings, R., and Kleinman, J.E. (1989). A quantitative investigation of hippocampal cell size, shape, and variability of orientation in schizophrenia. *Archives of General Psychiatry*, 46, 1027–1032.

Craik, K.H. (1959). *The Cosans versus the Cnidians, or comments on diagnosis in general and diagnosis of schizophrenia in particular*. Unpublished manuscript. Berkeley, California: University of California.

Cutting, J. (1985). *The psychology of schizophrenia*. Edinburgh: Churchill Livingstone.

Dohrenwend, B.P. (1990). Socioeconomic status (SES) and psychiatric disorders: Are the issues still compelling? *Social Psychiatry and Psychiatric Epidemiology*, 25, 41–47.

Ellard, J. (1987). Did schizophrenia exist before the eighteenth century? *Australian and New Zealand Journal of Psychiatry*, 21, 306–314.

Fishman, D. (1990). The quantitative, naturalistic case study: A unifying element for psychology. *International Newsletter of Uninomic Psychology*, 9, 1–10.

Gottesman, J.J., and Shields, J. (1972). *Schizophrenia and genetics*. New York: Academic Press.

Gubrium, J., and Holstein, J.A. (1990). *What is family?* Mountainview, California: Mayfield Publishing Company.

Hays, P. (1984, June 16). The nosological status of schizophrenia. *Lancet*, pp. 1342–1345.

Jernigan, T.L., Zatz, L.M., Moses, J.A., and Berger, P.A. (1982a). Computed tomography in schizophrenics and normal volunteers, I. Fluid volume. *Archives of General Psychiatry*, 39, 765–770.

Jernigan, T.L., Zatz, L.M., Moses, J.A., and Berger, P.A. (1982b). Computed tomography in schizophrenics and normal volunters, II. Cranial asymmetry. *Archives of General Psychiatry*, 39, 771–777.

Juhasz, J.B., and Sarbin, T.R. (1966). On the false alarm metaphor in psychophysics. *Psychological Record*, 16, 323–327.

Kety, S.S. (1974). From rationalization to reason. *American Journal of Psychiatry*, 103, 957–962.

Kety, S.S., Rosenthal, D., Wender, P.H., and Shulsinger, P. (1968). The types and prevalence of mental illness in the biological and adoptive families of adoptive schizophrenics. In D. Rosenthal and S. Kety (Eds.), *The transmission of schizophrenia* (pp. 345–362). New York: Pergamon.

Kety, S.S., Rosenthal, D., Wender, P.H., Schulsinger, F., and Jacobsen, B. (1975). Mental illness in the biological and adoptive families of adoptive individuals who have become schizophrenic: A preliminary report based upon psychiatric interviews. In R. Fieve, D. Rosenthal, and H. Brill (Eds.), *Genetic research in psychiatry* (pp. 147–165). Baltimore: Johns Hopkins University Press.

Kringlen, E., and Cramer, G. (1989). Offspring of monozygotic twins discordant for schizophrenia. *Archives of General Psychiatry*, 46, 873–877.

Landrine, H. (1989). The social class–schizophrenia relationship: A different approach and a new hypothesis. *Social and Clinical Psychology*, 8, 288–303.

Lewontin, R.C., Kamin, L., and Rose, S. (1984). *Not in our genes: Biology, ideology, and human nature.* New York: Pantheon.

Lidz, T. (1990). Optimism in treatment of schizophrenia still premature, says expert. *Psychiatric News, 25,* 26–33.

Lidz, T., and Blatt, S. (1983). Critique of Danish-American studies of biological and adoptive relatives of adoptees who became schizophrenic. *American Journal of Psychiatry, 140,* 426–435.

Lidz, T., Blatt, S., and Cook, B. (1981). Critique of Danish-American studies of adopted-away offspring of schizophrenic parents. *American Journal of Psychiatry, 138,* 1063–1068.

Mancuso, J.C. (1989). Review of Porter, R. *A Social History of Madness: The World Through the Eyes of the Insane. Society,* July-August, 92–94.

Marshall, R. (1986). Hereditary aspects of schizophrenia: A critique. In N. Eisenberg and D. Glasgow (Eds.), *Current issues in clinical psychology* (pp. 109–125). Brookfield, Vermont: Gower.

Meehl, P. (1989). Schizotaxia revisited. *Archives of General Psychiatry, 46,* 935–944.

Mesulam, M.-M. (1990). Schizophrenia and the brain. *New England Journal of Medicine, 322,* 842–845.

Nasrallah, H.A., Jacoby, C.G., McCalley-Whitters, and Kuperman, S. (1982). Cerebral ventricular enlargement in subtypes of chronic schizophrenia. *Archives of General Psychiatry, 39,* 774–777.

Paterson, T.T. (1966). *Management theory.* London: Business Publications, Ltd.

Pavkov, T.W., Lewis, D.A., and Lyons, J.S. (1989). Diagnosis and racial bias: An empirical investigation. *Professional Psychology, Research and Practice, 20,* 364–368.

Rosenberg, C.E. (1989). Disease in history: Frames and framers. *Milbank Quarterly, 67* (Supplement 1), 1–15.

Rosenhan, D. (1973). On being sane in insane places. *Science, 179,* 250–258.

Sarbin, T.R. (1967). The concept of hallucination. *Journal of Personality, 35,* 359–380.

Sarbin, T.R. (1969). Schizophrenic thinking: A role-theory interpretation. *Journal of Personality, 37,* 190–206.

Sarbin, T.R. (1972a). Imagining as muted role-taking: A historico-linguistic analysis. In P. Sheehan (Ed.), *The function and nature of imagery* (pp. 333–354). New York: Academic Press.

Sarbin, T.R. (1972b). Schizophrenia: From metaphor to myth. *Psychology Today,* June, pp. 18–27.

Sarbin, T.R. (1986). *Narrative psychology: The storied nature of human conduct.* New York: Praeger.

Sarbin, T.R. (1990). Metaphors of unwanted conduct: A historical sketch. In D. Leary (Ed.), *The history of metaphor in psychology* (pp. 300–330). New York: Cambridge University Press.

Sarbin, T.R., and Juhasz, J.B. (1967). The historical background of the concept of hallucination. *Journal of the History of the Behavioral Sciences, 3,* 339–358.

Sarbin, T.R., and Juhasz, J.B. (1970). Toward a theory of imagination. *Journal of Personality, 38,* 52–76.

Sarbin, T.R., and Juhasz, J.B. (1975). The social psychology of hallucination. In R. Siegel and L. West (Eds.), *Hallucination: Theory and research* (pp. 241–256). New York: Wiley.

Sarbin, T.R., and Juhasz, J.B. (1978). The social psychology of hallucinations. *Journal of Mental Imagery, 2,* 117–144.

Sarbin, T.R., and Juhasz, J.B. (1982). The concept of mental illness: A historical perspective. In I. Al-Issa (Ed.), *Culture and psychopathology* (pp. 71–110). Baltimore: University Park Press.

Sarbin, T.R., and Mancuso, J.C. (1980). *Schizophrenia: Medical diagnosis or moral verdict?* Elmsford, New York: Pergamon Press.

Sarbin, T.R., Mancuso, J.C., and Podczerwinski, J. (in preparation). *A critical review of research on schizophrenia reported in the Journal of Abnormal Psychology, 1959–1988.*

Schneider, K. (1959). *Clinical psychopathology.* New York: Grune and Stratton.

Scull, A. (1987). Desperate remedies: A Gothic tale of madness and modern medicine. *Psychological Medicine, 17,* 561–577.

Siegler, M., and Osmond, H. (1973). Aesculapian authority. *Hastings Center Studies, 1,* 41–52.

Singer, M.T., and Wynne, L.C. (1963). Differentiating characteristics of the parents of childhood neurotics and young adult schizophenics. *American Journal of Psychiatry, 120,* 234–243.

Valenstein, E.S. (1986). *Great and desperate cures: The rise and decline of psychosurgery and other radical treatments for mental illness.* New York: Basic Books.

van den Brink, W., Koeter, M.W.J., Ormel, J., Dijkstra, W., Giel, R., Sloof, C.J., and Woolfarth,

T.D. (1989). Psychiatric diagnosis in an outpatient population: A comparative study of PSE-Catego and DSM-III. *Archives of General Psychiatry, 46*, 369–372.

Warner, R. (1985). *Recovery from schizophrenia: Psychiatry and political economy*. Boston: Routledge & Kegan Paul.

Weinberger, D.R., Torrey, E.F., Neophytides, A., and Wyatt, R.J. (1979). Lateral cerebral ventricular enlargement in chronic schizophrenia. *Archives of General Psychiatry, 36*, 935–939.

White, H. (1972). The forms of wildness: Archeology of an idea. In E. Dudley and M. Novick (Eds.). *The wild man within* (pp. 3–38). Pittsburgh: University of Pittsburgh Press.

Willis, J.H., and Bannister, D. (1965). The diagnosis and treatment of schizophrenia: A questionnaire study of psychiatric opinion. *British Journal of Psychiatry, 111*, 1165–1171.

Wing, J., Cooper, J., and Sartorius, N. (1974). *The description and classification of psychiatric symptoms: An instruction manual for PSE and Catego system*. London: Cambridge University Press.

©1990 The Institute of Mind and Behavior, Inc.
The Journal of Mind and Behavior
Summer and Autumn 1990, Volume 11, Numbers 3 and 4
Pages 285 [39] – 300 [54]
ISSN 0271-0137
ISBN 0-930195-05-1

Institutional Mental Health and Social Control: The Ravages of Epistemological Hubris

Seth Farber

Network Against Coercive Psychiatry

I argue in this essay that the phenomena we classify as "mental illness" result largely from the refusal of socially authorized "experts" to recognize — and thus to constitute — the Other (the developing person, the social deviant) as a subject. I suggest that Institutional Mental Health refuses to do this not merely because it seeks to aggrandize its own power but also because it fears to acknowledge that we are all participants in a process of historical development. It denies this because it is historically conditioned by its own moment of origin in the project of the Enlightenment. It is consequently wed to an ethos of rationalized order that does not accommodate, much less support, the unpredictable creative power of the Other (the individual) and that sustains instead the project of mastery, of domination, of discovering eternal laws that will (supposedly) enable Reason to master history and to master the Other. For this reason Institutional Mental Health and its diverse ideologies, ranging from the psychoanalytic to genetic defect models, constitute a major obstacle to the evolution of humanity.

One cannot step into the same river twice.

Heraclitus

There is a widespread misconception in society that Institutional Mental Health (this term is intended to cover psychiatrists, psychologists and other "mental health" professionals) provides valuable services to individuals in need of help and generally attempts to foster personal change or "growth." I argue in this paper that the praxis of Institutional Mental Health is based on a model that is not oriented primarily toward generating change, but toward maintaining social control. Thus, this model is problematic on ethical as well as on epistemological grounds: it *underestimates* the individual's capacity for change and it consequently *undermines* this very capacity.

Requests for reprints should be sent to Seth Farber, Ph.D., 172 West 79th Street, Apt. 2E, New York, New York 10024.

The term "medical model" will be used here in a sense general enough to subsume a number of more specifically articulated models; the two most popular in the field today are the psychoanalytic model and the "genetic defect" model. Scheff's (1966) comment on psychoanalysis succinctly points to the fundamental premise (expressed through a number of different idioms) that underlies all medical models. "The basic model upon which psychoanalysis is constructed is the disease model, in that it portrays neurotic behavior as unfolding relentlessly out of a defective psychological system contained within the body" (p. 9).

The Mental Health Worker as a Social Control Agent

The contemporary disease model in psychology has its roots in a bureau-cratic, industrial society that promoted the idea of an increasingly rational-ized world-order as a solution to the ills of the world. The historian Scull (1975) has noted that the hegemony of the medical model in psychology and the increasing power of psychiatry to redefine any aspect of life in medical terms is merely one important example of a general trend in modern societies. "Elites in such societies over about the past century and a half have increas-ingly sought to rationalize and legitimize their control of all sorts of deviant and troublesome elements by consigning them to the ministrations of experts. No longer content to rely on vague cultural definitions of, and informal responses to deviation, rational-bureaucratic western societies have delegated this task to groups of people who claim, or who are assumed to have, special competence in these areas" (p. 219).

Many of these experts call themselves "psychotherapists" but they have in fact the orientation and values of social control agents within a rationalized world-order. Haley (1980) has defined the difference between the two social roles:

> The goal of a therapist is to introduce more complexity into people's lives, in the sense that he breaks up repetitive cycles of behavior and brings about new alternatives. He does not wish to have a problem person simply conform, but wants to place in that per-son's hands the initiative to come up with new ideas and acts that the therapist might not even have considered. In that sense a therapist encourages unpredictability. The therapist's job is to bring about change, and therefore new, often unanticipated behavior.
> The social control agent has quite the opposite goal. His task is to stabilize people for the community, thus he seeks to reduce unpredictability. He wants problem people to behave in respectable ways, like others in the community so that no one is upset by them. It is not change and new behavior that he seeks, but rather stability and no complaints from citizens. (pp. 54–55)

The medical model, the model of the social control agent, exemplifies an "objectivist" approach, to borrow Gadamer's (1976) term. It is based on the premise that patients are objects who are not influenced by the way in which they are understood and interpreted by Institutional Mental Health. Today, psychology, fueled by positivist aspirations, apes the natural sciences in a futile attempt to delineate transhistorical laws of human behavior that it imagines will allow it to achieve the ideal of total predictability. This is ultimately the project of Reason, which seeks to escape from its historical moorings by totally objectifying history − and by objectifying persons.

The hermeneutic approach provides the tools for exposing the limitations of objectivism. Hermeneutics recovers history. The observer is implicated in the act of observation, what he or she observes is not independent of this act. This is the fundamental hermeneutical insight. Objectivism obscures this reality, it pursues the illusory Enlightenment ideal of the "detached" scientist, unmindful of the historical roots of this ideal, unmindful of the social consequences of the futile attempt to realize it. Gadamer wrote, "In this objectivism the understander is seen . . . not in relationship to the hermeneutical situation and the constant operativeness of history in his own consciousness, but in such a way as to imply that his own understanding does not enter into the event" (p. 28).

Institutional Mental Health acts as if its own understanding does not enter into the event. It focuses its lenses upon the Others, the deviants, and professes to possess objective knowledge about their situation and their destinies. It fails to see how its own way of understanding the Other enters into the event. It is as if its particular way of understanding has no historical or social ramifications. It is as if psychiatrically labeled individuals are deaf to the discourse that Institutional Mental Health articulates through a variety of media, institutions, groups and individuals. Mental illness is a cultural artifact, the end result of a particular kind of highly structured dialogue between socially empowered experts and socially disenfranchised, psychiatrically stigmatized individuals.

To state that Institutional Mental Health is oriented toward social control is not to imply that its hegemony can be completely explained by economic and political motives. In the last analysis, its maintenance depends on a preference for a particular set of aesthetic values: uniformity, predictability, familiarity, orderliness. Institutional Mental Health consistently follows a particular narrative imperative: it seeks to banish history from its midst, to banish chance, *to banish the unexpected*. It secretly fears the creative autonomy of the Other which it regards as a threat to its attempt to control the process of change. It seeks to subordinate change to method and formula, to discover invariant laws, untouched by history, governing human behavior. To use a current metaphor it seeks to secure the domination of the left brain over the historical process.

This project is bound to fail. As Scheibe (1979) has written, "Because certain scholars start to view human beings as automatons or as very intelligent ants, the facts of human unpredictability do not suddenly change. . . . Full human predictability is impossible in principle" (p. 149). A willingness to accept human unpredictability, to encourage "unanticipated behavior" would spell the end of the disease model with its emphasis on diagnostic classifications and prognoses. The failure of this model (in human terms) is demonstrated by the draconian measures Institutional Mental Health has relied upon to maintain order, ostensibly to protect patients from their illnesses.

In the first half of this century the popular psychiatric "treatments" included: bleeding mental patients to the point of syncope, poisoning them with cyanide, inducing comas with insulin, performing lobotomies and freezing them into a state of nearly fatal coma by packing them in ice. Fifty thousand lobotomies were performed in America mostly during the 1940s and 1950s (Coleman, 1984). Electroconvulsive therapy was first introduced in the late 1930s and is currently being promoted by the American Psychiatric Association [APA]. The APA estimated in 1978 that 100,000 to 200,000 individuals received at least one battery of ECT a year (Coleman, 1984). (Most writers agree that the reliance on ECT is increasing. This is reflected also by the promotional campaign that APA has been leading to convince the population that ECT in its improved version is safe and harmless.) A treatment that has now become standard practice is pressuring "mental patients" to take neuroleptic drugs that are known to cause serious neurological damage when used for more than a brief period of time (Breggin, 1983); psychiatrists typically encourage long-term dependence on these drugs.

The Stability Orientation

There are two variants of the medical model that are dominant in the "mental health" field today; the neopsychoanalytic model (this term refers to the various revisions of classical psychoanalytic thought, including ego psychology and "object relations" theory) and the biochemical imbalance model. Both exemplfy what Gergen (1977) has termed the "stability orientation" which emphasizes the stability of behavior patterns over time and which implies that the individual is predictable. The neopsychoanalytic model assumes that individuals are programmed in the first few years of their lives. They will continue to reenact those early programs for the rest of their lives unless psychoanalysts intervene. As Gergen has put it, "Without massive intervention, ideally through psychoanalysis, the same psycho-behavioral patterns relentlessly repeat themselves throughout the life-cycle" (p. 141). Psychoanalysts claim to be able to change the programs of individuals who are "neurotic" through long-term psychoanalysis. A larger number of individuals are believed to be more pathological; these encompass "personality disorders" as well as such "severely mentally ill" types as "schizophrenics" and individuals with "bipolar disorders." Most psychoanalysts feel that the most they can offer these individuals in good conscience are supportive psychotherapy and psychiatric drugs (termed medication). This form of therapy cannot significantly alter the original program or, to use a popular psychoanalytic idiom, "correct the damage done to the ego," but it can help individuals to adjust to their pathology and thus to live somewhat more comfortable lives. In many intellectual circles such psychoanalytic dogmas are accepted uncritically.

For example in an article published in the *New York Times Book Review*, Trilling (1986) criticized Gloria Steinem for giving the reader the impression in her biography of Marilyn Monroe that the actress was in psychoanalysis rather than in "psychodynamically [i.e., psychoanalytically] derived supportive treatment." Trilling claims "The distinction is important. Patients with her emotional affliction are not available to orthodox psychoanalysis. Unhappily medicine has not yet found a cure or even a confident therapy for Marilyn Monroe's personality disorder" (p. 23). Unhappily modern intellectuals are credulously willing to accept psychoanalytic lore as scientific truth.

Gergen (1977) reviewed a number of studies that belie the psychoanalytic contention that events in early childhood predetermine the individual's later development. The work of Kagan (1970, 1984) provides a decisive refutation of psychoanalytic dogma. Both Gergen (1977, 1980) and Kagan agree that behavior patterns in the first six years of life have virtually no predictive validity in relation to behavior shown during adulthood. The major variable neo-psychoanalysts stress is anxiety over "object loss" in the first few years of life. As Kagan (1970) noted, "the variation in degree of anxiety over loss of access to attachment figures during the first three years of life predicted no significant behavior in adolescence or adulthood" (p. 60). Although current research supports a more optimistic interpretation of the effect of early childhood experience on later development there has not been a modification of psychoanalytic theory or practice. Nor has this research had any impact on contemporary culture which Gergen (1977) notes has "almost fully accepted the assumption that early experience is vital in shaping adult behavior" (p. 142).

Psychoanalysis accepts the premise, as do the various other medical models, that individuals can be placed in diagnostic classes that will predict their future development. But Gergen (1980) shows how the data collected by life-span development researchers indicate that development is idiosyncratic and unpredictable. "The individual seems fundamentally flexible in most aspects of personal functioning. Significant change in the life course may occur at any time. . . . An immense panoply of developmental forms seems possible; which particular form emerges may depend on a confluence of particulars, the existence of which is fundamentally unsystematic" (p. 43). As argued below, the intractability that Institutional Mental Health finds among "the severely mentally ill" is an artifact of its own practices.

The other main example of the stability orientation is the biochemical imbalance theory. This theory now dominates the field (Cohen and Cohen, 1986); its utility lies in the fact that it provides a justification for prescribing psychiatric drugs which in turn seem to lend credibility to the theory. In furtherance of the goal of social control, the majority of psychoanalysts adhere to an amalgam of psychoanalytic theory and the biochemical imbalance theory. According to the latter view, "mentally ill" individuals suffer from "genetic defects" that will cause their biochemical metabolism to become persistently and frequently "unbalanced"; this imbalance will manifest itself in predictably irrational and unmanageable behavior. If not for neuroleptic drugs the individual would be forced to relive the same nightmare, subject to the cruel decree of fate, the eternal law of return. The drugs ostensibly keep the "illness" under control; they also reduce the risk of unanticipated behavior or genuine novelty, as noted below.

It should be noted that contrary to a common misconception, it has not been established that "genetic defects" *cause* "mental illnesses" or "biochemical imbalances." The most that has been established is that certain individuals have a genetic *predisposition* to have certain experiences (usually precipitated by a crisis) that violate particular norms and that are "diagnosed" as "severe mental illnesses" (see the critical survey by Cohen and Cohen, 1986). The outcome of the predisposition obviously depends upon a complex of social, cultural and environmental factors.

Nonetheless, adherents to the biochemical imbalance theory maintain that once the disease appears it will recur in the same fashion at regular intervals. As Polantin and Fieve (1971) write about "manic depression" − a "disease" which seems to be replacing "schizophrenia" as the "sacred symbol of psychiatry" (to borrow Szasz's [1976] apt phrase): "The patient who cannot accept the fact that he is suffering from a chronic recurrent illness, analogous to diabetes, tends to deny the threat of recurrence and therefore refuses to accept the ingestion of lithium carbonate for the rest of his life" (p. 865). Patients are invariably indoctrinated to believe that they have a "chronic recurrent illness." Their lives become oriented around defending themselves against the recurrence of the original experience that led to the diagnosis. As the above quote indicates they are told they must take lithium for the rest of their lives.

Two advocates of lithium (Dyson and Mendelson, 1968) have described its effects as follows: "It's as if (patients') 'intensity of living' dial had been turned down a few notches. Things do not seem so very important or imperative; there is greater acceptance of everyday life as it is rather than as one might want it to be; their spouses report a much more peaceful existence" (p. 545).

The social control agent is not interested in exploring the idea that such "biochemical imbalances" might have adaptive value for the evolution of society, as Laing suggested about schizophrenia 25 years ago. Rather he or she mobilizes all his or her resources to make sure "manic depressives" accept life as it is "rather than as one might want it to be."

But the fact is that a number of individuals refuse to accept the disease metaphor and are able to turn these "imbalances" to their advantage once they become familiar with these unusual states of consciousness and learn not to be overwhelmed by them. Even such strong adherents to the disease model as Polantin and Fieve (1971) describe several such cases. One woman, a writer, felt "inhibited" on lithium. She discontinued taking it "and is now finishing her next novel, which her editors state appears very favorable. She is now relaxed, comfortable, happy, and says that for the first time in a long time she is really enjoying life. She remains at present in a mild hypomanic state" (p. 865). It is a strange disease that can manifest itself in enhanced creativity and joy and it is a strange sensibility that sees such joy as a symptom ("hypomania") of an illness. As Blake wrote in his poem *The Garden of Love,* "And the Priests in black gowns were walking their rounds, and binding with briars my joys and desires" (1974, p. 111).

Interpreting the Signs

The disease model in psychology is based on the presumption that individuals who manifest particular behavioral signs can be expected to behave in accordance with Institutional Mental Health's expectations. The fact that some individuals who manifest these signs consequently act counter to expectation refutes the model. It demonstrates that Institutional Mental Health has not discovered invariant transhistorical laws that enable it to make reliable predictions. Adherents to the disease model might counter that their expectations are based, if not on laws, then at least on probabilities. What this assertion tragically neglects to notice is that the historically conditioned expectations of the disease model are a significant factor *constituting* the probabilities it claims to discover. These expectations will determine for example whether a person "diagnosed" as schizophrenic will or will not remain incapacitated for life.

Certain individuals seem to have a predisposition, particularly when experiencing developmental crises, to manifest behavior that is socially deviant. These behaviors are invariably interpreted by Institutional Mental Health as signs that these individuals are mentally defective and must learn to drastically constrict the horizon of possibilities that they might otherwise believe are open to them. We come to the crux of the issue now: the way in which Institutional Mental Health's own understanding enters into the historical event. It does so by creating and sustaining a set of expectations that are fixed, uniform and limited. The expectations of Institutional Mental Health inevitably enter into the historical process. *These expectations constitute the covert discourse of psychology, its unexamined social text.*

In this connection the research on experimental bias is unequivocal. After reviewing the literature on this topic, Frank (1974) wrote, "To recapitulate the chief findings, an experimenter's expectations can strongly bias the performance of his subject by means of cues so subtle that neither experimenter nor subject need be aware of them." Furthermore, "A therapist cannot avoid biasing his patient's performance in accordance with his own expectations, based on his evaluation of his patient and his theory of therapy. His influence is enhanced by his role and his status, his attitude of concern, and his patient's apprehension about being evaluated" (pp. 127–128). Seen from this perspective the so-called epidemic of mental illness is a self-fulfilling prophecy created by Institutional Mental Health. It is an artifact of the set of uniform and limited expectations maintained about individuals who have been psychiatrically labeled — and an artifact of mental health workers' expectations about their own ability to genuinely help individuals who act in socially deviant ways.

A Dialectic of Domination

The dialectic that currently exists between Institutional Mental Health and individuals labeled "mentally ill" is one characterized by domination. Individuals seeking help are scoured for particular signs deemed relevant by the experts. On the basis of the presence or the imagined presence of particular signs, these individuals are placed in a particular "diagnostic" class. The class placement will determine Institutional Mental Health's expectations about these individuals' possibilities. These expectations are refracted throughout society and are encoded in a variety of social institutions.

Individuals in modern society are subjected to a constant barrage — from pop psychology books to TV talk shows to psychoanalytic journals — instructing them what behaviors ought to be interpreted as symptoms of "mental illness" or neurosis. Even in the best of cases — relatively rare — the individual seeking help will be defined as being mentally ill, as pathological or as neurotic. In these cases the expectation is that with *proper treatment* the damage can be undone or almost undone.

All individuals experience problems during the course of their lives. The claim that certain problems are signs of "mental illness" implies that persons with these problems are ontologically defective. In other words (1) their lives are lacking in authentic meaning or significance; (2) they are unworthy of being loved; and (3) they are incapable of judging what is in their own best interests (they are objects, not subjects).

The "mentally ill" are, in other words, fundamentally unworthy. One need only consult any standard psychiatric text or *The Diagnostic and Statistical Manual of Mental Disorders* (any edition) and examine the metaphors that are used to describe the psyche (the Greek word for soul) of an individual who is defined as a patient: "damaged ego," "deeply-rooted pathology," "basic fault," etc. It is useful to remember that terms such as psyche or ego do not refer to an actual corporeal body. Rather they are metaphors that attempt to convey something about the core, the essence of a person's being.

Epistemologists (Cua, 1982) have demonstrated that a scientific or philosophical theory depends on a root metaphor that provides the theory with a set of categories for classifying and interpreting diverse phenomena. Institutional Mental Health is based on the premise that a vast range of unusual or distressing human experiences can best be understood by fitting these experiences into the categories provided by the disease metaphor (Sarbin and Mancuso, 1980). From this perspective, aspiring persons, persons who are facing obstacles, are *necessarily* damaged beings (unless they have already achieved a certain social status).

Other metaphors could be used that would not lead to the conclusion that individuals seeking help are ontologically deficient. One might look at a troubled person as an artist attempting to create a life in harmony with his or her own innate sense of truth or beauty. We do not feel sorry for a painter who is struggling with his or her *oeuvre*. We might look at an individual in distress as a pioneer daring to explore uncharted territory of the psyche, as Laing suggested. Different metaphors would entail different social consequences.

An individual who "discovers" that he or she is "mentally ill" will typically go to a mental health worker who will usually prescribe a course of treatment. Should the person wish to terminate the treatment at a time that the therapist deems "premature," he or she will be told that this is a sign of his or her resistance to getting well, i.e., to remedying his or her ontological deficiency. Only the experts know if and when "mentally ill persons" are well enough to make authentic choices.

As long as people continue to grant experts the power to define them as "mentally ill," as ontologically defective, there will be perpetuated a dialectic of domination and dependency. As Szasz (1987) has argued there can be no viable democracy without faith in the individual's capacity to make his or her own choices about issues concerning his or her welfare — even if these lead to "mistakes." In short, defining individuals as mentally ill threatens the foundation of democracy.

By perpetuating the idea that certain kinds of deviant behavior are signs of ontological deficiency Institutional Mental Health perpetuates and aggrandizes its own power; it impedes the cultural evolution and democratization of society by creating and sustaining the polarities of Mental Health and mental illness, Truth and error, the experts who possess objective scientific knowledge and their charges, "the mentally ill."

These categories are absurd unless one accepts the premise that Institutional Mental Health constitutes an absolute standard by which all else is to be judged. That is to say it implies that the society we live in is an ideal, or at least that no improvement is possible. If on the other hand, a process of cultural evolution is taking place then the standards of any generation must be regarded with skepticism. (In the last century when the standard of sexual normality was different from the present standard, masturbation was regarded as an evident symptom of psychopathology.) Institutional Mental Health denies that it is conditioned by history and that we are all involved in a process of historical development and change.

In creating these polarities Institutional Mental Health follows here in the tradition of Institutional Christianity. Pagels (1988) has documented that St. Augustine radically revised Christian thought with his innovative interpretation of the myth of the Fall. Whereas Christians before Augustine had used this myth to illustrate to their contemporaries the danger of freedom, Augustine claimed that human beings had totally lost their capacity for free will as a result of Adam's original sin. Their souls were severely damaged and they were totally dependent on external intevention for any possible hope of redemption. Augustine developed his interpretation at a time when Christianity unexpectedly attracted the "blessing" of imperial power. "By insisting that humanity, ravaged by sin, now lies helplessly in need of outside intervention, Augustine's theory could not only validate secular power but justify as well the imposition of church authority – by force if necessary – as essential for human salvation" (p. 125). The parallel with Institutional Mental Health is chilling. Whereas Institutional Christianity impressed upon individuals the sense that they were helplessly damaged as a result of original sin, Institutional Mental Health now impresses upon individuals that they are helplessly "mentally ill" as a result of "bad" child-rearing or "bad" genes.

The enormous prestige of psychoanalysis among intellectuals has almost completely prevented the intelligentsia from taking a critical stance toward the idea of mental illness. For example, Jurgen Habermas accepts the psychoanalytic dogma that as a result of early childhood trauma individuals' communications are so "pathologically distorted" that they must go to psychoanalytic experts who can teach them how to communicate in an authentic fashion (Habermas, 1980). Habermas fails to see that a dialectic of domination is perpetuated by the ascription of "pathology" to the Other and by experts' arrogation of the right to decide on the basis of their own *conventional* criteria which individuals are capable of "true" communication. Habermas' argument demonstrates that if one does not believe that the possibility for *development* exists within the democratic process itself — which includes direct action and political struggle — one ends up advocating undemocratic elitist practices as a means of fostering democracy.

A New Dialectic

The fact that the behaviors that are interpreted as signs of "mental illness" in this culture do not have unequivocal meaning is demonstrated by looking at other cultures: that is to say, the same signs can be *interpreted* in radically different ways. Silverman (1967) has noted that whole societies have been known to conduct their everyday activities in such a way that from a psychiatric point of view one would have to regard them as "communities of psychotics" (p. 22). The attempt to create a cross cultural theory of "psychopathology" founders absurdly on this fact.

Two psychiatrists, (Billig and Burton, 1978) for example, recently wrote, "a belief in sorcery and ghosts may not be unusual unless it develops in an individual who never placed any trust in apparitions and if the beliefs are accompanied by a personality change, in which case they may be of pathological significance" (p. 49). One would not say that the symptoms of tuberculosis were pathological only if they occurred in an individual who had never experienced them before! The relevant lesson from anthropology teaches that adaptive and creative cultures existed (and exist) in which individuals normally exhibit the kinds of behaviors that Institutional Mental Health views a univocal signs of psychopathology when they are manifested in our culture.

Benedict's prescient remarks on this subject are as follows:

> It is clear that culture may value and make socially available even highly unstable human types. If it chooses to treat their peculiarities as the most valued variants in human behavior, the individuals in question will rise to the occasion and perform their social roles without reference to the ideas of the usual types who can make social adjustments and those who cannot. Those who function inadequately in any society are not those with certain fixed "abnormal" traits, but may well be those whose responses have received no support in the institutions of their culture. The weakness of these aberrants is in great measure illusory. It springs not from the fact that they are lacking in necessary vigor, but that they are individuals whose native responses are not reaffirmed by society. They are as Sapir phrases it, "alienated from an impossible world." (1934, p. 270)

It is typically a crisis that inaugurates the dialogue between Institutional Mental Health and psychiatrically labeled individuals. An individual in crisis goes to Institutional Mental Health for help. His or her sense of identity is in question. The psychodiagnostic procedure is the ritual in which Institutional Mental Health reaffirms its own identity and confers a new identity on the being in distress. Because the psychiatrist or psychologist making the diagnosis acts under the extraordinarily powerful authority of medicine and science, and because the individual in crisis is in a particularly impressionable state, this ritual is an effective force in stabilizing the identity of the two parties. The person in crisis may be said to have experienced a spiritual death; one finds a death/rebirth scenario in religious conversions and in the rites and initiations of many premodern societies (Eliade, 1975; Sarbin and Adler, 1971). In this society, the nature of rebirth is less felicitous. Institutional Mental Health examines the individual in crisis — the crisis is immediately assumed to be a symptom of *some* kind of "mental illness" — interprets the signs and then rechristens the individual: "You are a schizophrenic," or "You have a bipolar disorder," or "You are severely mentally ill." The crisis is now resolved, the individual is reborn, he or she now knows who he or she really *is*. All further interactions will take place within the parameters established in the diagnostic procedure in which the roles are ascribed, and in which the identitites are clarified.

What we take as evident signs of "mental illnesses" can be interpreted in an altogether different way, which would lead to an entirely different dialogue. In a society that values smooth operations above all else, it seems natural to interpret crises as symptoms of "mental illnesses." In premodern societies, crises, i.e., breakdowns, were valorized. They were believed to be necessary to the process of spiritual development. Mircea Eliade wrote, "The true knowledge, that which is conveyed by the myths and symbols, is accessible only in the course of or following upon, the process of spiritual regeneration realized by initiatory death and resurrection. . . . The future shaman, before becoming a wise man, must first know madness and go down into darkness. . . (1975, pp. 225–226).

Indeed, Silverman (1967) argued that the initiatory crisis of the future shaman is phenomenologically and behaviorally indistinguishable from the psychotic crisis. However as Silverman notes, "One major difference is emphasized — a difference in the degree of cultural acceptance of a unique resolution of a basic life crisis. In primitive cultures in which such a unique life crisis resolution is tolerated, the abnormal experience (shamanism) is typically beneficial to the individual cognitively and affectively; the shaman is regarded as one with expanded consciousness. In a culture that does not provide referential guides for comprehending this kind of crisis experience, the individual 'schizophrenic' typically undergoes an intensification of this suffering over and above his initial anxieties" (p. 21). *What was previously interpreted as signs that one was called upon to assume a leadership position in one's culture are now interpreted as symptoms of chronic disorders.*

The Hermeneutic Approach

It is not clear what kinds of new dialogues will develop today if individuals in positions of power and authority give up the stance of social control agents, if they relinquish the attempt to objectify the Other. But it is clear that new possibilities will be actualized.

It is beyond the scope of this essay to explore all of the epistemological implications of the hermeneutical insight. Nonetheless in conclusion I want to note that psychology must choose between two different epistemological approaches, reflective of two different modes of being in the world. By continuing to pursue the ideal of the objective scientist who can stand outside of history and subject humanity to methodical control, psychology is only succeeding in tightening the "mind-forged manacles" that prevent human beings from realizing their innate potential. This idolatry of scientific method represents the most tragic kind of epistemological hubris. Its claim to validity is belied by the findings of experimenter bias.

The alternative epistemology has been explored by Heidegger and by Gadamer (1976). It is exemplified by the therapist Haley, who — as the quote near the beginning of this essay reveals — "encourages unpredictability," evokes the creative autonomy of his clients. In this epistemology there is a continually renewed appreciation of the value of love and chance. The knower or the therapist participates in history, and in the midst of flux, of what he or she accepts as unpredictable events, is guided by his or her imagination and intuition. Certainly the therapist will use methods that have worked in the past but he or she also appreciates the value of experimentation. The process of change inevitably involves crises, mistakes, relapses. This approach does not seek to banish history, to achieve full predictability. On the contrary it is based on the realization that human creativity — freedom — manifests itself through the mysterious phenomenon we term chance. If this is so then it must be because the universe is "friendly," as Einstein once remarked. If we fail to find this the case then that is because *we* have alienated ourselves from the universe, by our efforts to dominate it rather than to dwell within it.

Gadamer believed that the project of understanding is undertaken as a means of overcoming our alienation as modern men and women, and finding our way back home. The attempt to banish the unpredictable — chance — precludes the completion of this project. The universe is so constituted that frequently we "come across," happen upon, the path that leads home, as Einstein happened upon the theory of special relativity. We can intuitively recognize this path when we discover it because we are accessible to truths that elude methodical prediction and control. We are not machines in a mechanical universe but artists in a wonder-land where God (i.e., meaning) is continually assuming unexpected guises, startling us with unpredictable revelations and opportunities.

If we forget to remember that we dwell in a universe that is continually changing, we will probably overlook the unexpected path that leads home. If we remember, we can remain ever present to new possibilities. As psychotherapists, as researchers, as scientists, as persons, our maps will prove of no avail unless we are also willing to discern the unpredictable signs of opportunity (of God?) as they reveal themselves in the nuances of a universe that is continually evolving.

Conclusion

The findings in experimenter bias, though published decades ago, have radical implications that have not yet been appreciated — there is not and cannot be a detached observer. If we *expect* individuals to fail we will increase the chances that they *will* fail. The fact that most therapists proceed as usual and ignore these findings is testimony to the ignorance and moral depravity of which human beings are capable.

To describe a person as "mentally ill," "schizophrenic," "manic-depressive," etc., means operationally that therapists hold low expectations for these individuals. We cannot help human beings to solve their developmental crises if we insist on defining these crises as symptoms of chronic mental illnesses. If we verbally encourage human beings to succeed while expecting them to fail, our encouragement is facile.

Haley (1980) described the attitude of one of his own teachers. "He believed that there was nothing wrong with a person diagnosed as schizophrenic. It was inspiring to watch him work with a mad offspring who was an expert at failing. I recall one who would not speak. She would sit pulling at her hair like an idiot. Yet Jackson treated her as if she was perfectly capable of normality, given a change in her family and treatment situation. The family was forced to accept her normality, partly because of Jackson's certainty" (p. 22).

The question arises: On what should therapists base their expectations of success? Since these expectations are *constitutive* they must not be based on the presence or absence of specific behaviors. Either the expectation is a gratuitous act of love or it is based on faith in the creative power of the human spirit. This power is manifesting itself today in the pioneering efforts of a growing number of individuals who have succeeded in responding adaptively to the challenges of life, in spite of the efforts of Institutional Mental Health to consign them to the ranks of the doomed, i.e., the severely mentally ill. To these individuals humankind owes a debt of gratitude.

References

Benedict, R. (1934). *Patterns of culture.* New York: Houghton-Mifflin.

Billig, O., and Burton, B. (1978). *The painted message.* New York: Schenkmann Publishing.

Blake, W. (1974). Songs of experience. In A. Kagin (Ed.), *The portable Blake* (pp. 99–120). New York: Viking Press.

Breggin, P.R. (1979). *Electroshock: Its brain-disabling effects.* New York: Springer.

Breggin, P.R. (1983). *Psychiatric drugs: Hazards to the brain*. New York: Springer.

Cohen, D., and Cohen, H. (1986). Biological theories, drug treatments, and schizophrenia: A critical assessment. *Journal of Mind and Behavior, 7*, 11–36.

Coleman, L. (1984). *The reign of error: Psychiatry, authority, and law*. Boston: Beacon Press.

Cua, A. (1982). Basic metaphors and the emergence of root metaphors. *Journal of Mind and Behavior, 3*, 251–256.

Dyson, W., and Mendelson, M. (1968). Recurrent depressions and the lithium ion. *American Journal of Psychiatry, 125*, 544–548.

Eliade, M. (1975). *Myths, dreams and mysteries*. New York: Harper and Row.

Frank, J. (1974). *Persuasion and healing*. New York: Schocken Books.

Gadamer, H. (1976). *Philosophical hermeneutics* [D. Linge, Trans]. Berkeley, California: University of California Press.

Gergen, K. (1977). Stability, change and chance in understanding human development. In N. Datan and H. Reese (Eds.), *Life span developmental psychology: Dialectical perspectives* (pp. 135–158). New York: Academic Press.

Gergen, K. (1980). The emerging crisis in life-span developmental theory. In P. Baltes and O. Brim (Eds.), *Life-span development and behavior* (pp. 31–63). New York: Academic Press.

Habermas, J. (1980). The hermeneutic claim to universality. In J. Bleicher (Ed.), *Hermeneutics as method, philosophy and critique* (pp. 181–213). London: Routledge and Kegan Paul.

Haley, J. (1980). *Leaving home*. New York: McGraw-Hill.

Kagan, J. (1970). Perspectives on continuity. In O. Brim and J. Kagan (Eds.), *Constancy and change in human development* (pp. 26–74). Cambridge: Harvard University Press.

Kagan, J. (1984). *The nature of the child*. New York: Basic Books.

Pagels, E. (1988). *Adam, Eve and the serpent*. New York: Random House.

Polantin, P., and Fieve, R. (1971). Patient rejection of lithium carbonate prophylaxis. *Journal of the American Medical Association, 218*, 864–866.

Sarbin, T.R., and Adler, N. (1971). Self-reconstitutive processes: A preliminary report. *The Psychoanalytic Review, 57*, 599–616.

Sarbin, T.R., and Mancuso, J.C. (1980). *Schizophrenia: Medical diagnosis or moral verdict?* New York: Pergamon.

Scheff, T. (1966). *Being mentally ill*. Chicago: Aldine.

Scheibe, K., (1979). *Mirrors, masks, lies and secrets*. New York: Praeger.

Scull, A. (1975). From madness to mental illness. *Archives of European Sociology, 16*, 219.

Silverman, J. (1967). Shamans and acute schizophrenia. *American Anthropologist, 69*, 21–31.

Szasz, T.S. (1976). *Schizophrenia: Sacred symbol of psychiatry*. New York: Basic Books.

Szasz, T.S. (1987). *Insanity: The idea and its consequences*. New York: John Wiley.

Trilling, D. (1986, December 21). Marilyn Monroe. *New York Times Book Review*, pp. 23–24.

©1990 The Institute of Mind and Behavior, Inc.
The Journal of Mind and Behavior
Summer and Autumn 1990, Volume 11, Numbers 3 and 4
Pages 301 [55] – 312 [66]
ISSN 0271-0137
ISBN 0-930195-05-1

Deinstitutionalization:
Cycles of Despair

Andrew Scull

University of California, San Diego

Examining the period from the rise of the asylum in the nineteenth century through the current debates about the failures of deinstitutionalization, this paper provides a critical perspective on the history of Anglo-American responses to chronic mental disability. It concludes with a pessimistic assessment of the prospects for the future evolution of public policy in this area.

As modern Western societies have grappled with the scourge of mental disorder, debates about how to deal with the chronically mentally disabled have periodically erupted into the political arena. At various times over the past two centuries, both public and professional sentiment have swung to one extreme or the other: embracing, at certain historical moments, an extraordinary optimism about the likely impact of new approaches to treatment; at others, relapsing into a numbing pessimism, hopelessness, and despair. On the whole, I shall argue that the historical record unfortunately makes the latter position the most plausible prognosis for both the present and the foreseeable future, and certainly we seem presently to be in one of those periods when informed opinion is on the brink of despair about our prospects. But I say this with great reluctance, since one of the effects of even realistic pessimism is that it tends to worsen an already grim outlook, for who can summon the energy to fight an essentially hopeless battle?

An earlier version of this paper was presented at a conference on "Fostering Useful Knowledge About What To Do With/For The Chronically Mentally Ill" held at UCLA on February 12 and 13, 1988. I am very grateful to David Cohen for his incisive comments on that early draft. Requests for reprints should be sent to Andrew Scull, Ph.D., Department of Sociology, C-002, University of California at San Diego, La Jolla, California 92093.

Asylums for the Mad

While from one point of view, specialized institutions for the mad have
a long ancestry in the Western world — one we can trace back, for example,
to the monastic foundation of Bethlem (Bedlam) in the English-speaking world,
and to the Arab-inspired asylums of medieval Spain — in another, the centrality of the asylum dates only from the early nineteenth century. In one
of those surges of optimism to which I previously referred, Victorian lunacy
reformers were captured by a utopian vision of what reformed, purpose-built
monuments of moral architecture could accomplish, engaging in a kind of
therapeutic Dutch auction in which expectations about the curability of insanity were built up to quite extraordinary heights. The sense, as Dwyer (1987)
recently put it, that there was "an economics of compassion" seized the imagination of a generation of reformers and philanthropists, and prompted
the construction of vast networks of publicly supported asylums in Britain,
Western Europe, and the United States. To invest substantial capital sums
in the construction of state hospitals, and to provide therein for the application of the powerfully restorative techniques of the new moral treatment,
was, if the proponents of reform were to be believed, to opt for the cheapest
of all policies in the long run — for the initally sizeable investiment in treatment facilities would all but guarantee the restoration of seventy, eighty, ninety
per cent of the mad to sanity, swiftly reducing the burden of serious mental
disorder to almost vanishingly small proportions.

Sadly, of course, in the face of these utopian fantasies, reality proved more
than a little recalcitrant. It was recognized at the outset of the reform process
that previous neglect and mismanagement had rendered a sizeable fraction
of the first patients the new institutions would admit beyond hope of cure,
for even the most enthusiastic proponents of moral treatment held that its
impact diminished sharply if therapy was delayed and the disordered allowed
to become chronic. But the assumption was that once the new system of
asylums permitted early recognition and intervention, the problem of chronicity would assume quite minor proportions. Suggestions by the less sanguine
that plans should be drawn to care for a population of the permanently disabled met with little support. In England, for example, the 1844 Report of
the wonderfully named Metropolitan Commissioners in Lunacy — the foundation for the legislation making construction of state funded asylums compulsory — had noted that

the disease of Lunacy . . . is essentially different in character from other maladies. In a
certain proportion of cases, the patient neither recovers nor dies, but remains an incurable
lunatic, requiring little medical skill in respect to his mental disease and frequently living
many years. A patient in this state requires a place of refuge, but his disease being beyond
the reach of medical skill it is quite evident that he should be removed from Asylums
instituted for the cure of insanity in order to make room for others whose cases have

not yet become hopeless. If some plan of this sort be not adopted the Asylums admitting
paupers will necessarily continue full of incurable patients . . . and the skill and labour
of the physician will thus be wasted upon improper objects. (Report, 1844, p. 92)

The legislation of the next year accordingly licensed local authorities to make
separate provision for the chronic. But, as in the United States, no one pressed
for its implementation, and no such facilities were erected – at least until
much later in the century.

The emerging profession of psychiatry was particularly vocal in its opposition to such schemes. On both sides of the Atlantic, alienists argued that
such receptacles for the chronic, while superficially attractive, would necessarily be productive of a repetition of the very abuses of the mentally ill that
the new asylums had been set up to avoid. In particular, they urged that it
would be difficult, if not impossible, to recruit suitable staff, and to maintain
the requisite morale and dedication in institutions that were avowedly
custodial, and since there remained a possibility of cure, however remote it
might seem, in even the most confirmed cases of lunacy, it would be both
cruel and unwise to consign the chronic to places where efforts directed toward
their restoration would cease. Public authorities, reluctant to incur the expense of erecting and providing for two separate institutions, happily opted
for the immediate capital savings of a single asylum for curable and incurable
alike.

Warehouses for the Unwanted

Cures, of course, if not quite as rare as hen's teeth, proved far more elusive
than the asylum's proponents had advertised. And as asylums steadily silted
up with the chronic and incurable, exactly the conditions predicted by the
opponents of separate facilities for the permanently mad began to characterize
the asylum system as a whole. Morale plummeted; the quality of the attendants (never particularly high) fell further still; funding levels declined, as
politicians saw little reason to invest "extravagant" sums in a holding operation; and the insitutions grew ever larger and more unmanageable. At the
theoretical level, psychiatrists responded by adopting grimly deterministic
hereditarian and somatic accounts of mental disorder which explained away
their failures to cure (and indeed such theorizing had an additional virtue,
in that it provided a eugenic argument for the seclusion of the mad); but
such "scientific" reinforcement of an existing pessimism came at the cost of
adding a vicious further twist to the downward spiral that now gripped public
asylums.

In a few jurisdictions, there was even a revived flirtation with the idea of
separate institutions for the chronically ill. In the late 1860s, the authorities
in London, for instance, constructed two institutions for the permanently

mad — at Caterham and Leavesden — huge, cheerlesss establishments housing between two and three thousand inmates (Scull, 1979). And New York
State, in a move heavily criticized by the American psychiatric establishment,
opened the Willard Asylum for the Chronic Insane in 1869 (Dwyer, 1987).
But the attempt to shunt aside the chronic, and reestablish the primarily
curative mission of the other asylums, proved a dismal failure. Within a few
years, in fact, it became difficult to distinguish the institutions for the chronic
from their supposedly therapeutic brethren. In both sets of institutions, more
inmates left each year in coffins than walked out of the gates restored to sanity.
The immense, decaying buildings in which thousands of patients now endured a dreary and monotonous existence, themselves offered mute testimony
to the fact that the asylum had become, as it was to remain for three quarters
of a century, "a mere refuge or house of detention for a mass of hopeless and
incurable cases" (Granville, 1877a, p. 8). Within these warehouses of the
unwanted,

> the classification generally made is for the purpose of shelving cases; that is to say, prac-
> tically it has that effect. . . . In consequence of the treatment not being personal, but
> simply a treatment in classes, there is a tendency to make whole classes sink down into
> a sort of chronic state. . . . They come under a sort of routine discipline which ends
> in their passing into a state of dementia. (Granville, 1877b, pp. 388; 396–397)

By the closing decades of the nineteenth century, some of the best informed
critics of mental health policy had become convinced of the pernicious effects of incarceration. S. Weir Mitchell, for example, the dean of American
neurologists, came before the annual meeting of American state hospital
superintendents to issue an indictment of their practices. Deeply affected by
his encounter with the harsh realities of the American mental hospitals, he
complained that "in the sadness . . . of the wards . . . the insane, who have
lost even the memory of hope, sit in rows, too dull to know despair, watched
by attendants; silent, grewsome [sic] machines which eat and sleep, sleep and
eat" (Mitchell, 1894, p. 19). Henry Maudsley characteristically rounded upon
those inclined to protest the proposition that asylums were "monstrous evils":
"[those] who advocate and defend the present asylum system . . . should not
forget that there is one point of view from which they who organize, superin-
tend, and act, regard the system, and that there is another point of view from
which those who are organized, superintended, and suffer, view it" (1871, p.
427). For visitors who lacked the peculiar blindness induced by a position
as superintendent of such an insitution, few things could be more depressing
than "the sight of so many patients in the prime of life sitting or lying about,
moping idly and listlessly in the debilitating atmosphere of the wards, and
sinking gradually into a torpor, like that of living corpses" (Massachusetts
State Board of Charities, 1867, p. xl).

Worse still, such publicly acknowledged therapeutic impotence threatened to reward psychiatrists with an even more marginal professional status than they had previously enjoyed, for it coincided with a marked upturn in the fortunes of their fellow medical practitioners, as the antiseptic revolution in surgery, the bacteriological revolution in medicine, and the reform of medical education and training came together to produce a sharp improvement in the profession's public image and position in the marketplace. The isolation of the syphilitic spirochete in the early twentieth century created a false dawn of hope that similar breakthroughs were at hand for a biological psychiatry, but state hospitals soon lapsed back into their slumbering state – and psychiatrists, despite spasmodic experiments with a variety of somatic treatments (convulsive therapies, insulin coma therapy, lobotomies), continued to preside over medical backwaters.

Indeed, from many points of view, the first half of the twentieth century witnessed a worsening of the situation in the asylums (and, concomitantly, a deterioration in the standard of care for the chronic). In the first place, the closure of the state almshouses brought with it an influx of the senile and the decrepit, for whom the mental hospital now became the only refuge. Between 1904 and 1923, the proportion of asylum inmates in residence for more than five years grew from 39.2 per cent to 54 per cent. In Massachusetts, the average length of hospital confinement had risen to 9.7 years by the late 1930s, and nearly 80 per cent of the beds were occupied by chronic patients (Grob, 1983, pp. 196–197). Nationwide, the total number of mental patients increased almost fourfold between 1900 and 1940, from 150,000 to 445,000, with the largest fraction of the increase coming in the ranks of the elderly. In New York State, for instance, 18 per cent of first admissions in 1920 suffered from senility or arteriosclerosis; by 1940, this had risen to 31 per cent (pp. 180–182). Clearly, these were not patients who posed threats to public order, or who could be expected to benefit from therapeutic interventions.

Secondly, despairing of making therapeutic progress with such recalcitrant raw materials, and conscious that their claims to professional competence, in the words of an internist at Harvard Medical School, "seemed so evanescent to most [medical] practitioners as to border on the ludicrous. . . (Bock, 1933, p. 1092), organized psychiatry increasingly attempted to establish a base for itself outside the institution, at as great a remove as possible from contact with the chronic patients who cluttered up the dormitories and dayrooms of the state hospitals. Psychopathic hospitals, research institutes, outpatient wards in general hospitals, mental hygiene clinics, child guidance centers, all offered the prospect of some respite, an "escape from the seemingly insoluble and depressing problems of the traditional mental hospital" (Grob, 1983, p. 240). As Grob further notes (p. 287), by 1956, only 17 per cent of the membership of the American Psychiatric Association were employed by state hospitals. And as they broadened their own occupational base and sought to acquire a more tractable and treatable clientele, psychiatrists silently attenuated their commitment to institutional care, and abandoned the chronically crazy to their fate. Mental hospitals, as Albert Deutsch (1973) put it, became "the shame of the states": a set of institutions characterized, in the words of another critic from the 1940s, by

> Inadequacy, Ugliness, Crowding, Incompetence, Perversion, Frustration, Neglect, Idleness, Callousness, Abuse, Mistreatment, Oppression. (Wright, 1947, p. 123)

At the nadir of their public regard, such psychiatric snakepits came under a new form of assault in the 1950s, as sociologists honed in on their therapeutic inadequacies and failings. A series of critical studies, reaching a crescendo in Erving Goffman's *Asylums* (1961), with its indictment of the baneful effects of the "total institution," recast the image of the mental hospital and forced home the message that "in the long run the abandonment of the state hospitals might be one of the greatest humanitarian reforms and the greatest financial economy ever achieved" (Belknap, 1956, p. 212). So far from being a positive force, hospitalization was now portrayed as having profound iatrogenic effects, its grossly deforming environment serving only to manufacture and stabilize chronicity.

The Panacea of Community Treatment

But a new panacea was lurking in the wings. Deinstitutionalization and treatment in the community could rapidly reverse the ill-effects of a badly mistaken century-old innovation in social policy. "By bringing [the mentally ill and other deviants] back into the community, by enlisting the good will and the desire to serve, the ability to understand which is found in every neighborhood, we shall meet the challenge which such groups of persons present, and at the same time ease the financial burden of their confinement in fixed institutions" (Alper, 1973, pp. vii-viii). Community care, and the social management of mental illness,[1] it was confidently predicted in the 1950s and 1960s, would revolutionize the outlook for the mentally ill, and finally resolve the nagging problems posed by chronicity.

---

[1] The introduction of the term "mental illness" is perhaps the proper occasion to comment briefly on some terminological issues. Embedded in whatever vocabulary one elects to use in discussing mental alienation is a whole complex of claims and presuppositions. One ventures here into what Steven Lukes has called "essentially contested terrain" where one can find no neutral ground. The use of such terms as "mental illness" invites accusations that one has thoughtlessly swallowed psychiatry's claims to rationality and disinterested benevolence, and uncritically accepts the so-called "medical model" of mental disorder. Yet the selfconscious avoidance of this terminology is linguistically awkward, and besides, it has unfortunately come to be associated with

How innocent and naive this all seems now. The mental hospital census, having declined slowly between 1955 and 1965, dropped precipitously over the next two decades — not primarily, as some have alleged, because the phenothiazines provided a technological fix for the psychoses, but rather in response to a broad expansion of social welfare programs, growing fiscal pressures on the states, and the opportunity to transfer costs away from the state budget, helped along, in a more minor key, by the interventions of public interest lawyers who sought to make it more difficult to employ the police power of the state to compel the mentally ill to enter psychiatric treatment facilities (see reviews of evidence on this point in Aviram, Syme, and Cohen, 1976; Gronfein, 1983, 1985; Lerman, 1982; Scull, 1984, pp. 79-94; 169-172).

This transfer of care was supposed to mark a glorious Paradise Regained for the denizens of the backwards, and to preserve future generations of "mental patients" from the damaging effects of institutionalization. Instead, as we are now all too acutely aware, the outcome has been "the wholesale neglect of the mentally ill, especially the chronic patient and the deinstitutionalized" (Langsley, 1980, p. 815). State and federal payments to the burgeoning entrepreneurial class "servicing" the chronically mentally disabled are scarcely munificent, and at best could be expected to purchase the most basic forms of custodial care. Worse still, under the conditions which now prevail, market failure is structurally guaranteed. A large number of atomized, uninformed consumers, whose mental condition renders them all-but-capable of initiative or of exercising meaningful choice, has been discharged into a hostile community and these people have been left to cope as best they can — in the

---

two equally unsatisfactory positions: either that one has embraced the romantic nonsense propounded by sociologists under the guise of labelling theory or that one accepts the equally pernicious Szaszian argument that mental illness is myth. I find none of these choices appealing. The medical personnel who claim the ability to decide for the rest of us what constitutes "mental illness" suffer from embarassing intellectual vulnerabilities, to say nothing of an all-too-visible therapeutic impotence; and psychiatrists are, of course, deeply and inextricably involved in the definition and identification of what consitutes madness in our world — in ways which render the notion that mental illness is a purely naturalistic category, devoid of contamination by the social, a patent absurdity. But to recognize that, at the margin, what consitutes madness is fluctuating and ambiguous, indeed theoretically indeterminate, is very different from accepting the proposition that mental alienation is simply the product of arbitrary social labelling or scapegoating. Such views play down the degree to which behavior recognized as mad is genuinely problematic. To ignore the enormity of the human suffering and the devastating character of the losses sustained by the victims of this form of communicative breakdown, or, alternatively, to lay blame for their plight simply and solely on the shoulders of a misguided or actively harmful profession is to embrace a romanticism with which I can have no truck. In the absence of a vocabulary that is neutral in these respects, reasoned discussion of our underlying difficulties, at least among persons of different theoretical persuasions, remains exceedingly elusive and difficult, the various factions all too often simply talking past one another. Faced with this problem, I have chosen to refer almost interchangeably to madness, mental illness, mental disturbance, and the like. Though this leaves no one wholly satisfied, I hope it at least reminds us that real issues lie behind our choice of words, issues that remain problematic and ought not to be rendered invisible through any linguistic sleight of hand.

virtual absence of state supported aftercare or follow-up services. Their plight has created fertile ground for the emergence of a new trade in lunacy, resembling the private madhouses of eighteenth century England (Parry-Jones, 1972), an industry almost wholly unregulated by the state. (Indeed, in a double sense, the state can hardly *afford* to regulate this industry in anything but a cosmetic fashion: a serious attempt at regulation would demand the commitment of substantial resources; and if any state attempted to insist on adequate standards of care, given current reimbursement levels, it would simply dry up the supply of beds.) Since the income of those speculating in this species of human misery is almost wholly inelastic (being fixed by the welfare payments that are their "clients' " principal source of income) profits are strictly dependent on paring costs. With the volume of profit inversely proportional to the amount expended on the inmates, the logic of the marketplace ensures that the operators of the board and care homes, the nursing homes, and the "welfare" hotels (which now form the primary locus of care for the seriously psychiatrically disabled in our society) have every incentive to warehouse their charges as cheaply as possible. It ill behooves us to protest if such places subsequently turn out to be a poor alternative to living; or to express surprise that decarceration "has not succeeded in ameliorating precisely those alleged results of institutionalization that [supposedly] led to it: the sociocultural and interpersonal isolation, degeneration and stigmatization of patients; the assymetrical [sic] dependency and vast power differences between patients and non-patients; the encouragement of chronicity contained in the treatment system and related social policies" (Estroff, 1981, pp. 116–117).

Prospects for the Future

That the new programs marked, not a humanitarian reform, but "the demise of state responsibility for the seriously mentally ill and [a] crisis of abandonment" (Gruenberg and Archer, 1979, p. 458) was already apparent to many as the seventies drew to a close. Reaganite callousness and fiscal conservatism has, of course, subsequently made a terrible situation worse. Chronicity has always implied indigence, and in modern capitalist societies necessarily prompts reliance on the public sector. But the state welfare apparatus is a demoralized, disorganized, fragmented, and increasingly underfinanced entity, beyond all question incapable of responding in any adequate fashion to the need. And even in the "kinder, gentler America" we now allegedly occupy, run by a Republican administration that displays a somewhat less visceral ideological hostility to the unfortunate, the realities of the budgetary catastrophe Reagan has left for his successor largely preclude the possibility of serious initiatives to palliate the situation.

And here, it seems to me, is the nub of the problem we confront. Those who speak of "fostering useful knowledge about what to do with/for the chronically mentally ill" [the title of a recent NIMH sponsored conference held at UCLA] invoke a rational model of policy formation at odds with what we know of the real world: if only we can foster some useful knowledge, the research community suggests, the situation of the chronically crazy (or whomever) can be expected to improve — a comforting notion for academic researchers. But the reasons for our current difficulties lie only partially, *very* partially, in the shortage of good ideas or workable programs. More seriously, one must question whether the issue of adequately responsive care for the seriously mentally ill is ever likely to have sufficient crowd appeal to stand out from the throng of supplicants seeking to feed at the public trough.

Let me itemize some of the difficulties: even the most compassionate and dedicated psychiatrists are now close to despair, and many of them have already joined the exodus of their less scrupulous colleagues to the greener pastures provided by less disturbed patients with private insurance coverage. Work with the chronically crazy is not only poorly paid, frustrating, and all-too-often lacking in intrinsic rewards, it is also professionally *declassé* and stigmatized. Chronic schizophrenics are mostly an unattractive lot, statistically unlikely to become more than marginally contributing members of society even under the best of circumstances. In a large fraction of the population, their condition attracts fear, loathing, and hostility, and such sympathy as their plight evokes scarcely weighs heavily enough in the balance sheet to offset the liability their persistent and permanent dependency represents in the competition for scarce resources. Perhaps their families can form a more effective lobbying group on their behalf. Certainly, in recent years, such family lobbies as the *National Alliance for the Mentally Ill* have been acquiring a growing measure of influence, helping to set research and practice agendas for the mental health bureaucracy. But here, too, the difficulties are great: the interest of the families and the psychotic by no means entirely coincide, and one must therefore have real concerns about the biases family activists may introduce into public policy-making. Nor is it clear that such activist groups are even broadly representative of the constituency they most obviously seem to represent. Given the social ecology of mental illness, many of the families of patients have few political or organizational skills and are unlikely to join such lobbying efforts; for others, the sheer burdens of coping with a mentally disabled or hallucinating relation are often such as to preclude public action; and the stigma attached to mental illness remains so strong that still others are reluctant to draw public attention to its presence in their family.

Biological psychiatry, as always, promises us that a medical solution is almost within our grasp. It would be nice if one could believe it. I fear one might as well be waiting for Godot. After almost two centuries of medical assurances on this front, psychiatrists' credibility ought to be wearing rather thin. Aside from its role as the monopolistic provider of the ambiguous blessings of psycho-pharmacology (a form of intervention whose iatrogenic effects are the subject of increasingly worried commentaries in the professional literature), psychiatry makes only marginal contributions to the management of the chronically crazy. The illusion that curative care is available, or on the brink of becoming available, serves to distract us from recognizing the essential irrelevance of expensive medical personnel when it comes to the provision of the supportive social care most mental patients need.

Meanwhile, the overall budgetary situation is close to calamitous, so that serious new initiatives on any number of politically *attractive* fronts are having a hard time securing a hearing. Chronic mental patients have never ranked very highly in political beauty contests. Their poverty, persistent dependency, and the seemingly ineradicable stigma attached to their condition combine to send them to the back of the queue, needy but essentially friendless. The sidewalk psychotic may be esthetically offensive to the sensibilities of the more fortunate, destructive of some of the remaining civilities of urban existence, and occasionally a real threat to the economic or physical well-being of the community as a whole. The mentally disturbed hidden from view in more domestic surroundings may impose all-but-intolerable burdens on family members. But neither set of problems seems acute or threatening enough to prompt collective responses proportional to the gravity of the need.

I think the parable for our times is the NIMH Community Support Program. An initiative designed to damp down the rising public clamor about the deficiencies of deinstitutionalization, this program was allegedly a response to the problem of how to deliver improved services to the chronically mentally ill. In the first seven years of its existence, it disposed of the munificent total of some 34.4 million dollars for the entire country. If one may judge by the number of large scale projects devoted to monitoring its progress,[2] expenditures to *study* the program must not fall all that far short of the money used to fund it. Yet as a fig leaf for the failures of public policy, the Community Support Program is so tiny as to leave the obscenity of our current circumstances in full view.

References

Alper, B. (1973). Foreword. In Y. Bakal (Ed.), *Closing correctional institutions* (pp. vii-x). Lexington, Massachusetts: Lexington Books.
Aviram, U., Syme, S.L., and Cohen, J. B. (1976). The effects of policies and programs on reduction of mental hospitalization. *Social Science and Medicine, 10,* 571-577.
Belknap, I. (1956). *Human problems of a state mental hospital.* New York: McGraw-Hill.

[2]I know of two of these in California alone, both absorbing large amounts of highly trained (and very expensive) professional labor: at UCLA, under the supervision of Dr. Oscar Grusky, and at Stanford University, run by Dr. W. Richard Scott.

Bock, A.W. (1933). Psychiatry in private practice. *New England Journal of Medicine, 208,* 1092–1094.

Deutsch, A. (1973). *The shame of the states.* New York: Arno. (originally published in 1948)

Dwyer, E. (1987). *Homes for the mad: Life inside two nineteenth century asylums.* New Brunswick, New Jersey: Rutgers University Press.

Estroff, S. (1981). Deinstitutionalization: A socio-cultural analysis. *Journal of Social Issues, 37,* 116–132.

Goffman, E. (1961). *Asylums: Essays on the social situation of mental patients and other inmates.* Garden City, New York: Doubleday.

Granville, J.M. (1877a). *The care and cure of the insane* (Volume 1). London: Harwicke and Bogue.

Granville, J.M. (1877b). Testimony before the *House of Commons Select Committee on the Operation of the Lunacy Law, 1877.*

Grob, G. (1983). *Mental illness and American society, 1875–1940.* Princeton: Princeton University Press.

Gronfein, W. (1983). *From madhouse to main street: The changing place of mental illness in post World War II America.* Unpublished doctoral dissertation, SUNY Stony Brook.

Gronfein, W. (1985). Psychotropic drugs and the origins of deinstitutionalization. *Social Problems, 32,* 437–454.

Gruenberg, E., and Archer, J. (1979). Abandonment of responsibility for the seriously mentally ill. *Millbank Memorial Fund Quarterly, 57,* 485–506.

Langsley, D.G. (1980). The community mental health center: Does it treat patients? *Hospital and Community Psychiatry, 31,* 815–819.

Lerman, P. (1982). *Deinstitutionalization and the welfare state.* New Brunswick, New Jersey: Rutgers University Press.

Massachusetts State Board of Charities. (1867). *Annual Report* (Volume 4).

Maudsley, H. (1871). *The physiology and pathology of mind.* New York: Appleton.

Mitchell, S.W. (1894). *Address before the Medico-Psychological Association.* Philadelphia.

Parry-Jones, W. (1972). *The trade in lunacy.* London: Routledge and Kegan Paul.

Report of the Metropolitan Commissioners in Lunacy for 1844. (1844). London.

Scull, A. (1979). *Museums of madness: The social organization of insanity in nineteenth century England.* London: Allen Lane; New York: St. Martin's Press.

Scull, A. (1984). *Decarceration: Community treatment and the deviant: A radical view* (2nd edition). New Brunswick, New Jersey: Rutgers University Press.

Wright, F.L., Jr. (1947). *Out of sight, out of mind.* Philadelphia: National Mental Health Foundation.

©1990 The Institute of Mind and Behavior, Inc.
The Journal of Mind and Behavior
Summer and Autumn 1990, Volume 11, Numbers 3 and 4
Pages 313 [67] – 322 [76]
ISSN 0271-0137
ISBN 0-930195-05-1

Twenty Years Since *Women and Madness:*
Toward a Feminist Institute of Mental Health and Healing

Phyllis Chesler

College of Staten Island, CUNY

This article reviews the development of a feminist analysis of female and male psychology from 1970 to 1990; the acceptance, rejection or indifference to feminist theory and practice by women in general and by female patients and mental health practitioners in specific. The article describes what feminist therapy ideally is and discusses the need for a Feminist Institute of Mental Health.

In 1969, I helped found The Association for Women in Psychology (AWP). I was a brand-new Ph.D., a psychotherapist-in-training, an assistant professor and a researcher. And I knew almost nothing about how to help another woman save her own life.

Most of what we take for granted today was not even whispered about twenty years ago. For example, none of my teachers ever mentioned that women (or men) were oppressed or that people suffer when they are victimized – and then blamed for their own misery. None of my clinical supervisors ever suggested that I review my own experience as a woman in order to understand women and mental health. In fact, no one ever taught me to administer a test for mental health – only for mental illness.

No matter. With feminism afoot in the land, I had been attending meetings almost nonstop for two years. I was surrounded by women who were passionate, confident, vocal, well-educated. I was studying what women "really wanted" from psychotherapy and planned to present my findings at the annual convention of the American Psychological Association (APA) in 1970, in Miami.

This paper is adapted from the Preface of *Women and Madness* [1989, second edition], Harcourt, Brace Jovanovitch, New York. Requests for reprints should be sent to Phyllis Chesler, Ph.D., College of Staten Island, CUNY, 715 Ocean Terrace, Staten Island, New York 10301.

I did my research and went to the convention, but decided not to deliver the paper that people were expecting. Instead, on behalf of AWP, I asked APA members for one million dollars "in reparations" for those women who had never been helped by the mental health professions but who had, instead, been further abused by them: punitively labeled, overly tranquilized, sexually seduced while in treatment, hospitalized against their will, given shock therapy, lobotomized, and, above all, disliked as too "aggressive," "promiscuous," "depressed," "ugly," "old," "disgusting," or "incurable." "Maybe AWP could set up an alternative to a mental hospital with the money, " I said, "or a shelter for runaway wives." The audience laughed at me. Loudly. Nervously. Some of my two thousand colleagues made jokes about my "penis envy." Some looked embarrassed, others relieved. Obviously, I was "crazy."

I started writing *Women and Madness* on the plane back to New York. I immersed myself in the psychoanalytic literature, located biographies and autobiographies of women who had been psychiatrically diagnosed or hospitalized; read novels and poems about sad, mad, bad women; devoured mythology and anthropology, especially about Goddesses, matriarchies, and Amazons. I began analyzing the "mental illness" statistics and the relevant psychological and psychiatric studies. I also began interviewing the experts: women patients.

Women and Madness was published in October 1972 to generally very positive reviews, including one on the front page of *The New York Times Book Review*. Over the years it was to sell more than a million and a half copies and it was translated into many European languages and into Japanese and Hebrew. I was interviewed a lot. Women began telling me that I had "saved their lives": they also deluged me with questions and requests. Would I be their therapist? If not, would I recommend one? Could I get them *out* of a mental hospital or into a *better* one? Would I testify for them in court, supervise their doctoral dissertation, conduct a workshop at their clinic? Would I be willing to talk to their husbands, mothers and children or lecture at their universities?

Since 1972 I've received more than 10,000 letters about *Women and Madness*, mainly from women but also from men. I have them still. Most confirm what I have written. Some letters are angry: I have offended God and Society and deserve to be punished — severely. Some letters are thoughtful: Now that I have "said it," what was I planning to "do about it?" Was I going to educate women (and men) or only talk to those who already agreed with me? A letter I received in January of 1989 begins:

> Please forgive my responding to your book almost 20 years late — but I never got around to reading it until now. I just hope you're still out there somewhere and will receive and answer this letter, the gist of which is, Boy, were you right, in spades, times ten, and

how I wish I knew nothing firsthand about the grim trick that is called "mental illness" in women.

Not only am I "still out there"; so are many other feminists in psychiatry, psychology, social work, nursing, and counseling. And so too is the book, which remains, unfortunately, quite up-to-date.

Changes

What has really changed since I wrote *Women and Madness?* The answer is: too little — and quite a lot.

Too little. Despite the existence of a vibrant and visionary feminism (see, for example, Chesler, 1972, 1976, 1978, 1979, 1986, 1988, 1990; Dworkin, 1974, 1982, 1987; Firestone, 1971; Friedan, 1963; Greer, 1971; Hooks, 1981, 1984; Johnson, 1988; Millett, 1970; Rich, 1976; Spender, 1982), women continue to experience childhood in father-dominated, father-absent and mother-blaming families. Although women differ in terms of class, race, and sexual preference, female psychology is still shaped by the almost universal belief that God is a (white) man, not a (black) woman; by the preference for sons, not daughters; by the parental policing of daughters into "Daddy's Girls"; by the punishment of girls who veer, even slightly, from their "feminine" roles; by an arbitrary system of rewards for girls when they are "good"; by the lack of strong heroic female role models; by the continuing epidemic of incest and sexual molestation; by the absence of group bonding among girls or among girls and boys; by women's fear of being raped or trapped into systems of pornography and prostitution — and then blamed for it; and by women's inability to defend ourselves against male or adult violence.

Women still behave as if they have been colonized. As I noted in *Women and Madness*, mental health professionals — and everyone else — devalue the way women either express or protest their colonization. For example, a "normal" woman is still supposed to be passive, dependent, emotional, and not good at math or science; as such, she commands little respect. However, a woman who is aggressive, independent, emotionless and good at physics commands as little respect and is also without a clean bill of mental health. ("She's not married. She's not a mother. She's not normal. She can't be happy.")

The image of women as colonized is a useful one. It explains why some women cling to their colonizers the way a child or a hostage clings to an abusive parent or captor; why many women blame themselves (or other women) when they are captured (she really "wanted" it, she freely "chose" it); and why most women defend their colonizers' right to possess them (God or Nature has "ordained" it). Like others who are colonized, women are harder on themselves. Women expect a lot from each other — but rarely forgive another woman when she fails even slightly. Women are emotionally intimate with each other, but tend to take their intimacy for granted. Almost unilaterally, women do the work of creating similar intimacy with men — and prize male reciprocity very highly.

Despite women's real ability to connect with others, women tend to disassociate themselves from both female victims and female rebels. We are often the first to denounce or ostracize other women who step out of line, even slightly. Most women experience our differences as potentially murderous. Like men, we have little nurturing compassion for women. Like "brotherhood," "sisterhood" is a powerful ideal, not an institutionalized reality.

Can mere words help us "overcome" this? Can psychoanalysts or psychotherapists perform such word magic? I did not address this question in *Women and Madness*. However, I observed the obvious: the traditional mental health professionals had, as yet, neither understood nor liberated women.

Today, the mental health professions are essentially the same patriarchal institutions I once described. Structually, they still tend to mirror or support the institution of marriage (especially for women), and to reinforce our belief in private, individual solutions (see Chesler, 1972, 1986, 1988, 1989).

Many male (and anti-feminist) therapists still pay no attention to what "women's libbers" are saying. Most do not read the feminist literature or invite feminists (even those with degrees in social work, medicine, psychology, counseling, or nursing) to address them as authorities. Whenever I or other feminists lecture professionally, we are usually received by the same women and/or feminists who fought to have us invited. Their male and anti-feminist colleagues appear in very token numbers. This is truly astounding — given that contemporary mental health professionals did not learn about incest, rape, wife-beating or child abuse from graduate or medical school textbooks but from feminist consciousness-raising; from grass-roots counselors, with and without degress; and from the victims themselves, empowered to speak, not by psychoanalytic but by feminist liberation.

It is very important, psychologically, for both women and men to learn how to listen to women as authorities. This is especially true for those who are themselves mental health professionals. Some male therapists have been educated by their female patients and by their daughters and wives. These men attend feminist conferences and are familiar with the feminist literature. Some are powerful courtroom advocates of mothers and children, especially when sexual abuse is involved; some are even more radically feminist than many of their female counterparts. (They can afford to be — but still it is nice when they are sincere.) However, such men are in the minority.

Interestingly, some non-feminist male and female therapists are more interested in studying or "helping" rapists and batterers — than in healing their female or child victims — more interested in appearing as expert custody witnesses for previously absent or exceptionally violent fathers than for "good enough" mothers. This is partly a matter of "going where the money is," and partly a continuation of our professions' (and our culture's) pro-man and anti-woman biases.[1]

Feminists have usually questioned the desirability of seeing a male therapist. According to 20 feminist therapists whom I recently interviewed, women increasingly prefer women as their therapists. When should a woman see a male therapist? In *Women and Madness* and in a later work (1976), I discussed women's preference for a male rather than a female therapist in terms of women's belief that God is a man. In a sense, a woman's "career" as a psychiatric patient (or as a wife), in addition to all else, is a way of getting close to God or to God's representatives here on earth.

So what did I mean when I said that *quite a lot* had changed since I began to write *Women and Madness*? In 1969 there were few feminist theories of psychology and virtually no feminist therapists. Now, we are everywhere. Feminists have established journals, referral networks, annual conferences and workshops within and outside the professions. They have also published many wonderful and important books and articles (e.g., Armstrong, 1978, 1983; Caplan, 1985;, Herman 1981; Miller, 1976; Rush, 1980; Walker, 1989; Weisstein, 1971). However, in *Women and Madness*, I wrote:

> The ideas and alternative structures of a "radical" or feminist psychotherapy both excite and disturb me. I don't know how much "professionalization" of either ideology might come to parallel hippie capitalism or limited social reformism or authoritarianism with a new party line. Part of the difficulty that a "service" profession faces in being "revolutionary" is that people won't voluntarily patronize what isn't already palatable to them — and shouldn't be forced to do so. Also, the difficulty of translating one's ideology into action remains a problem for clinicians and people, whether traditional, radical, or feminist. For example, what happens to us as children in families may be very difficult to "will" away psychologically, even in the best of peer-group structures, even by the most scrupulous "contracts" between a therapist and her patient, or between a group and an individual. (1989, pp. 112–113)

Despite my own early critique of institutional psychiatry and of private patriarchal therapy geared to high-income clients, I have come to believe that women can and do benefit from feminist therapy. Some feminists have questioned whether *any* therapy, including feminist therapy, is desirable. They have noted, correctly, that "therapism" may siphon off radical political

---

[1]Many feminist theorists and clinicians do not have the "stomach" for working with violent women-haters — especially since we do not have the legal, social or financial power to do so effectively. Perhaps we know too much about how dangerous these men are — and how reluctant "society" is to control them. Perhaps such men simply frighten us too much. We also know that no one knows how to "rehabilitate" such men. As feminists, we are unwilling to spend our energies in developing "compassionate" therapies for Jack the Ripper or Bluebeard. Our resources are very limited; why not concentrate on healing the victims who have at least lived to tell the tale?

energies. Individual, group or family therapy can — just as feminist consciousness-raising groups or revolutionary struggles can — also maintain the status quo, blame-the-victim, settle for what is comfortable and ultimately mirror reactionary family structures.

However, an incest survivor with insomnia or panic attacks often cannot sit in a room long enough to have her consciousness raised; an anorexic or "overweight" woman who is primarily concerned with losing weight or looking "pretty" may not be able to *notice* others long enough to engage in political struggle with them; a battered woman on a window ledge may not have the time to wait for an affinity group to choose *her* salvation as their political project; a rape victim who is also starved for affection or encouragement will not necessarily find it in a group of similarly starved revolutionaries: egos colliding, enemy-shadows everywhere, hostility horizontal, all looking for the Great Black Mother, no one willing to become Her without first having Her, all looking for the Great White Father — no one willing to put up with Him in female form.

Often, those who condemn institutional psychiatry, Freudian psychoanalysis, grassroots feminist shelters and feminist therapies — all in the same breath — do not feel responsible for the female casualties of patriarchy and do not know how to *listen* to others — especially to women. Such critics, even if well-intentioned, do not comprehend how healing it is to be listened to in a loving and skillful "holding" environment; or how psychologically wounded women, men or politically active people also are. Such critics may also be confusing the fact that quality mental health care is not available to all who *want* it with the question of whether or not quality mental health care exists at all.

What does a feminist therapist *do* that is different? A feminist therapist tries to *believe* what women say. Given the history of psychiatry and psychoanalysis, this is a radical act. When a woman begins to remember being sexually molested as a child, a feminist does not conclude that the woman's "flashbacks" or "hysteria" prove that she is lying or "crazy."

A feminist therapist believes that a woman needs to be told that she is "not crazy"; that it is normal to feel sad or angry about being overworked, undervalued and underpaid; that it is healthy to harbor fantasies of running away when the needs of others (aging parents, needy husbands, demanding children) threaten to overwhelm her.

A feminist therapist believes that women need to hear that men "do not love enough" *before* they are told that women "love too much"; that fathers are *as* responsible for their children's "problems"; that absolutely no one will rescue a woman but herself; that self-love is the basis for love of others; that it is hard to "break free" of patriarchy; that the struggle to do so is both miraculous and life-long; that very few of us know how to support women in flight from – or at war with – low self-esteem and violence against women and children.

A feminist therapist tries to *listen* to other women respectfully rather than in a superior or contemptuous way. A feminist therapist does not minimize the extent to which a woman has been wounded. Experiencing life as a second- or third-class citizen is not a minor occurrence with only minor consequences. However, a feminist therapist believes that with the right support, every woman has the power to give birth to herself.

To give birth to oneself against all odds, and after sustaining mortal wounds, is not easy. A feminist therapist is more like a midwife than like a surgeon, more like a teacher than a scientist, more like a priestess than a priest, more intuitive than objective. Such therapists believe that any attempt to integrate mind and body is "healing"; that body work is as important as (or *is*) political work; that women need to be touched and nurtured in a gentle and non-invasive way, both physically and spiritually, especially by other women (role models) who themselves have access to the great female archetypes, or the "goddesses within."

It is no accident that I wrote about goddesses in *Women and Madness*: great Earth Mothers like Demeter who rescued her daughter, Persephone, from male kidnapping, rape and incest; great Amazons like Diana, who protected women in childbirth and communed with the "wild beasts." Such goddess images are our collective legacy, our dangerously repressed role models. Both women and men are strengthened by examples of women who embody *all* the human (not merely the "feminine") possibilities.

I previously criticized (1972, 1978, 1986, 1988) traditional mental health professionals for their gender-, sexual-preference-, class-, and raced-based double standards of mental health and for the way in which they punitively label women. A feminist therapist does not label a woman as mentally ill because she expresss strong emotions or is at odds with her "feminine" role. Feminists do not view women as mentally ill when they engage in sexual, reproductive, economic, or intellectual activities outside of marriage – for example, when they have full-time careers, are lesbians, refuse to marry, commit adultery, want divorces, choose to be celibate, have abortions, use birth control, have an "illegimate" baby, choose to breastfeed against expert advice, or expect men to be responsible for 50% of the child care and housework. Women often lose custody of their children for these exact reasons – pronounced unfit by courtroom psychiatrists, psychologists or social workers.

What if a woman really is "crazy" – say, suicidally depressed or actively psychotic? Feminist (and the best non-feminist) therapists try not to experience such a woman as *malevolently* resisting our efforts to help her, try not to hospitalize her against her will, if at all. (As I pointed out in *Women and Madness*, unless someone is very wealthy, that person will probably be forcibly and improperly medicated, denied both psychiatric and non-psychiatric medical care, and forever burdened with the shame and punishment of having a psychiatric "record.")

In the last twenty years, we have learned that psychotropic drugs — all of which have negative side effects and should be very carefully prescribed and monitored — may be helpful in some cases, enabling verbal or other supportive therapies to take place. However, medication by itself is never enough. Women who are depressed or anxious also need access to feminist information and support.

Feminist therapists know that we possess crucial and lifesaving information that all women, especially those in crisis, need. Women often need immediate sanctuary, employment, child care, and orders of protection; they also require more "crisis management" than most high-status, high-income therapists can provide. Some feminist therapists try to provide women with the kinds of advocacy and support networks that most families routinely provide for their sons, fathers, and brothers — but withhold from their female members. Feminist therapists develop referral lists of lawyers, physicians, and others who are at least committed to *struggling* against their own double standards.

Some feminist therapists believe that women must understand and/or engage in "politics" in order to engage in psychological transformations; that participation in feminist consciousness-raising is therapeutic; that our mental health will improve only as the feminist agenda is implemented; that no feminist government-in-exile, and no sovereign space yet exists to make our struggle any easier; that we have to create such spaces as a way of creating ourselves.

In *Women and Madness*, I asked us to value the devalued "female" ways of being and to expand also our definition of "female." Since then, feminists have focused either on valuing women's "relational" and "nurturing" abilities or on women's ability to incorporate both "male" and "female" behavior — that is, "human" behavior. The first approach is gender-specific; the second is gender-neutral. Both approaches are important; neither is necessarily radical. Women's deepest longings for love and family may only be realized when women (or feminists) control the means of production and of reproduction; nothing less will do. I wrote that in order for this to happen:

> Woman's ego-identity must somehow shift and be moored upon what is necessary for her own survival as a strong individual. Such a radical shift in ego-focus is extremely difficult and very frightening (but) women need not "give up" their capacity for warmth, emotionality, and nurturance. They do not have to forsake the "wisdom of the heart" and become like "men."
>
> They need only transfer the primary force of their "supportiveness" to themselves and to each other — and never to the point of self-sacrifice. Women need not stop being tender, compassionate, or concerned with the feelings of others. They must start being

tender and compassionate with themselves and with other women, including their daughters and mothers. (1989, pp. 299–301)

Today, most feminist theorists and therapists would agree that a woman's ability to nurture others must first focus on herself and not be limited to her own family. A woman's ability to create and sustain *non-traditional* relationships — especially to the larger world — is as important as her ability to keep one man (or one woman) at any price.

Some feminist theorists and therapists have been moved by the radical liberation theology in *Women and Madness*. Thus, they agree that women's control of our bodies is as important as sexual pleasure, and that we must be able to defend "our bodies, ourselves" against violent or unwanted invasions — like rape, battery, unwanted pregnancy or unwanted sterilization. In order to defend ourselves, women must do things that both men and women view as "unfeminine," such as take risks, think "big," express anger. Women must learn how *not* to become paralyzed when we are verbally baited. ("Yes, we are all kikes, niggers, commies, and dykes. Now let's get back to the subject at hand.") Women must also learn how to confront others *directly*, and having done so, how to "let it go."

At the precise moment that women are developing strong selves, they must simultaneously begin to cooperate with each other — not to maintain the status quo but to change it. How can we do this and at the same time take care of our wounded? How can we attend to the next generations and also take care of our own evolving needs? As feminists, how can we do what we have already been doing — but in ways that will touch the world more deeply?

We need a Feminist Institute of Mental Health and Healing that is both local and global, a learning community that lasts beyond our lifetimes, a clinical training program that is not patriarchal, a spiritual retreat with an intellectual and political agenda, a place where feminists can come together to both learn and teach in ways that are inspired, rigorous, humane, and healing.

References

Armstrong, L. (1978). *Kiss daddy goodnight: A speak-out on incest.* New York: Pocket Books.

Armstrong, L. (1983). *The home front: Notes from the family war zone.* New York: McGraw-Hill.

Caplan, P.J. (1985). *The myth of women's masochism.* New York: E.P. Dutton.

Chesler, P. (1972). *Women and madness.* New York: Doubleday.

Chesler, P. (1976). *Women, money and power.* New York: Morrow/Bantam.

Chesler, P. (1978). *About men.* New York: Simon & Schuster.

Chesler, P. (1979). *With child: A diary of motherhood.* New York: Lippincott-Crowell.

Chesler, P. (1986). *Mothers on trial: The battle for children and custody.* New York: McGraw-Hill.

Chesler, P. (1988). *Sacred bond: The legacy of Baby M.* New York: Times Books.

Chesler, P. (1989). *Women and madness* [Second edition]. New York: Harcourt, Brace Jovanovitch.

Chesler, P. (1990). *About men* [Second edition]. New York: Harcourt, Brace Jovanovitch.

Dworkin, A. (1974). *Women hating*. New York: Dutton.

Dworkin, A. (1982). *Pornography: Men possessing women*. New York: G.P. Putnam.

Dworkin, A. (1987). *Intercourse*. New York: The Free Press.

Firestone, S. (1971). *The dialectics of sex*. New York: William Morrow.

Friedan, B. (1963). *The feminine mystique*. New York: Dell.

Greer, G. (1971). *The female Eunuch*. New York: McGraw-Hill.

Herman, J. (1981). *Father-daughter incest*. Cambridge: Harvard University Press.

Hooks, B. (1981). *Ain't I a woman: Black women and feminism*. Boston: South End Press.

Hooks, B. (1984). *Feminist theory from margin to center*. Boston: South End Press.

Johnson, B. (1988). *Lady of the beasts: Ancient images of the Goddess and Her sacred animals*. San Francisco: Harper & Row.

Lorde, A. (1982). *Sister outsider: Essays and speeches*. Trumansburg, New York: The Crossing Press.

Miller, J.B. (1976). *Toward a new psychology of women*. Boston: Beacon Press.

Millett, K. (1970). *Sexual politics*. New York: Doubleday.

Rich, A. (1976). *Of woman born: Motherhood as experience and institution*. New York: Prentice-Hall.

Rush, F. (1980). *The best-kept secret: The sexual abuse of children*. New York: Prentice-Hall.

Spender, D. (1982). *Women of ideas and what men have done to them*. London: Routledge & Kegan Paul.

Walker, L.E. (1979). *The battered woman*. New York: Harper & Row.

Walker, L.E. (1989). *Terrifying love: Why battered women kill and how society responds*. New York: Harper & Row.

Weisstein, N. (1971). Psychology constructs the female. In V. Gornick and M. Moran (Eds.), *Woman in sexist society* (pp. 133–146). New York: Basic Books.

©1990 The Institute of Mind and Behavior, Inc.
The Journal of Mind and Behavior
Summer and Autumn 1990, Volume 11, Numbers 3 and 4
Pages 323 [77] – 336 [90]
ISSN 0271-0137
ISBN 0-930195-05-1

The Ex-Patients' Movement:
Where We've Been and Where We're Going

Judi Chamberlin

Ruby Rogers Advocacy and Drop-In Center

The mental patients' liberation movement, which started in the early 1970s, is a political movement comprised of people who have experienced psychiatric treatment and hospitalization. Its two main goals are developing self-help alternatives to medically-based psychiatric treatment and securing full citizenship rights for people labeled "mentally ill." The movement questions the medical model of "mental illness," and insists that people who have been labeled as "mentally ill" speak on their own behalf and not be represented by others who claim to speak "for" them. The movement has developed its own philosophy, and operates a variety of self-help and mutual support programs in which ex-patients themselves control the services that are offered. Despite obstacles, the movement continues to grow and develop.

A complete history of the mental patients' liberation movement is still to be written. Like other liberation struggles of oppressed people, the activism of former psychiatric patients has been frequently ignored or discredited. Only when a group begins to emerge from subjugation can it begin to reclaim its own history. This process has been most fully developed in the black movement and the women's movement; it is in a less developed stage in the gay movement and the disability movement (of which the ex-patients' movement may be considered a part).

The "madman," as defined by others, is part of society's cultural heritage. Whether "madness" is explained by religious authorities (as demonic possession, for example), by secular authorities (as disturbance of the public order), or by medical authorities (as "mental illness"), the mad themselves have remained largely voiceless. The movement of people who call themselves variously, ex-patients, psychiatric inmates, and psychiatric survivors is an attempt to give voice to individuals who have been assumed to be irrational — to be "out of their minds."

Requests for reprints should be sent to Judi Chamberlin, Ruby Rogers Advocacy and Drop-In Center, 2336 Massachusetts Avenue, Cambridge, Massachusetts 02140.

The ex-patients' movement began approximately in 1970, but we can trace its history back to many earlier former patients, in the late nineteenth and early twentieth centuries, who wrote stories of their mental hospital experiences and who attempted to change laws and public policies concerning the "insane." Thus, in 1868, Mrs. Elizabeth Packard published the first of several books and pamphlets in which she detailed her forced commitment by her husband in the Jacksonville (Illinois) Insane Asylum. She also founded the Anti-Insane Asylum Society, which apparently never became a viable organization (Dain, 1989). Similarly, in Massachusetts at about the same time, Elizabeth Stone, also committed by her husband, tried to rally public opinion to the cause of stopping the unjust incarceration of the "insane."

In the early part of this century, Clifford Beers, a wealthy young businessman, experienced several episodes of confused thinking and agitation which caused him to be placed in a mental hospital. Following his recovery, Beers (1953) wrote a book, *A Mind that Found Itself*, which went through numerous editions and which led to the formation of the influential National Committee on Mental Hygiene (later the National Association for Mental Health). Dain (1989) states that

> . . . Beers was outspoken about abuse of mental patients and passionate in defending their rights and damning psychiatrists for tolerating mistreatment of patients. But he eventually toned down his hostility to psychiatry as it became obvious that for his reform movement to gain the support he sought at the highest levels of society it would have to include leading psychiatrists. Although he envisioned that eventually fomer mental patients and their families would be recruited into the movement, the public's persistent prejudice against mentally disturbed people and Beers' own doubts and inclinations, plus pressures from psychiatrists, drew him away from this goal. (pp. 9–10)

Dain also notes, in passing, the formation of the Alleged Lunatics' Friend Society in 1845 by former patients in England. On the whole, however, this early history is obscure, and the development of modern ex-patient groups in the United States at the beginning of the 1970s occurred primarily without any knowledge of these historical roots.

Although the terms have often been used interchangeably, "mental patients' liberation" (or "psychiatric inmates' liberation") and "anti-psychiatry" are not the same thing. "Anti-psychiatry" is largely an intellectual exercise of academics and dissident mental health professionals. There has been little attempt within anti-psychiatry to reach out to struggling ex-patients or to include their perspective. The focus in this paper is on ex-patient (or ex-inmate) groups. I identify the major principles that have guided the development of the ex-patients' movement, sketch the recent history of this movement, describe its major goals and accomplishments, and discuss the challenges facing it in this decade.

Stigma and discrimination still make it difficult for people to identify themselves as ex-mental patients if they could otherwise pass as "normal," reinforcing public perceptions that the "bag lady" and the homeless drifter are representative of all former patients. Like the exemplary black persons of a generation or two ago — who were held to be "a credit to their race" and, by definition, atypical of black people generally — so the former mental patient who is successfully managing his or her life is widely seen as the exception that proves the rule.

Guiding Principles of the Movement

Exclusion of Non-Patients

In the United States, former patients have found that they work best when they exclude mental health professionals (and other non-patients) from their organizations (Chamberlin, 1987). There are several reasons why the movement has grown in this direction — a direction which began to develop in the early 1970s, influenced by the black, women's and gay liberation movements. Among the major organizing principles of these movements were self-definition and self-determination. Black people felt that white people could not truly understand their experiences; women felt similarly about men; homosexuals similarly about heterosexuals. As these groups evolved, they moved from defining themselves to setting their own priorities. To mental patients who began to organize, these principles seemed equally valid. Their own perceptions about "mental illness" were diametrically opposed to those of the general public, and even more so to those of mental health professionals. It seemed sensible, therefore, not to let non-patients into ex-patient organizations or to permit them to dictate an organization's goals.

There were also practical reasons for excluding non-patients. Those groups that did not exclude non-patients from membership almost always quickly dropped their liberation aspects and became reformist. In addition, such groups rapidly moved away from ex-patient control, with the tiny minority of non-patient members taking on leadership roles and setting future goals and directions. These experiences served as powerful examples to newly-forming ex-patient organizations that mixed membership was indeed destructive.

In attempting to solve these organizational problems, group members began to recognize a pattern they referred to as "mentalism" and "sane chauvinism," a set of assumptions which most people seemed to hold about mental patients: that they were incompetent, unable to do things for themselves, constantly in need of supervision and assistance, unpredictable, likely to be violent or irrational, and so forth. Not only did the general public express mentalist ideas; so did ex-patients themselves. These crippling stereotypes became recognized as a form of internalized oppression. The struggle against internalized oppression and mentalism generally was seen as best accomplished in groups composed exclusively of patients, through the process of consciousness-raising (borrowed from the women's movement).

Consciousness-Raising

The consciousness-raising process is one in which people share and examine their own experiences to learn about the contexts in which their lives are embedded. As used by the women's movement, consciousness-raising helped women to understand that matters of sexuality, marriage, divorce, job discrimination, roles, and so forth were not individual, personal problems but were instead indicators of society's systematic oppression of women. Similarly, as mental patients began to share their life stories, it became clear that distinct patterns of oppression existed and that our problems and difficulties were not solely internal and personal, as we had been told they were. The consciousness-raising process may be hampered by the presence of those who do not share common experiences (e.g., as women or as mental patients). As the necessity for consciousness-raising became more evident, it provided still another reason for limiting group membership.

Consciousness-raising is an ongoing process, with people and groups constantly recognizing deeper levels of oppression. Within an ex-patient group, various activities often lead to further consciousness-raising experiences. For example, a group may approach a local newspaper or television reporter to write a story about the group's work or to give its viewpoint on a current mental health issue. If the group's representatives are treated respectfully and their opinions listened to, no consciousness-raising issue arises. If, however, the reporter is unwilling to listen to the group's representatives or seems to disbelieve them or makes comments about their mental status, it can become an occasion for further consciousness-raising. Whereas, before the advent of the patients' liberation movement, the group might have altered its strategy or even disbanded after such a discouraging incident, armed with the knowledge that they have run into systematic discrimination they can decide how to proceed. They may complain to the reporter's superior. They may raise questions about discrimination against mental patients. Because of consciousness-raising, they will have a clear idea of what they are facing.

Historical Development of the Movement

Like many new developments in the United States, mental patients' liberation groups began primarily on the east and west coasts and then spread inland. Among the earliest groups were the Insane Liberation Front in Portland, Oregon (founded in 1970), the Mental Patients' Liberation Project in New York City, the Mental Patients' Liberation Front in Boston (both founded in 1971), and the Network Against Psychiatric Assault in San Francisco (founded in 1972). Local groups took a long time to establish ongoing communications, because they were not funded and membership consisted mostly of low income individuals. The development of two major means of communication, the annual Conference on Human Rights and Psychiatric Oppression, and the San Francisco-based publication, *Madness Network News*, helped the movement to grow. Interestingly, both the Conference and *Madness Network News* began as mixed groups but later were operated and controlled solely by ex-patients (see below).

The first Conference on Human Rights and Psychiatric Oppression was held in 1973 at the University of Detroit, jointly sponsored by a sympathetic (non-patient) psychology professor and the New York City-based Mental Patients' Liberation Project (MPLP). Approximately fifty people from across the United States (and Canadian representatives) met for several days to discuss the developing philosophy and goals of mental patients' liberation. The leadership role of ex-patients was acknowledged; for example, the original name proposed by the sponsoring professor for the conference ("The Rights of the Mentally Disabled") was roundly rejected as stigmatizing. Although no plan was made in Detroit to continue the conference, the practice later developed of designating an attending group to sponsor the next year's conference. The conference became limited to patients and ex-patients only in 1976. Conferences were held annually through 1985 (see below for later developments).

Madness Network News began as a San Francisco-area newsletter in 1972 and gradually evolved into a newspaper format covering the ex-patients' movement in North America as well as worldwide. *Madness Network News'* original core group included both self-styled "radical" mental health professionals and ex-patients, but within a few years a major struggle ensued and the paper was published solely by ex-patients. There were also struggles between women and men ex-patients resulting in special women's issues edited by all-women, all-ex-patient staffs. *Madness Network News* existed solely on subscription income, which was sufficient to cover printing and mailing costs, but did not allow for salaries. For many years this publication was the voice of the American ex-patients' movement, a journal which published personal experiences, creative writing, art, political theory, and factual reporting, all from the ex-patient point of view. *Madness Network News* ceased publication in 1986.

The heart of the movement, however, continued to be the individual local group. Although some groups existed for only short periods, the overall number of groups continued to grow. Most groups were started by a small number of people coalescing out of a shared anger and a sense that through organization they could bring about change. Groups were independent, loosely linked through *Madness Network News* and the annual Conference. Each group developed its own ideologies, terminology, styles and goals. Groups were known by an astonishing variety of names, from the straightforward (Mental Patients' Alliance; Network Against Psychiatric Assault) to the euphemistic (Project Acceptance; Reclamation, Inc.). Some groups were organized as traditional hierarchies with officers and held formal meetings while other groups moved toward more egalitarian structures with shared decision-making and no formal leadership. Groups were united by certain rules and principles: mental health terminology was considered suspect; attitudes that limited opportunities for mental patients were to be discouraged and changed; and members' feelings — particularly feelings of anger toward the mental health system — were considered real and legitimate, not "symptoms of illness."

The activities of various groups included organizing support groups, advocating for hospitalized patients, lobbying for changes in laws, public speaking, publishing newsletters, developing creative and artistic ways of dealing with the mental patient experience, etc. The two primary thrusts were advocacy and self-help alternatives to the psychiatric system, as it quickly became clear to each group that its own membership's needs largely fell into these two areas.

Different groups developed different terminologies to describe themselves and their work. "Ex-patient" was a controversial term because it appeared to embrace the medical model; *Madness Network News* promoted the use of "ex-psychiatric inmate," which became widespread. Other groups referred to themselves as "clients," "consumers," or "psychiatric survivors." Differences in terminology stressed differing emphases and priorities; clearly the individuals labelling themselves "inmates" or "survivors" took the more militant stance.

Because most groups existed with little or no outside funding they were limited in their accomplishments. The question of funding generated numerous controversies, as did the question of reimbursement for organizational labor. Even if the group decided it had no objection in principle to receiving outside funding, obtaining such funding was difficult. Potential funding sources tended to look askance on ex-patient groups — especially groups that rejected psychiatric ideology and terminology. Moreover, foundations which funded community organizing efforts did not view ex-patient groups as falling within their purview. Finally, state departments of mental health were seldom approached because of their role in running the very institutions in which group members had been oppressed. And those mental health departments that were approached were highly skeptical of the ability of ex-patient groups to run their own projects.

Gradually, however, inroads were made. Members of ex-patient groups demanded involvement in the various forums from which they were excluded — conferences, legislative hearings, boards, committees and the like. Although at first in only the most token numbers, ex-patients were slowly invited to take part in such forums. Often groups had to insist on being invited, however.

Once involved in such meetings, ex-patients could move in two different tactical directions: cooperation or confrontation. Clearly, much was said in these forums which directly contradicted the movement's developing ideology. While most such meetings featured a reliance on psychiatric terminology and diagnosis, and on the assumption that patients existed in a lifetime dependency relationship, the patients' movement stood in opposition to the medical model and in support of self-reliance and self-determination. Although ex-patients' objections to such mentalist assumptions were often used as a reason to exclude ex-patients from future meetings, it is to the movement's credit that the ex-patients did speak up and object to much of what was being said. Frequently-heard objections from professional participants were that the ex-patients "polarized the discussion" or were "disruptive." Professionals sometimes chose to work with non-movement identified ex-patients who were much more likely to be compliant. For example, the most publicly visible post to go to an ex-patient in the 1970s — as one of the twenty-member President's Commission on Mental Health — went to a woman who had never worked with an ex-patient group but who had written about her patienthood experience in professional journals.

However, from this forum, as from others, the movement refused to be excluded. Movement activists packed many of the Commission's public hearings, testifying eloquently about the harmfulness of the psychiatric treatments they had experienced while pleading for enforcement of patients' rights and funding of patient-run alternatives to traditional treatment. The Commission's final report acknowledged the role of alternative treatments, stating that many of the latter "are wary of being classified as mental health services, convinced that such a classification entails a medical perspective and implies authoritarian relationships and derogatory labeling" ("Report," 1978, p. 14). The report went on to note that "groups composed of individuals with mental or emotional problems are in existence or are being formed all over the United States" (pp. 14–15).

The movement also demanded its inclusion in a series of conferences organized by the Community Support Program (CSP), a small division of the National Institute of Mental Health (NIMH). CSP, which began in the late 1970s, focused on providing assistance to programs in community settings. However, in the movement's view, these programs often perpetuated many of the worst features of institutionalization, including labeling, forced drugging, and paternalistic control. The participation of ex-patients in CSP conferences (even though the movement activists were vastly outnumbered by mental health professionals) forced CSP to acknowledge the importance of funding patient-run programs as a part of community support. Such recommendations would not have been made — indeed, would not even have been considered — without the tenacity of movement activists who insisted on being heard.

Participation in professionally-sponsored conferences and meetings produced an additional unintended benefit. It enabled ex-patients to meet each other and learn from one another. Such contacts, especially by people from different geographical areas, were previously difficult but later became a source of inspiration and support during the exercise of an otherwise thankless task — to present the patient viewpoint to audiences that were often indifferent or even hostile toward that view.

Self-Help and Empowerment

Gradually, the movement began to put some of its principles into action in the operation of self-help programs as alternatives to professional treatment. Although the Mental Patients' Association (MPA) in Vancouver, Canada, began operating its drop-in center and residences within months of its founding in 1971, the first such projects did not appear in the United States until the late 1970s, largely because funding was unavailable.

Programs that developed out of the ex-patients' movement tend to be skeptical about the value of the mental health system and traditional psychiatric treatment (Chamberlin, Rogers, and Sneed, 1989). Members usually gravitate to these groups because they have had negative experiences in the system. Often, members are angry, and their anger is seen by the group as a healthy reaction to their experiences of abuse by the mental health system. At the same time, members, despite their distrust of the system, may simultaneously be involved in professionally-run programs. Members of user-run services are free to combine their participation in self-help groups with professionally-run services, in whatever proportion and combination each member determines.

Through successes experienced in self-help groups, members are enabled to take a stronger role in advocating for their own needs within the larger mental health system. Empowerment means that members have a voice in mental health matters generally — they reject the role of passive service recipient. Group members found themselves moving naturally into the role of advocate, representing the needs of clients on panels, boards, and committees. This may require accommodation on the part of other groups and group members such as administrators, policy makers, legislators, and family members, who typically have listened to everyone but the client about client needs.

Self-help groups do not exist in a vacuum. Even a group that sees itself as totally separate from the mental health system will, of necessity, have some interactions with it, while groups that have been aided or brought into existence by mental health professionals will need to devise their own ways of making themselves autonomous from the larger system. By taking on a role other than that of the passive, needy client, self-help group members can change the systems with which they interact, as these systems adjust to respond to clients in their new roles as advocates and service providers.

Self-help is a concept, not a single program model. The concept is a means by which people become empowered and begin to think of themselves as competent individuals as they present themselves in new ways to the world. By its very nature, self-help combats stigma, because the negative images of mental patients ultimately must give way to the reality of clients managing their own lives and their own programs. The successes of self-help groups have been striking. Groups are handling annual budgets that may be in the hundreds of thousands of dollars; producing newsletters, books, and pamphlets; educating other clients and professionals about group work; influencing legislation and public policy; publicizing and advocating on their own behalf in the media; and, in general, challenging stereotypes and creating new realities. At the same time, individual group members may still be battling the particular manifestations that led to their being psychiatrically labeled in the first place. Self-help is not a miracle nor a cure-all, but it is a powerful confirmation that people, despite problems and disabilities, can achieve more than others (or they themselves) may have ever thought possible.

Advocacy

Self-help is one of two co-equal aspects of the ex-patients' movement; the other is advocacy, or working for political change. Unlike groups such as Recovery Inc. or Schizophrenics Anonymous, patient liberation groups tend to address problems that go beyond the individual. The basic principle of the movement is that all laws and practices which induce discrimination toward individuals who have been labeled "mentally ill" need to be changed, so that a psychiatric diagnosis has no more impact on a person's citizenship rights and responsibilities than does a diagnosis of diabetes or heart disease. To that end, all commitment laws, forced treatment laws, insanity defenses, and other similar practices should be abolished.

Ending involuntary treatment is a long-term goal of the patients' liberation movement. Meanwhile, movement activists work to improve conditions of people subjected to forced treatment, and to see that their existing rights are respected, keeping in mind that these are interim steps within a basically unjust system.

Existing laws have the power to compel people to receive treatment for mental illness. This almost never occurs in the case of physical illness, except in the rare instances when courts overrule parents who refuse medical treatment for a child. The courts in these instances assume the *parens patriae* role, acting in lieu of parents in what the court defines as the child's best interest. When a person of whatever age is ordered by a court to undergo psychiatric treatment, this same *parens patriae* power comes into effect. This connection between the legal and medical systems places the mental patient at a disadvantage that is not faced by patients with physical illnesses.

In addition to the *parens patriae* doctrine, which assumes that a mentally ill individual is incapable of determining his or her own best interest, an additional doctrine, the police power of the state, is used to justify the involuntary confinement of individuals labeled mentally ill. This doctrine is based on the assumption that mentally ill people are dangerous and may do harm to themselves or to others if they are not confined. The belief in the dangerousness of the mentally ill is firmly rooted in our culture. It is especially promoted by the mass media, which frequently run stories in which crimes of violence are attributed to mental illness. If the alleged criminal has been previously hospitalized, the fact is prominently mentioned; if not, frequently a police officer or other authority figure will be quoted to the effect that the accused is "a mental case" or "a nut." In addition, unsolved crimes are often similarly attributed. Both the *parens patriae* power and the police power relate to the stereotyped view of the prospective patient — that he or she is sick, unpredictable, dangerous, unable to care for himself or herself, and unable to judge his or her own best interest.

The movement's advocacy has focused on the right of the individual *not* to be a patient, rather than on mere procedural safeguards before involuntary treatment can be instituted. A major lawsuit testing this right was filed by seven patients at Boston State Hospital in 1975, many of whom had been members of a patients' rights group that met weekly in the hospital with the aid of the Mental Patients' Liberation Front. The suit, originally known as *Rogers v. Macht*, was called, in later stages, *Rogers v. Okin* and *Rogers v. Commissioner of Mental Health* (1982). It established a limited right-to-refuse-treatment (i.e., psychiatric drugs) for Massachusetts patients.

Since *Rogers v. Commissioner*, right-to-refuse-treatment cases have been decided in a number of states, including New York (*Rivers v. Katz*, 1986) and California (*Reise v. St. Mary's Hospital*, 1987), and the right has been established administratively in some other states. While the movement first greeted these decisions as victories, it has become clear that, in practice, these reforms do little to change the power relationship between patient and psychiatrist. Each procedure (varying from state to state) provides one or more methods to override the patient's decision to refuse drugs; and whether the procedure is administrative or judicial, the end result is that most drug-refusing patients whose cases are heard are forced, ultimately, to take the drugs, despite the

ostensible right to refuse them (Appelbaum, 1988). Many movement activists
have become discouraged and no longer believe that the courts will help people
avoid involuntary patienthood through the mechanism of the right to refuse
treatment.

Many individuals in the ex-patients' movement first encountered a critique
of the mental health system — a critique which confirmed their feelings — in
the works of Thomas Szasz. In such books as *The Myth of Mental Illness* (1961)
and *The Manufacture of Madness* (1970), in a career spanning more than thirty
years, Szasz has always spoken powerfully about the essential wrongness of
forced psychiatric treatment, and the fallacy of defining social and behavioral
problems as illnesses. In a recent paper, Szasz (1989) provides a devastating
critique of the mental patients' "rights" movement, which has been guided
largely by lawyers and non-patients.

> Rallying to the battle cry of "civil rights for mental patients," professional civil libertarians,
> special-interest-mongering attorneys, and the relatives of mental patients joined conven-
> tional psychiatrists demanding rights for mental patients — *qua* mental patients. The
> result has been a perverse sort of affirmative action program: since mental patients are
> ill, they have a right to treatment; since many are homeless, they have a right to hous-
> ing; and so it goes, generating even a special right to reject treatment (a right every non-
> mental patient has *without* special dispensation). In short, the phrase "rights of mental
> patients" has meant everything but according persons called "mental patients" the same
> rights (and duties) as are accorded all adults *qua* citizens or persons. (p. 19)

The National Association of Psychiatric Survivers (NAPS), founded in 1985
as the National Alliance of Mental Patients, promotes the same ideals Szasz
espouses. The first item in its *Goals and Philosophy Statement* reads:

> To promote the human and civil rights of people in and out of psychiatric treatment
> situations, with special attention to their absolute right to freedom of choice. To work
> towards the end of involuntary psychiatric intervention, including civil commitment and
> forced procedures such as electroshock, psychosurgery, forced drugging, restraint and
> seclusion, holding that such intervention against one's will is not a form of treatment,
> but a violation of liberty and the right to control one's own body and mind. We em-
> phasize freedom of choice for people wanting to receive psychiatric services through true
> informed consent to treatment which includes the right to refuse any unwanted treatments.
> We will also work to assure the rights of all people who have been psychiatrically labeled
> including but not limited to people in halfway houses, day treatment, residential facilities,
> vocational rehabilitation, nursing homes, psycho-social rehabilitation clubs as well as
> psychiatric institutions. (NAPS, no date, p. 1)

This is the essence of "mental patients'" liberation. NAPS was formed
specifically to counter the trend toward reformist "consumerism," which
developed as the psychiatric establishment began to fund ex-patient self-help.
Ironically, the same developments which led to the movement's growth and
to the operation of increasing numbers of ex-patient-run alternative programs,
also weakened the radical voices within the movement and promoted the

views of far more cooperative "consumers." The very term "consumer" implies an equality of power which simply does not exist; mental health "consumers" are still subject to involuntary commitment and treatment, and the defining of their experience by others.

It is not surprising that once the Community Support Program at NIMH began funding "consumer" conferences, the International Conference on Human Rights and Psychiatric Oppression disbanded. The first CSP-funded conference, "Alternatives '85," was held in Baltimore in June, 1985; the last International Conference in Burlington, Vermont, in August of that year. The dissolution was aided by a group of "consumers" who may have seen the liberation perspective as a threat. At the same time, some extreme radicals opposed any form of organization as oppressive, believing that a totally decentralized and unstructured movement could accomplish its goals.

Madness Network News disintegrated the next year. Its all-volunteer staff became exhausted by the effort of putting out the newspaper with no funds but member subscriptions, and they were succeeded by a very small group of extreme radicals who published only one issue — critical of anyone attempting to develop organizational structure or sources of funding for movement activities. The paper then ceased publication, leaving a gap in movement communication that went unfilled for several years. Although *Dendron*, a newsletter published by the Clearinghouse on Human Rights and Psychiatry in Eugene, Oregon, began publishing shortly thereafter, only recently has it become as visible within the movement as had been *Madness Network News*.

Where the Movement Stands Now

At present, many groups exist that claim to speak "for" patients, that is, to be patients' advocates. Even the American Psychiatric Association claims this role, as does the National Alliance for the Mentally Ill (NAMI), a group primarily composed of relatives of patients, which enthusiastically embraces the medical model and promotes the expansion of involuntary commitment and the lifetime control of people labeled "mentally ill." However, a basic liberation principle is that people *must* speak for themselves.

Former patients recognize numerous currents of opinion within their community (which, after all, numbers in the millions). There are groups whose members promote the illness metaphor (e.g., National Depressive and Manic-Depressive Association); groups whose members promote self-help in conjunction with treatment for illness (e.g., Recovery, Inc.); groups whose members see themselves as consumers (e.g., the National Mental Health Consumers' Association); and groups whose members see themselves as liberationists (e.g., National Association of Psychiatric Survivors). However, it is safe to say that by far the largest number of patients and ex-patients are those who identify with *none* of these organizations — indeed most patients and ex-patients have probably never even heard of these groups.

The movement continues to face formidable obstacles. The psychiatric/medical model of "mental illness" is widely accepted by the general public. Indeed, new psychiatric "illnesses" are being "discovered" all the time, and psychiatry now claims that social deviants — from rapists to repetitive gamblers — are suffering from a variety of newly defined "mental illnesses." Psychiatry is entrenched, as well, in the courts, the prisons, the schools, and all major institutions of society.

At the same time, there are many hopeful signs for the movement. The ex-patients' movement is developing alliances with the physically disabled, with the poor, and with ex-patients in other countries. Physically disabled people have organized their own self-help programs, using the model of independent living. According to the principles of independent living, any person — no matter how physically disabled he or she may be — can live independently if provided with the proper supports. Such supports must be individualized — a person may need special equipment, personal care attendents, modified transportation vehicles, and so forth. The particular mix of supports is determined by the individual, in consultation with an independent living specialist (who is also a physically disabled person). As the disability rights movement has grown, it has become a powerful force for legal change as well. For more than ten years, this movement has lobbied in favor of the Americans with Disabilities Act, the so-called civil rights bill for the disabled. The bill was signed into law on July 26, 1990. Although the ex-patients' movement entered that struggle late, the final version of the Act does include persons with "psychiatric disabilities" under its protections.

Linkages of the ex-patients' movement with the impoverished include efforts at affordable housing, campaigns for universal medical insurance, and involvement in the Rainbow Coalition. It has proved extremely useful for ex-patient activists to become involved in these activities — not only do ex-patients require the services being advocated but demystification in the eyes of one's allies can serve an invaluable purpose. When labeled as "mentally ill" — a nameless, faceless person — the "mental patient" may be seen as the enemy; as a co-worker and a colleague, facing the same problems and struggling for the same solutions, the ex-patient becomes an individual: knowable and understandable.

The growing internationalization of the ex-patients' movement is another sign of the movement's growth and strength. As groups exchange newsletters, and attend meetings and conferences, a shared ideology is developing. Although the lack of a solidifying terminology continues to be troubling, such variety does not necessarily indicate wide variations in viewpoints and activities. Whether group members call themselves clients, consumers, ex-patients, users, or psychiatric survivors, groups throughout the world are united by the goals of self-determination and full citizenship rights for their members.

It is true that the vast majority of former patients remain unorganized, but this challenge is being met. As groups become more visible, they recruit more members. This occurs because ex-patient groups speak to a truth of the patienthood experience: that people's anger and frustration are real and valid, and that only by speaking out can individuals who have been harmed by the entrenched power of psychiatry mount a challenge against it.

References

Appelbaum, D. (1988). The right to refuse treatment with antipsychotic drugs: Retrospect and prospect. *American Journal of Psychiatry, 145,* 413–419.

Beers, C. (1953). *A mind that found itself.* Garden City, New York: Doubleday.

Chamberlin, J. (1979). *On our own: Patient-controlled alternatives to the mental health system.* New York: McGraw-Hill.

Chamberlin, J. (1987). The case for separatism. In I. Barker and E. Peck (Eds.), *Power in strange places* (pp. 24–26). London, England: Good Practices in Mental Health.

Chamberlin, J., Rogers, J.A., and Sneed, C.S. (1989). Consumers, families, and community support systems. *Psychosocial Rehabilitation Journal, 12,* 93–106.

Dain, N. (1989). Critics and dissenters: Reflections on 'anti-psychiatry' in the United States. *Journal of the History of the Behavioral Sciences, 25,* 3–25.

National Association of Psychiatric Survivors. (No date). *Goals and philosophy statement.* Unpublished manuscript.

Report to the President for the President's Commission on Mental Health. (1978). Volume I. Washington, D.C.: United States Government Printing Office.

Riese v. St. Mary's Hospital, 209 Cal. App. 3rd, 1303, 1987.

Rivers v. Katz, 67 N.Y., 2nd, 485, 1986.

Rogers v. Commissioner of Mental Health, 390 Mass. 498, 1982.

Szasz, T. (1961). *The myth of mental illness.* New York: Hoeber-Harper.

Szasz, T. (1970). *The manufacture of madness.* New York: Dell.

Szasz, T. (1989, July). The myth of the rights of mental patients. *Liberty,* pp. 19–26.

©1990 The Institute of Mind and Behavior, Inc.
The Journal of Mind and Behavior
Summer and Autumn 1990, Volume 11, Numbers 3 and 4
Pages 337 [91] – 352 [106]
ISSN 0271-0137
ISBN 0-930195-05-1

AIDS and the Psycho-Social Disciplines:
The Social Control of "Dangerous" Behavior

Mark S. Kaplan

University of Illinois at Urbana-Champaign

AIDS provides society an opportunity to expand and rationalize control over a broad range of psychological phenomena. Social control today is panoptical, involving dispersed centers and agents of surveillance and discipline throughout the whole community (as exemplified by workplace drug testing). The control of persons perceived as "dangerous" is effected partly through public psycho-social discourse on AIDS. This reproduces earlier encounters with frightening diseases, most notably the nineteenth-century cholera epidemic, and reveals a morally-laden ideology behind modern efforts at public hygiene.

The hospital psychiatrist, noticing Marcus' effeminate mannerisms, immediately decided to administer an HIV antibody test. And in fact, the boy tested positive. Instantly he became a pariah. When it became known that Marcus was currently sexually active, the professionals and officials began a steady campaign to get him out of town or locked up in a hospital or reformatory. (Epstein, 1988, p. 46)

AIDS today serves as an impetus and rationale for controlling marginal groups and their "dangerous" behavior. Marcus's story above illustrates that the interruption of the spread of the human immunodeficiency virus (HIV) occasions — like previous epidemics — measures for medical "policing" (Ergas, 1987). Social control today, however, is not only characterized by direct and punitive measures as suggested above. Instead, as Michel Foucault and others have argued, modern social control is "panoptical" in nature, involving widely dispersed centers and agents of surveillance and discipline throughout the whole community (Rodger, 1988). G. Marx (1985) put it this way: "the ethos of social control has expanded from focused and direct coercion [face-

Preparation of this article was supported by a fellowship from the National Cancer Institute, National Research Service Award T32-CA09492. Requests for reprints should be sent to Mark S. Kaplan, Dr.P.H., School of Social Work, University of Illinois at Urbana-Champaign, 1207 West Organ Street, Urbana, Illinois 61801.

to-face] used after the fact and against a particular target to anticipatory actions entailing deception, manipulation, planning, and a diffuse panoptic vision [to observe and normalize]" (p. 26). Social control is thus no longer exclusively aimed at keeping "criminal" or "dangerous" classes at bay. Instead, modern surveillance penetrates — at "multiple levels" (Ericson and Shearing, 1986) — a broad range of social and health phenomena deemed or construed as "threats" to the body politic.

Foucault (1979, 1988) and Turner (1984) argue that imperatives of discipline and surveillance began to take shape in the late eighteenth and early nineteenth centuries with the rise of industrial capitalism. As early as 1779 in Germany, Johan Peter Frank proposed in his six-volume *System for a Complete Medical Policing* a scheme "to prevent evils through wise ordinances" (cited in Ericson and Shearing, 1986, p. 154). This was at a time when concerns about the social consequences of individual behavior, morality, and disease were first expressed, when the health and physical well-being of entire populations came to figure as explicit political objectives, when the "policing" of public hygiene could ensure economic regulations and social order (Foucault, 1980).

In the twentieth century, the social control of hygiene has undergone a scientific and technological transformation. Today, such control is characterized by the intersection of three general mechanisms of power which have virtually consolidated an "inclusivist gaze" (Smart, 1985): disciplinary technologies (e.g., psychoactive drugs), disciplinary institutions, and scientific discourse (Conrad, 1979). This work looks at the role that discourse has had in framing and managing sexuality during the AIDS crisis. I will examine the extent to which the psycho-social sciences — via scientific discourse — have extended and rationalized controls over sexual beliefs, desires, and behaviors. Under the term psycho-social, I include psychiatry and psychology, clinical medicine, the human sciences, and the various pedagogical and clinical practices aimed at controlling sexuality (see Lemert and Gillan, 1982).

My line of inquiry follows Mort's (1987) argument that "AIDS is the contemporary moment in a much longer history, the extraordinarily complex interweaving of medicine and morality with surveillance and regulation — even the definition — of sex" (p. 2). In focusing on discourse, I attempt to answer the following question: How do psycho-social disciplines fit into the much broader, historically-influenced agenda bent on normalizing and individualizing what has been designated in scientific publications as "promiscuous" behavior in the AIDS era? The label "promiscuous," as we will see, is meaningful only on a wider, nonepidemiological level (Murphy and Pilotta, 1987; Padgug, 1989). The notion of "promiscuity" has given the psycho-social disciplines an opportunity to penetrate and conduct surveillance of a broad range of psychological phenomena associated with the transmission of HIV. I do not mean to suggest that all HIV/AIDS-related behaviors labelled "promiscuous" or "dangerous" are somehow epidemiologically spurious. Rather, these designations and the societal responses they evoke must be placed in some social-historical context in order to make sense of their ideologic components.

To help in this task, I first turn to two postulates from Turner's (1984) book, *The Body and Society*: (1) disease language is ideology and social practice, and (2) medicine is a political practice.

Disease Language as Ideology and Social Practice

The language of disease is not a value-neutral medium that communicates ideas and meanings independently formed. Instead language is a structure of sentiments and interests that frame and channel definitions, perceptions, and practices in certain directions (Connolly, 1983). In particular, the modern language of the psycho-social disciplines carries enormous institutional currency on what is to count as desirable or undesirable health-related behavior (Turner, 1984).

Acording to Mercer (1983), the AIDS epidemic has produced a "rewriting of the codes and grammar of pleasure, within our culture" (p. 85). Treichler (1988) put it this way: AIDS language "enact[s] and reinforce[s] deeply entrenched, pervasive, and often conservative cultural 'narratives' about sexuality" (p. 192). As with earlier medico-moral crises, AIDS has brought the concerns over "promiscuous" behavior to center stage. Therefore, to understand the deeper social structures of the crisis we must understand the language or discourse of AIDS.

Smith-Rosenberg (1985) distinguishes between two types of languages: "public language" – which appears in printed, formal sources – and "private language" – the thoughts of individuals found in less formal sources. Theories of sexuality can be read as public-symbolic language in which the individual body stands as a representation of the social body; the structure of cultural forms and social relationships merge with visions of the body (Smith-Rosenberg, 1985, p. 48). Hierarchical societies concerned with rigid maintenance of social hygiene and moral order will act out this concern upon the physical body. Words, conceptual categories, rituals, and codes are used in these societies to label and demarcate the boundaries between health and disease, order and disorder. Consequently, those who are perceived as vectors of the disease will be treated as simultaneously dangerous and physically polluting, and stern efforts will be made to "police" them. The "public language" of AIDS on "dangerous" sexuality, while infused with epidemiological realities, is aimed at controlling a broad range of behaviors and, ultimately, at the inculcation of sexual/behavioral self-restraint. Thus a combination of moral and empirical factors have been responsible for placing "promiscuity" at the heart of the concerns of the psycho-social disciplines (Mort, 1987). Borrowing from Gusfield's discussion in another context (1981, p. 9), on one side we have beliefs about the facts of the situation and events comprising the problem — for example, the probability of the transmission of HIV among heterosexuals. On the other side, we have beliefs about the morality which depicts the situation as abnormal, unnatural, and immoral. According to Gusfield (1981), the moral dimension is what makes eradication and social control desirable. With this formulation in mind, we can begin to see how medical constructs reproduce dominant socio-moral values, ranging from the older asceticism of Puritanism (purity = health = salvation) to the new sexual order (monogamy = health = salvation) [Foucault, 1979; Kyle, 1989].

Medicine Is a Political Practice

How does medicine, as a psycho-social discipline, fit into the administration of the body politic? We are not accustomed to thinking of medical discourse and practices as political, even when we recognize the inherently political nature of health care policy and research (Altman, 1986). In the twentieth century, the psycho-social disciplines have supplanted religion as the guardian of morality in the Western world (Turner, 1984). The management of the AIDS crisis provides the psycho-social disciplines with new surveillance opportunities and challenges. Writing in another context, Arney and Bergen (1984) could have been speaking of AIDS where they noted that "[s]een in this light, the care of the social body as a whole presents new and exciting challenges to the medical profession; it constitutes an enlargement of its calling" (p. 93).

Foucault more than any other author in recent times has brought to our attention the role psycho-social sciences play in the growth and maintenance of the disciplinary society. The utility of the Foucaultian framework is that it permits us to analyze the extensive disciplinary matrix which coordinates and subordinates individuals' bodies (Armstrong, 1983), their families (Donzelot, 1979), their work and leisure activities (Hecker and Kaplan, 1989), their sexual desires (Turner, 1984, p. 163), and even their "souls" (O'Neill, 1985, p. 25). In the case of medicine, a Foucaultian framework permits us to deconstruct the codes and the disciplinary matrix in which an individual who is ill resides (O'Neill, 1987, p. 33). A Foucaultian exposition requires that attention be given to broader socio-historical factors bound up with the development of this disciplinary matrix. For example, for Foucault, "[t]he hospital was born not of an inevitable or natural necessity but out of a set of practices resulting from the clinical gaze; namely, the internal demand for control, systematic observation, collections of cases and patient histories" (D'Amico, 1989, pp. 80–81). As for its potential social power, Foucault (1980) himself demonstrated that medicine assumes an increasingly important place in the administrative system and the machinery of power, a role which is constantly widened and strengthened throughout the eighteenth century. The doctor wins a footing within the different instances of social power. The administration acts as a point of support and sometimes a point of departure for the great medical enquiries into the health of populations, and conversely doctors devote an increasing amount of their activity to tasks, both general and administrative, assigned to them by power. A "medico-administrative" knowledge begins to develop concerning society, its health and sickness, its conditions of life, housing and habits, which serves as the basic core for the "social economy" and sociology of the nineteenth century. And there is likewise constituted a politico-medical hold on a population hedged in by a whole series of prescriptions relating not only to disease but to general forms of existence and behavior. . . . The doctor becomes the great advisor and expert, if not in the art of governing, at least in that of observing, correcting and improving the social "body" and maintaining it in a permanent state of health. (pp. 176–177)

Many of Foucault's ideas about social control revolve around the terms of knowledge and power. His conception of power constitutes a radical departure from Marxian and liberal interpretations. For Foucault, power is not a possession, won by one class that struggles to retain it against its acquisition by another. Rather, as suggested above, Foucault ". . . translates the problem of social control [i.e., surveillance and discipline] out of the terms of class conspiracy into the history of the scientization of power/knowledge produced in the double context of population policy and clinical medicine designed to administer the body politic. . ." (O'Neill, 1987, p. 24). The aim of power changed from the "visibility, excess and crudity" of punishment of earlier times to the "invisible, calculated refinement of discipline" which was transformed during the industrial revolution (Armstrong, 1980, p. 300). Modern power operates through inclusion of outcasts, rather than their exclusion (e.g., incarceration or quarantine). The modern practice of power is deployed by ". . . invent[ing] the individual [today's outcast] as an object to be measured and managed in a social space that no longer has a boundary since it incorporates *everything* in the name of 'scientific truth' " (Arney and Bergen, 1984, p. 126) [italics added]. Foucault, in *Discipline and Punish* (1979), dubs this modern control paradigm "panopticism."

Panopticism as the New Control Paradigm

The Panopticon is the "all-seeing eye" (Strub, 1989, p. 41). The *Oxford English Dictionary* defines "Panopticon" as "fully seen or visible" and adds that it was the name given in 1791 by Jeremy Bentham to a proposed form of prison of circular shape having cells built round and fully exposed toward a central "well," hence the prison officers could at all times observe the inmates. Bentham's original plan for the ideal prison serves as an eloquent symbol for the disciplinary sciences: "a system of knowledge whose radii penetrate into every corner of life, and thus make possible swift and effective control" (Ingelby, 1983, p. 164). Bentham's Panopticon represents the first stage in the introduction of individual pleasures into the field of social regulation (Mercer, 1983, p. 91). Each person's conduct stands within the reach of a central, invisible inspection. Individuals, not knowing when they are observed, have to behave at all times as though they were being watched. The ultimate effect is that they are brought to internalize the locus of discipline, to exercise self-restraint, and thus to act in accordance with the conventions and expectations of the disciplinary system in which they are caught (Hecker and Kaplan, 1989). An important feature of this control paradigm is that it enables whole populations to be observed and classified. Zuboff (1988), in her excellent analysis of modern surveillance, notes:

> Panopticism is the general principle of a new "political anatomy" whose object and end are not the relations of sovereignty but the relation of discipline. . . . What are required are mechanisms that analyze distributions, gaps, series, combinations, and which use instruments that render visible, record, differentiate and compare. . . . It is polyvalent in its application. . . . Whenever one is dealing with a multiplicity of individuals on whom a task or a particular form of behavior must be imposed, the panoptic schema may be used. (p. 322)

We can trace the imperative of panoptical control back to the challenge of transforming a predominantly agrarian, pre-capitalist population into a workforce more amenable to factory production. According to Gronfors and Stalstrom (1987, p. 55), with the advent of industrialization, capitalism saw the control and disciplining of thoughts and feelings of workers as one tool for supporting economic expansion. By the late nineteenth century, according to Arney and Bergen (1984, p. 65), "[t]o [further] improve worker control, managers had to look deeper and deeper into the production processes . . . . Managers could control the relationships within the walls of the factory and make adjustments as necessary; events outside remained out of their control but they were crucial nonetheless and demanded consideration and monitoring." By the early twentieth century, with the advent of industrial psychology (Taylorism) and medicine along with a new focus on the "ecology of the factory" (Arney and Bergen, 1984), leisure-time activity would now be seen as an indispensable part of the factory's production process. For example, certain expressions of sexuality, defined as leisure-time activity, were seen to fit poorly into the early labor-intensive capitalistic efforts. According to Greenberg (1988), "medical writings of the eighteenth and nineteenth centuries viewed men as having a limited amount of bodily energy; excessive discharge of their energy through sexual release . . . would deplete the supply available for other purposes and would thus lead to enervation and lethargy, if not more dire consequences" (p. 362). Homosexuality, as Weeks (1985) documents, became a particular target of a panoptic network of moral agencies, political interventions, and diverse social practices. The net effect of panopticism was the production of docility, utility and governability of the social body (O'Neill, 1987). According to Foucault (1979) and interpreters, the development of new techniques of industrial management – including Panopticism and Taylorism – laid the groundwork for a new kind of "disciplinary society," one in which the bodily discipline, regulation, and surveillance would soon be taken for granted (Zuboff, 1988, p. 319).

In the late twentieth century, we see the realization of panopticism throughout society in such forms as drug testing (i.e., urinalysis), pre-employment HIV testing ("60% of employers," 1989), pre-marital HIV testing (Mohr, 1988), and psychological evaluation of employees ("This is your life", 1989). In the workplace, drug testing as well as HIV testing give new and explanded means for probing and controlling the "inner environment" of individuals (Hecker and Kaplan, 1989). Bodily fluids tell tales not only about one's own "impairment," but about one's lifestyle, habits, and psyche. Drug, HIV, and other invasive probing constitute surveillance without interruption, induce "self-restraint" central to Panopticism, and transcend far beyond the legitimate concerns over threats to the public hygiene into the private and concealed domains of the individual body and mind. Put another way, testing of bodily fluids certainly appears to extend what Foucault identified as the exigencies of a developing industrial capitalist system: to ensure the mechanism and circulation of power through "progressively finer channels, gaining access to individuals themselves, to their bodies, their gestures, and all their daily action" (Foucault, 1979, cited in Hecker and Kaplan, 1989, pp. 26–27). In summary, the twentieth century has seen the deployment of a new and more penetrating surveillance and disciplining gaze, one that expands far beyond the confines of the body to its social sphere.

AIDS Language as Social Control:
The Regulation of Libidinal Impulses

There are some theoretical grounds for believing that the nature of homosexual coitus can cause immunosuppression. (Lacey and Waugh, 1983, p. 464)

At the beginning of the AIDS epidemic there was an almost immediate emphasis in the scientific and popular discourse on "fast lane" behavior and "profound promiscuity" (Bayer, 1987). The first report of AIDS appeared in the *New York Times* on July 3, 1981, and included the comment that "according to Dr. Friedman-Kien the reporting doctors said that most cases had involved homosexual men who have had multiple and frequent sexual encounters with different partners" (cited in Altman, 1986, p. 34). If this claim had been clearly linked to the argument that "promiscuity" was significant because it increased the risk of exposure to pathogens, it would have been self-evident. Unfortunately, readers were left with the distinct impression that "promiscuity" (as an adverse lifestyle behavior) *per se* was the cause of the disease, an idea seized upon by both scientific publications and mass media. For example Navarro and Hagstrom (1982) noted in the *New England Journal of Medicine* that "Promiscuous male homosexuals may therefore be repeatedly exposed to immosuppresive factors [in seminal fluid] as well as antigenic challenge during rectal intercourse" (p. 933). The reality constructed by this discourse is as follows: given the abnormally high "promiscuity" of gay men, some form of sexually transmitted virus (HIV) or exposure to a common lifestyle (i.e., the use of "poppers") played a critical role in establishing immunodeficiency. This interpretation directed attention to gay men as its victims and their sexuality as the problem. In the *Lancet* published in May 1982 a widely cited paper concluded that "amyl nitrate [poppers] exposure and sexual *promiscuity* were associated with development of Kaposi's sarcoma, as well as histories of mononucleosis and sexually transmitted diseases" (Marmor, Laubenstein, Williams, Friedman-Kien, Byrum, D'Onofrio, and Dubin, 1982, p. 1086) [italics added]. Pointing to salient links between the spread of the disease and promiscuity, the article drew attention to alarming differences between the sexual behavior of the infected homosexuals and a control group of non-infected heterosexuals. Fifty percent of the gay patients admitted to having sex with ten or more partners in an average month. The most promiscuous patient estimated he had intercourse with ninety different partners per month in the year before onset of the disease. Conclusions were tentative but an initial hypothesis was made clear — "promiscuous" behavior was an important factor in spreading this potentially killer disease (cited in Mort, 1987, p. 1).

A literature search through the National Library of Medicine MEDLINE Database reveals that a number of articles published as recently as 1988 and 1989 still implicate "promiscuity" in the transmission of HIV (see, for example, Couarvoisier, Tauber, and Luthy, 1989; Cruz, Dieguez, Fos, and Hierro, 1988; Duesberg, 1989; Fleming, 1988; Fouchard, Schmidt, and Krasnik, 1989; N'Galy and Ryder, 1988; Schroter, Nher, and Petzoldt, 1988; Seidlin, Krasinski, Bebenroth, Itri, Paolino, and Valentine, 1988; Soriano, Tor, Muga, Fernandez, Ribera, Balanzo, and Foz, 1989; Taylor, Taylor-Robinson, Jeffries, and Tyms, 1988; Titti, Rezza, Verani, Butto, Sernicola, Rapicetta, Sarrecchia, Oliva, and Rossi, 1988). All these articles specifically mention "promiscuity" as a HIV risk factor. For example, Fouchard et al. (1989) write that "HIV was introduced in Denmark toward the end of the nineteen eighties among *promiscuous* homosexual men in Copenhagen to a level in which ¼ – ⅓ were found to be infected in small selected materials" (p. 613) [italics added]. In the October 1988 issue of *Psychiatric Annals*, a psychiatrist could also write: "It is well known that promiscuity is a hallmark of homosexuality. It is also well-established that promiscuity promotes the spread of AIDS and has to be rejected on statistical, if not *moral*, grounds (Tanay, 1988, p. 596) [italics added]. According to another psychiatrist, to "cease dangerous [read promiscuous] activity . . . public health authorities may be forced to resurrect sanitaria [read "policing"] for the quarantine of *relentlessly* contagious carriers" (Eth, 1988, p. 575) [italics added].

Again, the problem with such textual constructions of reality, according to Altman (1986), is that they inevitably lead to the conclusion that "promiscuity" is a risk factor and that everyone with AIDS (or infected with HIV) has necessarily been and remains dangerously "promiscuous." Moreover, professional vocabulary and imagery on the number of sexual partners tends to reinforce anti-homosexual sentiment that gay men are morally depraved (Meredith, 1984, p. 58). The image of the homosexual male as a dangerous/promiscuous individual has existed since the nineteenth century, when such an individual was viewed as a ". . . [walking] time bomb who at some moment [would] explode, destroying those who let themselves be seduced" (Gilman, 1985, p. 71). Contained in nineteenth century discourse on sexual "dangerousness" (see, for example, Foucault, 1988), as well as in the late twentieth century concept of AIDS-related "promiscuity," is invariably the notion of an immediate threat to the social order. The vocabulary and imagery of "promiscuity" constructed in the scientific literature serves as a foremost instrument of disciplinary power for normalizing non-normative sexual practices (Levine and Troiden, 1988; Smart, 1985).

The Rise of Medico-Moral Discourse

The reactions evoked by AIDS are determined not only by its biological nature but by historically produced meanings attached to sex, health, and disease (Mort, 1987, p. 215). That is, social and moral ideologies along with biomedical realities define the meaning and management of epidemics both for its victims and the entire society. Therefore, the impact of AIDS, the fear of HIV, and the development of public and personal hygiene must all be seen within the larger context aimed at disciplining and civilizing (Goudsblom, 1986).

Nineteenth Century Cholera Epidemics

The framework guiding the societal interpretation and response (images and vocabulary) to AIDS has its roots in the nineteenth century cholera triangular relationship of morality, sexuality, and pathology. According to Rosenberg (1986), nineteenth century cholera is the closest modern analogy to AIDS. No other disease had a more terrifying impact in the nineteenth century than cholera, which reached Europe from Asia around 1830, and immediately unleashed panic as well as determined efforts to contain it. It was widely believed that cholera was a disease which would find its victims almost without exception among the poor — then referred to as "dangerous classes" (Goudsblom, 1986). The words of a popular German writer and physician, C. Reclam, captured the general fear of these marginal groups as the source of the disease in the following lines:

> Don't think that the foul air of the street, propelled by the wind, turns around and humbly recedes when it meets windows adorned with marble and sculpture. Be assured that the germs of disease from the dwellings of the proletarians can be easily transmitted through the air to the parlour and the bedroom of the first servant of the state. (cited in Goudsblom, 1986, p. 178)

The cholera epidemic in Europe and the United States fell disproportionately on marginal groups. During the nineteenth century, poverty and disease were viewed as a consequence of idleness and intemperance — the latter believed to make the individual more susceptible to cholera. In the United States, not only were the poor blamed but the new immigrants were accused of bringing the disease into the country. Prostitutes were accused of being reservoirs of disease and rounded up under social hygiene provisions even though cholera was not thought to be a venereal disease. Many felt that immigrants' and prostitutes' "moral corruption" caused them to develop cholera.

> Representations of sexual immorality were constructed through institutional programmes which linked the habits and environment of the urban poor with medical-moral pathology. Professional experts and groups targeted their therapeutic gaze at the specific domain of sexuality, attributing the spread of cholera to "excessive bouts of unnatural sex." (Mort, 1987, p. 215)

In Great Britain, the newly founded medical journal, *Lancet*, along with other leading periodicals, carried many articles on the causes of cholera and the steps to be taken for prevention (Mort, 1987). Evidence was conflicting and contradictory, reflecting current medical divisions on the origins and transmission of disease. But though there was little consensus about causation, physicans, clerics, bourgeois reformers and other local officials all agreed that the urban poor and their lifestyles, including their sexual behavior and morality, were responsibility for spreading contagion. According to Mort (1987),

> The logic which twinned poverty and immorality with contagion was made through a specific language — the discourse of early social medicine — and was circulated at key institutional sites within the central and local state. The intentions were clear: greater surveillance and regulation of the poor. . . . The proposed solution was twofold: to isolate the human sources of infection, subjecting them to a regime of compulsory inspection and detention, combined with propaganda to educate the poor into a regime of cleanliness and morality. (p. 16)

In the pamphlet, *The Moral and Physical Condition of the Working Classes Employed in the Cotton Manufacture in Manchester, 1832*, the British sanitarian Dr. James Phillips Kay set out his own early contribution to the debate on the immorality of the urban poor. As Kay put it, the development of a strategy for the "mitigation of suffering" had to take in fundamental questions of economic, political and moral causation (cited in Mort, 1987, p. 19). Reform of sexual conduct was an important part of Kay's schema. Sexuality — always referred to by Kay as sexual immorality — was constructed in relation to the themes and the perceived threat of an oppositional culture (p. 21). The strategic aim then was much broader, namely, the panoptic surveillance and regulation of the urban working-class culture (p. 25). In the following section I discuss how nineteenth century morality has infiltrated modern notions of disease causation.

Modern "Lifestyle" Disease

Nineteenth century discourse on sin, disease, and morality is still frequently translated into the etiological formulations of AIDS, while the reaction to the AIDS epidemic has implicated lifestyles, desires and sexual practices. With AIDS such schemes of disease etiology constitute a framework within which a blend of moral and social assumptions can be legitimated (Rosenberg, 1988). Since the late 1970s, the emphasis on disease-producing lifestyle decisions has been at the center of Americans' debate over health and government policy (Bayer, 1989). As far as lifestyle explanations of AIDS are concerned, both popular and some of the scientific literature emphasize that persons with AIDS are afflicted as a direct result of their lifestyle excesses — their sexual practices or their use of illegal drugs. These recent depictions of promiscuity serve to individualize responsibility for the disease. The individualization carries moral overtone and fits well into the goal of the panoptic vision — a shift from the punitive external control of behavior to the inculcation of disciplined self-restraint.

Individualization blames the individual and limits the responsibility of the larger society (Nelkin and Gilman, 1988). Rosenberg (1986) put the individualization of the disease this way:

> [T]he desire to explain sickness and death in terms of volition — of acts done or left undone — is ancient and powerful. The threat of disease provides a compelling occasion to find prospective reassurance in aspects of behavior subject to individual control. . . . In the nineteenth century epidemics of cholera . . . there was much talk of predisposition. The victims' behavior or place of residence explained why they, in particular, succumbed to a general epidemic influence. With decreasing fear of acute infectious disease in the mid-twentieth century, Americans have turned increasingly to a positive concern with regimen — to diet and exercise — as they seek to reduce their real or sensed risk, to redefine the mortal odds that face them. (p. 50)

"Dangerous" Sexuality

In an important essay, "About the Concept of the Dangerous Individual in 19th Century Legal Psychiatry," Foucault (1988) argues that the notion of "dangerousness" gave psychiatric medicine an opportunity to infiltrate the law: ". . . while for a long time, the criminal was no more than the person to whom a crime could be attributed and who could therefore be punished, today, the crime tends to be no more than the event which signals the existence of a dangerous element . . . in the social body. . . . The doctor must therefore be the technician of this social body, and medicine a public hygiene" (p. 134). This image of the doctor is akin to the "straightener" in Samuel Butler's *Erewhon* who was called upon at the first sign of immoral behavior (cited in Siegler and Osmond, 1974).

Foucault suggests that sexuality deemed "dangerous" has been repressed in the West, at least since the beginning of industrial capitalism. In his *History of Sexuality*, Foucault (1978) argues that this repression led to progressively more complex means of "policing" the person. As the deployment of surveillance expands today, so has the scope of what encompasses sexuality (see, for example, Lotringer, 1988). "It is no longer a question of simply saying what was done – the sexual act – and how it was done, but of reconstructing, in and around the act, the thoughts that recapitulated it, the obsessions that accompanied it, the images, desires, modulations, and quality of the pleasure that animated it" (Foucault, 1978, p. 63). As the contemporary moment in the history of sexuality and its repression, AIDS presents an opportunity for the imposition of what Goldstein (1988) calls "sexual retrenchment and libido shrinking" (p. 42). Seen from a critical perspective, the scientific formulations regarding the spread of the HIV – while promoting rigid sexual norms of monogamy on utilitarian grounds – are unwittingly upholding authoritarian and unegalitarian values.

Conclusion

While the official history of AIDS as a medical entity in the United States began in 1981, the beliefs and values responsible for the social reaction to the epidemic have deeper historical roots. In my analysis I identified the heavily moralized structure of AIDS discourse as well as the individualization, pathologification, and social regulation of lifestyle choices.

AIDS, like past epidemics, must be viewed not only as a medical crisis but as an opportunity for expanding panoptic surveillance and repressive modes of social control. The current political anatomy of AIDS, namely, the decision to analyze and intervene at the level of the individual body, has some additional undesirable consequences. This reductionist and fragmented analysis means that a number of critical issues are not being addressed. For example, we know that the epidemic is attaining particular virulence in the urban underclass (Ergas, 1988). Yet, very few psycho-social investigators have penetrated deeply enough to understand an array of overarching adverse socio-structural factors contributing to, and associated with, the transmission of HIV. Whether analyzing intravenous drug use behavior or sexuality, the time is ripe to focus on the potentially lethal effects that repressive cultures and economies have on the psyche. Most people's choices and behaviors are influenced by the conditions of the social relations in which they are caught. Our attention therefore must be aimed at identifying and changing the adverse social relations which often make "dangerous" choices appear optimal. Sexual minorities have been particular targets of this oppression. This brings to mind Berube's recent observation (1988, p. 16): "How do you rationally weigh risks when your shelters seem to threaten your life?"

References

Altman, D. (1986). AIDS in the mind of America. New York: Anchor Press.

Armstrong, D. (1980). Madness and coping. Sociology of Health and Illness, 2, 293–316.

Armstrong, D. (1983). Political anatomy of the body. Cambridge: Cambridge University Press.

Arney, W.R., and Bergen, B.J. (1984). Medicine and the management of living. Chicago: University of Chicago Press.

Bayer, R. (1987). Homosexuality and American psychiatry. Princeton: Princeton University Press.

Bayer, R. (1989). Private acts, social consequences. New York: Free Press.

Bersani, L. (1988). Is the rectum a grave? In D. Crimp (Ed.), AIDS: Cultural analysis/cultural activism (pp. 197–222). Cambridge: MIT Press.

Berube, A. (1988). Caught in the storm − AIDS and the meaning of natural disaster. Out / Look, 3, 8–9.

Connolly, W. (1983). The terms of political discourse. Oxford: Martin Robertson.

Conrad, P. (1979). Types of medical social control. Sociology of Health and Illness, 1, 1–11.

Couarvoisier, S., Tauber, M.G., and Luthy, R. (1986). Bisexuality and AIDS. Schweizerische Rundschau fur Medizin Praxis, 78, 486–493.

Cruz, M., Dieguez, A., Fos, E., and Hierro, F. (1988). Epidemiologic survey on hepatitis B in gypsy women. European Journal of Epidemiology, 4, 314–317.

D'Amico, R. (1989). Historicism and knowledge. London: Routledge and Kegan Paul.

Donzelot, J. (1979). The policing of families. London: Hutchinson.

Douglas, M. (1966). Purity and danger. London: Routledge and Kegan Paul.

Duesberg, P.H. (1989). Human immunodeficiency virus and Acquired Immunodeficiency Syndrome: Correlation, but not causation. Proceedings of the National Academy of Sciences, 86, 755–764.

Epstein, S. (1988). Nature vs. nurture and politics of AIDS organizing. Out / Look, 1, 46–53.

Ergas, Y. (1987). The social consequences of the AIDS epidemic. Social Sciences Research Council Items, 41, 33–39.

Ericson, R.V., and Shearing, C.D. (1986). The scientification of police work. In G. Bohme (Ed.), The knowledge society (pp. 129–159). Boston: D. Reidel Publishing Company.

Eth, S. (1988). AIDS, ethics, and psychiatry. Psychiatric Annals, 18, 577–581.

Fleming, A.F. (1988). Seroepidemiology of human immunodeficiency viruses in Africa. Biomedicine and Pharmacotherapy, 42, 309–320.

Foucault, M. (1978). The history of sexuality Vol. 1 New York: Pantheon.

Foucault, M. (1979). *Discipline and punish: The birth of the prison.* New York: Pantheon.
Foucault, M. (1980). *Power / knowledge.* C. Gordon (Ed.). New York: Pantheon.
Foucault, M. (1988). The dangerous individual. In L.D. Kritzman (Ed.), *Michel Foucault: Politics, philosophy, culture* (pp. 125–151). New York: Routledge.
Fouchard, J.R., Schmidt, K.W., and Krasnik, A. (1989). HIV infection among homosexual and bisexual men in Denmark. *Ugeskrift for Laeger, 151,* 613–616.
Gilman, S.L. (1985). *Difference and pathology: Stereotypes of sexuality, race, and madness.* Ithaca: Cornell University Press.
Goldstein, R. (1988, April 5). Fatal contraction. *Village Voice,* p. 42.
Goudsblom, J. (1986). Public health and the civilizing process. *The Milbank Quarterly, 64,* 161–168.
Green, B.S. (1983). *Knowing the poor: A case-study in textual reality construction.* London: Routledge and Kegan Paul.
Greenberg, D.F. (1988). *The construction of homosexuality.* Chicago: University of Chicago Press.
Gronfors, M., and Stalstrom, O. (1987). Power, prestige, and profit: AIDS and the oppression of homosexual people. *Acta Sociologica, 30,* 53–66.
Gusfield, J.R. (1981). *The culture of public problems.* Chicago: University of Chicago Press.
Hecker, S., and Kaplan, M.S. (1989). Workplace drug testing as social control. *International Journal of Health Services, 19,* 693–707.
Ingleby, D. (1983). Mental health and social order. In S. Cohen and A. Scull (Eds.), *Social control and the state* (pp. 141–188). Oxford: Martin Robertson.
Kyle, G.R. (1989). AIDS and the new sexual order. *The Journal of Sex Research, 26,* 276–278.
Lacey, C.J.N., and Waugh, M.A. (1983). Cellular immunity in male homosexuals. *The Lancet, 2,* 264.
Lemert, C.C., and Gillan, G. (1982). *Michel Foucault: Social theory and transgression.* New York: Columbia University Press.
Levine, M.P., and Troiden, R.R. (1988). The myth of sexual compulsivity. *The Journal of Sex Research, 25,* 347–363.
Lotringer, S. (1988). *Overexposed: Treating sexual perversions in America.* New York: Pantheon.
Marmor, M., Laubenstein, L., Williams, D.C., Friedman-Kien, A.E., Byrum, R.D., D'Onofrio, S., and Dubin, N. (1982). Risk factors for Kaposi's sarcoma in homosexual men. *Lancet, 1,* 1083–1087.
Marx, G.T. (1985). I'll be watching you: Reflections on the new surveillance. *Dissent,* Winter, 26–34.
Mercer, C. (1983). A poverty of desire: Pleasures and popular politics. In *Formations of pleasure* (pp. 84–100). London: Routledge and Kegan Paul.
Meredith, N. (1984, January). The gay dilemma: The AIDS threat has brought it up: Why are some homosexual men so promiscuous? *Psychology Today,* pp. 56–62.
Merquior, J.G. (1985). *Foucault.* London: Fontana Press.
Mohr, R.D. (1988). Mandatory AIDS testing. *Report from the Institute for Philosophy and Public Policy, 8,* 8–11.
Mort, F. (1987). *Dangerous sexualities.* London: Routledge and Kegan Paul.
Murphy, J.W., and Pilotta, J.J. (1987). Research note: Identifying "at risk" persons in community research. *Sociology of Health and Illness, 9,* 62–75.
Navarro, C., and Hagstrom, J.W.C. (1982). Opportunistic infections and Kaposi's sarcoma in homosexual men. *The New England Journal of Medicine, 306,* 933.
N'Galy, B., and Ryder, R.W. (1988). Epidemiology of HIV infection in Africa. *Journal of Acquired Immune Deficiency Syndrome, 1,* 551–558.
Nelkin, D., and Gilman, S.L. (1988). Placing blame for devasting disease. *Social Research, 55,* 361–378.
O'Neill, J. (1985). *Five bodies: The human shape of modern society.* Ithaca: Cornell University Press.
O'Neill, J. (1987). Sociological nemesis: Parson and Foucault on therapeutic disciplines. In M.L. Wardell and S.P. Turner (Eds.), *Sociological theories in transition* (pp. 84–100). London: George Allen and Unwin.
Oxford English Dictionary. (1984). Oxford: Oxford University Press.
Padgug, R.A. (1989). Gay villain, gay hero: Homosexuality and the social construction of AIDS. In K. Peiss and C. Simmons (Eds.), *Passion and power: Sexuality in history* (pp. 293–313). Philadelphia: Temple University Press.

Paternek, M.A. (1987). Norms and normalization: Michel Foucault's overextended panoptic machine. *Human Studies, 10,* 97–121.

Rodger, J.J. (1988). Social work as social control re-examined: Beyond the dispersal of discipline thesis. *Sociology, 22,* 563–581.

Rosenberg, C.E. (1986). Disease and social order in America: Perceptions and expectations. *The Milbank Quarterly, 64* (Supplement 1), 34–55.

Rosenberg, C.E. (1988). The definition and control of disease: An introduction. *Social Research, 22,* 563–581.

Ross, J. W. (1989). The militarization of disease. *Soundings, 72,* 39–55.

Ruse, M. (1988). *Homosexuality: A philosophical inquiry.* Oxford: Basil Blackwell.

Schroter, R. Nher, H., and Petzoldt, D. (1988). Skin manifestations of syphilis maligna in HIV infection. *Hautarzt, 39,* 463–466.

Seidlin, M., Krasinski, K., Bebenroth, D., Itri, V., Paolino, A.M., and Valentine, F. (1988). Prevalence of HIV infection in New York call girls. *Journal of Acquired Immune Deficiency Syndrome, 1,* 150–154.

Sheridan, A. (1980). *Michel Foucault: The will to truth.* London: Tavistock Publications.

Siegler, M., and Osmond, H. (1974). *Models of madness, models of medicine.* New York: Harper Tourchbooks.

60% of Employers Report AIDS Cases. (1989, June 14). *Los Angeles Times,* p. 2.

Smart, B. (1983). *Foucault, marxism and critique.* London: Routledge and Kegan Paul.

Smart, B. (1985). *Michel Foucault.* London: Tavistock Publications.

Smith-Rosenberg, C. (1985). *Disorderly conduct.* Oxford: Oxford University Press.

Soriano, V., Tor, J., Muga, R., Fernandez, J.L., Ribera, A. Balanzo, X., and Foz, M. (1989). Human immunodeficiency virus type 2 infection in Western Africans living in Catalonia. *Medicina Clinica, 92,* 161–163.

Strub, H. (1989). The theory of panoptical control: Bentham's panopticon and Orwell's nineteen eighty-four. *Journal of the History of the Behavioral Sciences, 25,* 40–59.

Tanay, E. (1988). Psychiatric reflections on AIDS education. *Psychiatric Annals, 18,* 594–597.

Taylor, D.L., Taylor-Robinson, D., Jeffries, D.J., and Tyms, A.S. (1988). Characterization of cytomegalovirus isolates from patients with AIDS by DNA restriction analysis. *Epidemiology and Infection, 101,* 483–494.

This is your life. (1989, December). *Harper's Magazine,* p. 19.

Titti, F., Rezza, G., Verani, P., Butto, S., Sernicola, L., Rapicetta, M., Sarrecchia, B., Oliva, C., and Rossi, G.B. (1988). HIV, HTLV-1, and HBV infections in a cohort of Italian intravenous drug abusers: Analysis of risk factors. *Journal of Acquired Immune Deficiency Syndrome, 1,* 405–411.

Treichler, P.A. (1988). AIDS, gender, and biomedical discourse: Current contests for meaning. In E. Fee and D.M. Fox (Eds.), *AIDS: The burden of history* (pp. 190–266). Berkeley: University of California Press.

Turner, B.S. (1984). *The body and society.* Oxford: Basil Blackwell.

Weeks, J. (1985). *Sexuality and its discontents.* London: Routledge and Kegan Paul.

Weeks, J. (1988). Love in a cold climate. In P. Aggleton and H. Homans (Eds.), *Social aspects of AIDS* (pp. 10–19). London: The Falmer Press.

Wright, P., and Treacher, A. (1982). *The problems of medical knowledge: Examining the social construction of medicine.* Edinburgh: Edinburgh University Press.

Zuboff, S. (1988). *In the age of the smart machine.* New York: Basic Books.

©1990 The Institute of Mind and Behavior, Inc.
The Journal of Mind and Behavior
Summer and Autumn 1990, Volume 11, Numbers 3 and 4
Pages 353 [107] – 368 [122]
ISSN 0271–0137
ISBN 0-930195-05-1

Therapeutic Professions and the Diffusion of Deficit

Kenneth J. Gergen

Swarthmore College

The mental health professions operate largely so as to objectify a language of mental deficit. In spite of their humane intentions, by constructing a reality of mental deficit the professions contribute to hierarchies of privilege, reduce natural interdependencies within the culture, and lend themselves to self-enfeeblement. This infirming of the culture is progressive, such that when common actions are translated into a professionalized language of mental deficit, and this language is disseminated, the culture comes to construct itself in these terms. This leads to an enhanced dependency on the professions and these are forced, in turn, to invent additional terms of mental deficit. Thus, concepts of infirmity have spiraled across the century, and virtually all remaining patterns of action stand vulnerable to deficit translation. Required within the professions are new linguistic formulations that create a reality of relationships without evaluative fulcrum.

How may I fault thee? Let me count the ways. . .

Impulsive personality	*Low self-esteem*
Malingering	*Narcissism*
Reactive depression	*Bulimia*
Anorexia	*Neurasthenia*
Hysteria	*Hypochondriasis*
Mania	*Dependent personality*
Psychopathia	*Frigidity*
Peter Pan syndrome	*Voyeurism*
External control orientation	*Authoritarianism*
Anti-social personality	*Transvestism*
Exhibitionism	*Agoraphobia*
Seasonal affective disorder. . .	

My central concern in this paper is with the effects of the mental health professions on the quality of cultural life. Judging from my many colleagues,

Requests for reprints should be sent to Kenneth J. Gergen, Ph.D., Department of Psychology, Swarthmore College, Swarthmore, Pennsylvania 19081.

students and friends engaged in therapeutic practices, I believe there is a strong and genuine commitment to a vision of human betterment. Further, although research results are interminably equivocal, I am convinced that at least from the standpoint of many who seek help, the therapeutic community plays a vital and humane role in cultural life. Yet, my concern in the present offering is with the paradoxical consequences of the prevailing vision of human betterment, and the pervasive dependency of people on these professions for improving their lot. For, there is reason to believe that in the very efforts to furnish effective means of alleviating human suffering, there are important respects in which mental health professionals simultaneously generate a network of increasing entanglements for the culture at large. Such entanglements are not only self-serving for the professions, but add exponentially to the existing sense of deficit. After exploring this progressive infirming of the culture, its causes and proliferating effects, I shall open discussion on possible alternatives to the existing condition.

Mental Language: Reified or Relational

In order to appreciate the nature and magnitude of the problems at stake, a prelude is required. In particular, a distinction must be drawn between existing views of the vocabulary of mind. We commonly employ such terms as "thinking," "feeling," "hoping," "fearing," and the like referentially. That is, we use such terms as if they depicted or reflected actual occurrences. The statement, "I am angry," is intended, by common convention, to describe a state of mind, differing from other states such as joy, embarrassment or ecstasy. The vast majority of therapeutic specialists proceed in much the same manner. Therapists listen for hours to people's accounts in an attempt to ascertain the quality and character of their "inner life" — their cognition, emotions, unarticulated fears, conflicts, illogicalities, blind spots, repressions, "the world as they experience it," and so on. As it is typically presumed, the individual's language provides a vehicle for "inner access" — revealing or setting forth to the professional the character of the not-directly-observed. And, as it is further reasoned, this task is essential to the therapeutic outcome — whether for reasons of furnishing the therapist with information about the problem domain (thus leading to remedial actions on the therapist's part), or for the client-provoking self-insight and clarification, enhancing the sense of autonomy or self-control, instigating a process of catharsis, reducing guilt and so on.

Whether in the therapeutic context or daily life, the presumption that the language of the mind reflects, depicts or refers to actual states may be termed *reificationist*. That is, such an orientation treats as real (as ontological existants) that to which the language seems to refer. As otherwise put, it is to engage in the *fallacy of misplaced concreteness*, treating as concrete the putative object rather than the sign. Certain readers will protest at this juncture at the demotion of what they believe to be a referential language (referring to actual states) to the status of reifying device. They may argue that, "It simply is the case that I have mental states, and when I say I am angry I do so because my state of mind is different from when I am sad or sexy. I speak of anger to reflect real states of anger." However, lest such resistance render the reader insensitive to all that follows, it is useful to make a rapid tour through the groves of intractable problems generated by a realist view of psychological language:

1. How can consciousness turn in upon itself to identify its own states? How can experience become an object to itself? Can a mirror reflect its own image?

2. What are the characteristics of mental states by which we can identify them? By what criteria do we distinguish, let us say, among states of anger, fear and love? What is their color, size, shape, or weight? Why do none of these attributes seem quite applicable? Because our observations of the states prove to us that they are not?

3. How can be we certain when we identify such states correctly? Could other processes (e.g., repression, defense) not prevent accurate self-appraisal? (Perhaps anger is eros after all.)

4. By what criterion could we judge that what we experience as "certain recognition" of a mental state is indeed certain recognition? Would not this recognition require yet another round of self-assessments, the results of which would require additional processes of internal identification, and so on in an infinite regress?

5. Although we may all agree in our use of mental terms (that we experience fear, ecstasy, or joy, for example, on particular occasions) how do we know that our subjective experiences resemble each other? By what process could we possibly determine whether my "fear" is equivalent to yours? How then do I know I possess what everyone else calls "fear"?

6. How are we to account for the disappearance from the culture of many mental terms popular in previous centuries, along with the passing fashions in mental terminology of the present century? (Whatever happened to melancholy, sublimity, neuralgia, the inferiority complex, and the adolescent identity crisis?) Have the words disappeared because such processes no longer exist in mortal minds?

7. How are we to account for the substantial differences in psychological vocabulary from one culture to another? Did we once have the same mental events as the primitive tribesman, for example, the emotion of *fago*, described by Lutz (1988) in her studies of the Ifaluk? Have we lost the capacity to experience this emotion? Is it lurking there within the core of our being, buried beneath layers of Westernized, industrialized acculturation?

Mental realists have yet to furnish viable and compelling answers to any of these perennial conundrums. Thus, although we need not go so far as to doubt that "something is going on" when we report a mental state, to treat the reports as descriptions, pictures or maps of identifiable events is essentially to reify the existing language practices.

Let us contrast the reificationist orientation to mental language with yet another. Following Wittgenstein (1963) in this case, let us abandon the view of mental language as a referential picture of inner states, and consider such language as a constituent feature of social relationships. That is, we may venture that psychological language obtains its meaning and significance from the way in which it is used in human interaction. Thus, when I say "I am unhappy" about a given state of affairs, the term "unhappy" is not rendered meaningful or appropriate according to its relationship to the state of my neurons or my phenomenological field. Rather, the report plays a significant social function. It may be used, for example, to call an end to a set of deteriorating conditions, enlist support and/or encouragement, or to invite futher opinion. Both the conditions under which the report can be used and the functions it can serve are also circumscribed by social convention. The phrase, "I am deeply sad" can be satisfactorily reported at the death of a close relative but not the demise of a spring moth. A report of depression can secure others' concern and support; however it cannot easily function as a farewell, an invitation to laughter, or a commendation. In this sense mental language is more like having a nine iron when shooting from a sandtrap than possessing a mirror of the interior, more like a strong grip between trapeze artists than a map of inner conditions. We shall call this orientation to mental language *relational*, in its emphasis on the use of mental language within ongoing relationships.

(It should be noted that the relational view of mental discourse does not commit one to a "skin deep" view of such language. Rather, mental terms are only constituent parts of full blown action patterns — patterns that may engage one fully. To "do anger" properly, for example, may require an enormous recruitment of bodily resources — with mental language playing but a minor part in the performance. For a more extended account, see Gergen and Gergen, 1988.)

Invitations to Infirmity

The pervasive stance toward psychological language in Western culture is decidedly reificationist. We generally accept persons' accounts of their subjective stats as valid (at least for them). If sophisticated, we may wonder if they are fully aware of their feelings, or have been misled in an attempt to protect themselves from what is "really" there. And, if scientific in bent, we may wish to know the distribution of various mental states (e.g., loneliness, depression) in the society more generally, the conditions under which they occur (e.g., stress, burnout), and the means for their alleviation (e.g., the comparative efficacy of differing therapies). However, we are unlikely to question the existence of the reality to which such terms seem to refer; and because the prevailing ontology of mental life remains generally unchallenged, we seldom inquire into the utility or desirability of such terms in daily life. If the language exists because the mental states exist, there is little reason to ask about preferences. To do so would be tantamount to asking whether we approve the roundness of the world.

Yet, if we view psychological discourse from a relational perspective, the language of the mind loses its rhetorical capacity as "truth bearing." One cannot claim rights to language use on grounds that existing terms "name what there is." Rather, significant questions are invited concerning the functions of existing terminologies in maintaining or changing the patterns of cultural life. What are the effects on human relationships of the prevailing vocabularies of the mind? Given our goals for human betterment, do these vocabularies facilitate or obstruct? And, most important for present purposes, what kinds of social patterns are facilitated (or prevented) by the existing vocabulary of psychological deficit? How do the terms of mental health professions, terms such as "neurosis," "cognitive dysfunction," "depression," "post-traumatic stress disorder," "character disorder," "repression," "narcissism" and so on, function within the culture more generally? Do such terms lend themselves to desirable forms of human relationship, should the vocabulary be expanded, are there more promising alternatives? There are no simple answers to such questions; however, neither is there at present a prevailing dialogue concerning such issues. My purpose here is not so much to develop a final answer as to generate a forum for continuing discussion.

Grounds for such discussion have been laid in several relevant arenas. In a range of pointed volumes Thomas Szasz (1961, 1963, 1987) has demonstrated that concepts of mental illness are not demanded by observation. Rather, he proposes they function much as social myths, and are used (or misused, from his perspective) largely as means of social control. Sarbin and Mancuso (1980) echo these arguments in their focus on the concept of schizophrenia as a social construction. Similarly, Ingelby (1980) has demonstrated the ways in which categories of mental illness are socially negotiated so as to serve the values or ideological investments of the profession. Kovel (1980) proposes that the mental health professions are essentially forms of industry that operate largely in the service of existing economic structures. Feminist thinkers have also explored the ways in which nosologies of illness, diagnosis and treatment have all been biased in favor a patriarchal system (Brodsky and Hare-Mustin, 1980; Hare-Mustin and Marecek, 1988).

Let us extend the implications of such discussions to consider the functioning of mental deficit language in social life. Again, there is much to be said on this matter, and not all of it is critical. On the positive side, for example, the vocabulary of the mental health professions does serve to render the alien familiar, and thus less fearsome. Rather than viewing non-normative activities as "the work of the devil" or "frighteningly strange," for example, they are given professional labels, signifying that indeed, they are perfectly reasonable by scientific standards. At the same time, this professional transformation of the unusual invites one to replace repugnance with more humane reactions – sympathetic reactions of the kind displayed toward the physically ill. Further, because the mental health professions are allied with science, and science appears to be a progressive or problem solving activity, such labels also invite a hopeful attitude toward the future. One need not labor under the belief that today's strangeness is forever.

For most of us these represent improvements of the present vocabulary of mental deficit over predecessors of yore. Yet, optimism on such matters is hardly merited. For there is a substantial "down side" to existing intelligibilities, and as I shall hope to demonstrate later in this paper, these problems are of continuously increasing magnitude. As an opening to the problem, we must consider the functioning of mental deficit vocabularies in engendering and facilitating each of the following processes.

Social Hierarchy

Although attempting to occupy a position of scientific neutrality, it has long been recognized that the helping professions are premised on certain assumptions of the cultural good (Hartmann, 1960; Masserman, 1960). Professional visions of "healthy functioning" are suffused with cultural ideals of personhood (London, 1986; Margolis, 1966). In this context we find, then, that mental deficit terms operate as evaluative devices, demarking the position of individuals along culturally implicit dimensions of good and bad. We may often feel a degree of sympathy for the person who complains of being incapacitated by depression, anxiety, or a Type A personality. However, such sympathies may often be tinged with a sense of self-satisfaction, for the complaint simultaneously casts us into a position of superiority. In each case the other reveals a failure – insufficient buoyancy, levelheadedness, calm, control – and thereby defines others as superior in these regards. While such results may seem inevitable, even desirable as a means of sustaining cultural values, it is vital to realize that (1) the existence of the terms invites such rituals of degradation (Goffman, 1961), and (2) other vocabularies could carry out the same descriptive work without such perjorative effects.

This is to say, that the existence of a vocabulary of deficit is akin to the availability of weapons; their very presence invites certain patterns of action, in this case the creation of implicit hierarchies. The greater the number of criteria for mental well-being, the greater number of ways in which one can be rendered superior (or inferior) in comparison to others. Further, the same events can be indexed in other ways, with far different outcomes. Through skilled language use one might reconstruct depression as "psychic incubation," anxiety as "heightened sensitivity," and Type A freneticism as "Protestant work ethic." Such use of language would either reverse or erase the existing hierarchies.

Reduced Interdependency

Because mental deficit terms imply the existence of "problems in need of attention," and the mental health professions are accorded a certain degree of expertise on such matters, the use of the vocabulary contributes to the institutionalization of treatment. In the same way that attributing teenage criminality to economic deprivation, deteriorated family conditions, or lack of recreational outlets would each have different behavioral or policy implications, attributing non-normative actions to mental deficits suggests that professional help is required. Yet, when such help is sought, the discussion of "the problem" is removed from its generating context and reestablished within the professional sphere. Or, in other terms, the mental health professions appropriate the process of realignment that would naturally occur in the non-professional context. One may venture that processes of natural realignment are often slow, anguished, brutal, or befuddled, and that life is too short and too precious to "wait and see." However, the result nevertheless is that problems otherwise requiring concerted participation of organically related persons are removed from their ecological niche. Marriage partners carry out more intimate communication with their therapists than with each other, even saving significant insights for revelation in the therapeutic hour. Parents discuss their children's problems with specialists, or send problem children to treatment centers, and thereby reduce the possibility for authentic (unselfconscious) communication with their offspring. Organizations placing alcoholic executives in treatment programs thereby reduce the kind of self-reflexive discussions that would elucidate their contribution to the problem. In each case, tissues of organic interdependency are injured or atrophy.

Self-Enfeeblement

Because of their reifying capacities, mental deficit terms are essentialist in character. That is, they operate so as to establish the essential nature of the person being described. They designate a characteristic of the individual perduring across time and situation, and which must be confronted if the person's actions are to be properly understood. The result of deploying mental deficit terms is thus to inform the recipient that "the problem" is not circumscribed, limited in time and space to a particular domain of his/her life, but that it is fully general. He or she carries the deficit, like a cancer, from one situation to another, and like a birthmark or a fingerprint, as the textbooks say, the deficit will inevitably manifest itself. In effect, once people understand their actions in terms of mental deficits, they are sensitized to the problematic potential in all their activities, the ways in which they are infected or diminished. The weight of "the problem" now expands manyfold; it is as inescapable as their own shadow. The sense of enfeeblement becomes complete.

There are other lamentable repercussions of mental deficit language. As existentialist theorists argue, because such language is embedded in a deterministic worldview, in which persons' actions are caused by their essences, people cease to experience their actions as voluntary (Bugenthal, 1965). They feel their actions to be outside the realm of choice, inevitable and unchangeable, unless they place themselves — dependently — in professional hands. Further, as Sparks (1989) has proposed, by conceptually placing problems within the personality structure of the individual, professionals suggest to people that their problems are virtually intractable.

The Process of Progressive Infirmity

It is a central contention of the present paper that problems of the preceding variety are not simply pervasive in modern culture; rather, they are expanding exponentially within the present century. This process of progressive infirmity now requires attention. The concept of neurosis did not originate until the mid-18th century. (Had such problems simply escaped general notice for so many centuries?) In 1769 William Cullen, a Scottish physician, elucidated the four major classes of *morbi nervini*. These included *Comota* (reduced voluntary movements, with drowsiness or loss of consciousness), the *Adynamiae* (diminished involuntary movements), *Spasmi* (abnormal movement of the muscles), and *Vesaniae* (altered judgment without coma) [see Lopez-Pinero's 1983 account]. Yet, even in 1840, with the first official attempt in the United States to tabulate mental disorder, categorization was crude. It proved satisfactory, indeed to use only a single category, in which idiotic and insane persons were grouped together (Spitzer and Williams, 1985). At present, the American Psychiatric Association's 1987 *Diagnostic and Statistical Manual of Mental Disorders*, third edition, revised [DSM-III-R] lists some 200 categories of mental disorder. Many additional "problematic behaviors" (e.g., stress, burnout, erotomania, etc.) are discussed and treated within the profession more generally. As the language of psychological deficit has expanded, so have we increased the culture's hierarchies of discrimination, damaged the naturalized patterns of interdependence, and expanded the arena of self-deprecation. In effect, as the language of deficit has proliferated, so has the culture become progressively infirmed.

On the optimistic side, one might propose that the increase in the language of deficit reflects an incremental sharpening of our capacities to distinguish among the existing array of psychological states and conditions. However, such a proposal grows from the same reificationist soil that proved so barren in our initial proceedings. There is little sense to be made of the supposition that the enormous proliferation in the language of psychological deficit represents a refinement in linkages between discourse and the mental world as it really is. How then are we to account for the proliferation of such language and the consequent infirming of the culture? Here again the relational view of language becomes useful, for as we consider the functions of discourse in human relationships it is possible to discern a pattern of formidable consequence. In particular, we may locate a cyclical process which, once activated, operates to expand the domain of deficit discourse in ever increasing degrees. We are not dealing, then, with an accidental surge in such discourse, but with a systematic process that feeds upon itself to engender an exponentially increasing infirmity.

For analytic purposes the cycle of progressive infirmity may be broken into four major stages. In actual practice, events in each of these stages may be confounded, with temporal ordering seldom smooth, and with exceptions at every turn. However for purposes of clarity, the cycle of progressive infirmity may be outlined as follows:

Deficit Translation

Let us view the situation of mental health professionals in the following way: they confront a client group whose lives are managed in terms of a common or everyday discourse. Because life management seems impossible in terms of everyday understandings individuals in the client group seek professional help. Or, in effect, they seek advanced (more objective, discerning, etc.) forms of understanding. In this sense it is incumbent upon the professional to (1) furnish an alternative discourse (theoretical framwork, nosology, etc.), and (2) translate the problem as presented in the daily language into the uncommon language of the profession. In terms of the preceding this means that problems understood in the profane or marketplace language of the culture must be translated into the sacred or professional language of mental deficit. A person whose habits of cleanliness are excessive by common standards becomes an "obsessive compulsive," one who rests the morning in bed becomes "depressive," one who feels he is not liked is redefined as "paranoid," and so on. (An extended treatment of the way in which the client's childhood memories are reformulated by the psychoanalyst in terms of Freudian theory of psychosexual development is furnished by Spence, 1982.) For the client such translations may be essential, for not only do they assure that the professional is doing a proper job, but that the problem is well recognized or understood within the profession.

Cultural Dissemination

The mental health professional generally follows a scientific mode of analysis in which the attempt is to establish systematic ontologies or inclusive categories for all that exists within a given domain (e.g., animal or plant species, tables of chemical elements). The DSM-III-R is perhaps the most apt exemplar within the field of mental health, in its attempt to reduce all existing problems to a systematic and finite array of categories. The result of this mode of procedure, however, is to universalize existing problems. It is to inform the client that his/her problem is but an isolated instance of a larger class. Other instances in the class may thus be presumed. It is partly for this reason that pressures are created for a broad dissemination of mental deficit language. In the same way that signs of breast cancer, diabetes or venereal disease should become common knowledge within the culture, so should citizens be able to recognize symptoms of stress, alcoholism, and depression. Thus, mental deficit information is featured in undergraduate curricula, popular magazines, television programming, newspaper features, and the like. (Because of the exotic and self-relevant character of such information, there is also a broad audience for such materials.) The result is, however, a continuous insinuation of the professional language into the sphere of daily relationships.

Cultural Construction

As intelligibilities of deficit are disseminated into the culture at large, they become absorbed into the common language. They become part of "what everybody knows" about human behavior. In this sense, terms such as neurosis, stress, alcoholism and depression are no longer "professional property." They have been "given away" by the profession to the public. Terms such as split personality, identity crisis, PMS (pre-menstrual syndrome) and mid-life crisis also enjoy a certain degree of popularity. And, as such terms make their way into the cultural vernacular, they become available for the construction of everyday reality. Shirley is not simply "too fat"; she has "obese eating habits"; Fred doesn't simply "hate gays," but is "homophobic"; and so on.

Nor is such construction limited to the redefinition of problems already recognized. That is, as deficit terms become increasingly available for making the social world intelligible, that world becomes increasingly populated by deficit. Events which passed unnoticed become candidates for interpretation; events once viewed as "good and proper" can now be reconceptualized as problematic, and in the extreme case recognized symptoms come to serve as cultural models. (Consider the spread of "bulimia" once it was recognized as a "common problem.") Once such terms as "stress" and "occupational burn-out" enter the commonsense vernacular, they become lenses through which any working professional can reexamine his/her life and find it wanting. What was valued as "active ambition" can now be reconstructed as "workaholic"; the "smart dresser" can be redefined as "narcissistic"; and the "autonomous and self-directed man" becomes "defended against his emotions." Furnish the population with hammers of mental deficit, and the whole world needs pounding.

Vocabulary Expansion

As individual actions are increasingly identified in terms of mental deficit terminology, so does the culture generate a new wave of candidates for professional help. Counseling, weekend self-enrichment programs, and programs of personality refurbishment may represent a first line of dependence; all allow people to escape the uneasy sense that they are "not all they should be." Others may seek more direct means of help for their "eating disorders," "incest victimization," or "post traumatic stress disorders." At this point, however, the stage is set for the final revolution in the cycle of progressive infirmity. For as the layperson approaches the profession with a now-appropriated professional discourse, the role of the professional is threatened. If the client has already identified the problem accurately, and knows (as in many cases) what is commonly to be done at the professional level, then the window of professional expertise is increasingly closed. (The worst case scenario would be that people learn to diagnose and treat themselves within their family and friendship circles, thus rendering the professional redundant.) In this way there is a constant pressure placed upon the professional to "advance" understanding, to spawn "more sophisticated" terminology, and to generate new insights and forms of therapy. It is not that the shift in emphasis from classic psychoanalysis to neo-analysis to object relations, for example, is required by an increasingly sensitive understanding of mental dynamics. Indeed, each wave sets the stage for its own recession and replacement; as therapeutic vocabularies become common sense the therapist is propelled into new modes of departure. The ever-shifting sea of therapeutic fads and fashions is no mere defect in the profession; rapid change is virtually demanded by a public whose discourse is increasingly "psychologized."

Progressive Infirmity: No Exit?

A recent circular invited participation in a San Diego conference on theory, research and treatment of addiction. As the circular announced, "Addictive behavior is arguably the number one health and social problem facing our country today." Among the "addictions" to be discussed were exercise, religion, eating, work, and sex. New domains of behavior now enter the ledger of deficit, subject to broad concern and professional treatment. The construction of infirmity expands again, and there is no principled means of termination. When the culture is furnished a language of mental deficit, and persons are increasingly understood in these ways, an increasing population of "patients" is created. This population, in turn, forces the profession to expand its vocabulary and thus the array of mental deficit terms available for cultural use. More problems are constructed, more help sought, and the array of deficit terms again presses forward. Again, one can scarcely view this cycle as smooth and undisrupted. Some schools of therapy remain committed to a single vocabulary; others have little interest in dissemination; some professionals attempt to speak with clients only in the "common language," and many popular concepts within the culture lose currency over time. Rather, we are speaking here of a general drift, an historical tendency of the kind, for example, that enables American psychiatric discourse to move from the restricted domain of a single journal (The *American Journal of Insanity*) in the mid-1800s to a three volume handbook − with over 50 chapters − a century later that has made therapeutic training an essential part of pastoral preparation, and that has made clinical psychology one of the fastest growing professions of the century.

I am in no way attempting to allocate blame for this trajectory. For the most part it is a necessary byproduct of the earnest and humane attempt to enhance the culture's life quality. With certain variations in the logic of the cycle, it is not unlike the trajectories spawned by both the medical and legal professions − toward increased medical needs on the one hand and the increased forms of litigation on the other. However, to the extent that the mental health professions are concerned with cultural life quality, discussion of progressive infirmity should become focal. Are there important limitations on the above arguments; are there signs of a leveling effect; are there means of reducing the proliferation of an enfeebling discourse?

I have no ready remedy in hand for the termination of the cycle. However, I do feel that the same logic that enables such a cycle to be articulated does invite a dialogue from which solutions might be derived. For, as we have seen, progressive infirmity is favored by the reificationist assumption of mental language. It is when we believe that the words for mental deficit stand in a referential relationship to processes or mechanisms in the head that the problem begins. It is when we believe that people actually possess mental processes such as repression, for example, that we can comfortably characterize them as repressed. At the outset, then, some form of generalized reeducation in the functions of language might be favored.

Of course it is absurdly optimistic to believe that either the formal or informal educational processes could significantly alter the picture theory of language, and the companionate assumption of mind-body dualism, both so central to Western tradition. More promising is the development of alternative vocabularies within the mental health profession, vocabularies that (1) do not trace problematic behavior to psychological sources within single individuals, and (2) ultimately erase the concept of "problem behavior" itself. I am speaking here first of the development of a vocabulary of relatedness that would come to equal the rhetorical power of individualized language in making the social world intelligible. We have innumerable terms for characterizing individuals; and when confronting the social world we rapidly and securely fall back on this vocabulary. For example, we see an individual acting in a particular way, and we can scarcely avoid characterizing these actions as outward signs of inner states of depression, fear, anxiety and the like. The individualized form of accounting is ready at hand. It is far more difficult, however, to view such behavior as indicative of processes of relatedness, signs of particular forms of interaction. Such conclusions are not conceptually impossible; we simply have little vocabulary at hand for making the world intelligible in this way. While we have a highly nuanced vocabulary of individual players we are virtually inarticulate regarding the games in which they are embedded. With an adequate vocabulary in hand, we might reconstruct depression as a constituent part of a relational form. In the same way that a serve is essential for the game of tennis, and the consumption of a wafer for Catholic mass, so are "depressed actions" essential constituents of certain kinds of interaction sequences (see Gergen and Gergen, 1988). The same kind of translation could be undertaken with the full body of psychological terminology available for common use.

The impetus toward relational intelligibilities is already manifest in the mental health professions. Harry Stack Sullivan's emphasis on the embeddedness of symptoms in interpersonal relations represented an important beginning. In varying degrees the work of theorists in family systems, second order cybernetics, social ecology, stragetic therapy, contextual therapy, and therapeutic communication processes (see Hoffman's 1981 summary) all extend and elaborate a relational perspective. For many social practitioners the language of mental deficit also stands inadequate, and means are sought to generate understandings of individuals-in-relationship (Kirk, Siporin, and Kutchins, 1989). And too, these ventures share much with present theorizing in social constructionism, discourse processes, parent-child interaction, conversational management, ethnomethodology, and organizational management. With cooperative efforts across these otherwise isolated endeavors, the possibilities for new and significant forms of intelligibility seem enormous.

With the development of relational intelligibilities may ultimately come the demise of the category "problem behavior" itself. As we come to see human actions as embedded within larger units, parts of wholes, such actions cease to be "of themselves." There are no problem behaviors independent of arrangements of social interdependency. However, we need not capitulate to the presently alluring move of shifting blame from individual to group. (The concept of "dysfunctional family" or "perverse triangle," for example, simply sets the stage for a new cycle of impairment.) For, it is also clear from a relational standpoint that the language of evaluation, blame, and thus problematics is born of relatedness; such language functions so as to coordinate the activities of individuals around ends they signify as valuable. Thus, the labeling of actions as in some way "problematic" is itself an outcome of relational process. In this way we see that there are no intrinsic or essential "goods" or goals to which individuals or groups should necessarily strive. There are only goods and goals (and concomitant failures) within particular systems of understanding. The professional need not be concerned, then, with "improvement" as a real-world challenge. (Depressive activity, for example, is not inherently problematic, and may serve an important function in maintaining the well-being of a group from its standpoint.) Rather, the emphasis may appropriately shift to enhancing consciousness of the larger system of interdependencies in which such evaluations are generated, and the capacity of relationships for coordinated integration into the larger network.

References

American Psychiatric Association. (1987). *Diagnostic and statistical manual of mental disorders* (third edition, revised). Washington, D.C.: Author.

Brodsky, A.M., and Hare-Mustin, R.T. (1980). *Women and psychotherapy: An assessment of research and practice.* New York: Guilford.

Bugenthal, J.F.T. *The search for authenticity.* New York: Hold, Rinehart & Winston.

Gergen, K.J., and Gergen, M.M. (1988). Narrative and the self as relationship. In L. Berkowitz (Ed.), *Advances in experimental social psychology* (pp. 17–56). New York: Academic Press.

Goffman, E. (1961). *Asylums: Essays on the social situation of mental patients and other inmates.* Garden City, New Jersey: Doubleday.

Hare-Mustin, R., and Marecek, J. (1988). The meaning of difference: Gender theory, postmodernism and psychology. *American Psychologist, 43,* 455–464.

Hartmann, H. (1960). *Psychoanalysis and moral values.* New York: International Universities Press.

Hoffman, L. (1981). *Foundations of family therapy.* New York: Basic.

Ingleby, D. (1980). Understanding mental illness. In D. Ingleby (Ed.), *Critical psychiatry: The politics of mental health* (pp. 23–71). New York: Pantheon.

Kirk, S., Siporin, M., and Kutchins, H. (1989). The prognosis for social work diagnosis. *Social Casework: The Journal of Contemporary Social Work, 70,* 295–304.

Kovel, J. (1980). The American mental health industry. In D. Ingleby (Ed.), *Critical psychiatry: The politics of mental health* (pp. 72–101). New York: Pantheon.

London, P. (1986). *The modes and morals of psychotherapy*. New York: Hemisphere Publishing.

Lopez-Pinero, J.M. (1983). *Historical origins of the concept of neurosis* [D. Berrios, Translator]. Cambridge: Cambridge University Press.

Lutz, C. (1988). *Unnatural emotions*. Chicago: University of Chicago Press.

Margolis, J. (1966). *Psychotherapy and morality*. New York: Random House.

Masserman, J. (1960). *Psychoanalysis and human values*. New York: Grune and Stratton.

Rose, N. (1985). *The psychological complex*. London: Routledge & Kegan Paul.

Sarbin, T.R., and Mancuso, J.C. (1980). *Schizophrenia: Medical diagnosis or moral verdict?* Elmsford, New York: Pergamon.

Sparks, P. (1989). *Causal attributions of personality*. Unpublished doctoral dissertation, Oxford University.

Spence, D. (1982). *Narrative truth and historical truth*. New York: Norton.

Spitzer, R.L., and Williams, J.B. (1985). Classification of mental disorders. In H.L. Kaplan and B.J. Sadock (Eds.), *Comprehensive textbook of psychiatry* (pp. 580–602). Baltimore: Williams & Wilkins.

Szasz, T.S. (1961). *The myth of mental illness: Foundations of a theory of personal conduct*. New York: Hoeber-Harper.

Szasz, T.S. (1963). *Law, liberty and psychiatry: An inquiry into the social uses of mental health practices*. New York: Macmillan.

Szasz, T.S. (1987). *Insanity: The idea and its consequences*. New York: John Wiley.

Wittgenstein, L. (1963). *Philosophical investigations* [G. Anscombe, Translator]. New York: Macmillan.

©1990 The Institute of Mind and Behavior, Inc.
The Journal of Mind and Behavior
Summer and Autumn 1990, Volume 11, Numbers 3 and 4
Pages 369 [123] – 384 [138]
ISSN 0271-0137
ISBN 0-930195-05-1

The Futility of Psychotherapy

George W. Albee

University of Vermont

While psychotherapy is helpful to individual clients, the slim cadre of therapists and the vast number of disturbed people precludes any hope that more than a relative few will receive help. Nowhere is the futility of psychotherapy as obvious as among the poor and powerless whose suffering, crowding, and despair will yield only to social and political solutions. In the United States the expansion of the number of psychiatric diagnoses and the demographic changes in populations will only make larger the gap in numbers between therapists and clients. Psychotherapy is an expensive oddity to the poor, but their taxes will help the affluent obtain prepaid care. Psychotherapy does reveal some of the social and economic factors, like bad parenting, homelessness and unemployment, that cause emotional disturbances. But one-to-one treatment, medical or psychological, does not, and cannot, affect incidence. The rightward movement of American psychiatry, supported by political conservatives and by activist parent-citizens groups, espouses an organic explanatory model for all mental disorders and for a wide range of human problems. Only effective primary prevention leading to social change will reduce future incidence.

Back at the beginning of the "Age of the Psychotherapist," Raimy (1950, p. 3) defined therapy as: an "unidentified technique applied to unspecified problems with unpredictable outcomes." And, he added, "for which long and rigorous training is required!" In the intervening decades a veritable flood of training programs, workshops, demonstrations, articles and books has modified only modestly this description. Now Strupp (1986) says: "Psychotherapy has become a billion-dollar industry . . . lacking clear boundaries, with hazy quality control and relatively vague ethical standards . . . the training of professional therapists remains fairly heterogenous, unsystematic, and in many cases, insufficiently thorough" (p. 121).

The most compelling arguments against psychotherapy do not start by questioning its effectiveness. The early, and frequently quoted, criticisms of therapy

Requests for reprints should be sent to George W. Albee, Department of Psychology, University of Vermont, Burlington, Vermont 05405.

by Eysenck (1952, 1964) have been adequately refuted (Meehl, 1965; Vanden-Bos, 1986). A major review of the efficacy of therapy was done by Saxe (1980) who found overall positive outcomes. Rather, a more critical problem, after accepting the evidence that psychotherapy is often effective in reducing anxiety and developing more effective and mature social relationships, is the unbridgeable gap between the enormous number of people with serious emotional problems and the small number of therapists available. The prospect is slim for developing a sufficiently large cadre of therapists to increase significantly the present barely perceptible impact on demand (see Kiesler and Sibulkin, 1987). Further, as the history of public health methods (that emphasize social change) has clearly established, no mass disease or disorder afflicting humankind has ever been eliminated by attempts at treating affected individuals. Changing the incidence of emotional disorders will require large scale political and social changes affecting the rates of injustice, powerlessness, and exploitation, none of which is affected by individual psychotherapy. These bed-rock facts make futile a reliance on therapy to affect directly the incidence of both physical and mental disorders. Yet individual treatment remains the focus of medicine, psychiatry, clinical psychology, and social work.

The American focus on psychotherapy was made "official" in the final report (*Action for Mental Health*) to the United States Congress of the Joint Commission on Mental Illness and Health (1960). The Commission proposed that hundreds of new Community Mental Health Centers be built, offering services focusing on individual treatment. Grudging acceptance in the report of psychotherapeutic practice by psychologists and social workers in the Centers was occasioned by the chronic shortage of psychiatrists. But it was psychotherapy that was to be the "backbone of treatment" (see Glasscote, Sanders, Forstenzer, and Foley, 1964). Fifteen years later Henderson (1975) was still arguing that ". . . help is therapy not prevention. Early therapy by all means, thorough therapy if at all possible, but above all *therapy*" (p. 243).

How Many Disturbed People?

A recent major epidemiological investigation funded by the National Institute for Mental Health (NIMH) illustrates the startling dimensions of the problems commonly defined as mental disorders (see Regier, Myers, Kramer, Robins, Blazer, Hough, Eaton, and Locke, 1984). On the basis of this study nineteen percent of the adult population of the United States is believed to have a diagnosable mental/emotional condition. The NIMH study is a major contribution of psychiatric epidemiology, but many of the problems remain that have always faced epidemiologists trying to count past the present mental conditions. Computer-generated DSM-III (American Psychiatric Association, 1980) diagnoses were made on the basis of what people could remember or were willing to reveal to interviewers about their use of alcohol and drugs, and about their fears, delusions, anxieties, depressions, and anger. Women — probably because they were more likely to be home when the interviewers visited, or were more willing to be interviewed — were overrepresented in the sample. Institutionalized people were not included, nor were the homeless. Other sources of error included the fact that older interviewees remembered fewer emotional crises than did younger persons; if someone could not complete an interview, the interviewer asked someone else about the person; no attempt was made to differentiate among the various kinds of organic mental disorders; there was a significant number of refusals.

The study did not explore the presence of many of the conditions contained in the DSM-III. For example, "psychosexual dysfunctions" that are said to affect nearly a quarter of the adult population were not investigated, probably because it was decided that people would be reluctant to discuss their sex problems with interviewers they were seeing only once. To push the adult prevalence figure to its ultimate absurdity, we could add in the well-established clinical observation that, on the average, three other people are strongly distressed by each person with a serious emotional problem. Pull all these numbers together and we might end up with more mental disorders, serious and otherwise, than there are people in the United States (see Albee, 1985).

The Expansion of Disorders and Diagnoses

Kramer (1983) has raised some important and alarming questions about what he calls "the rising pandemic of mental disorders" throughout the world. He points out that the United States faces, in the decades immediately ahead, a steadily increasing prevalence rate of both serious mental disorders like "schizophrenia" and diseases involving hypertension and cerebrovascular accidents. The growth in frequency of these conditions will result from the large increase in the numbers of persons in those age groups that are at highest risk for their occurrence, as well as the steadily increasing duration of chronic conditions resulting from the development of medical techniques for prolonging the lives of affected individuals. Further, more people, throughout the world, are living into middle and old age, and at the same time high birth rates continue to produce crowded cities, undernourishment, and despair, so physical and mental problems of both adults and children proliferate. And now we learn that the AIDS virus is attracted to brain tissue and often leads to dementia, with further demands for neuropsychiatric and neuropsychological interventions, in short supply or unavailable in much of the world.

A related problem involves the continuing expansion of the number of conditions identified as "psychiatric disorders." About every decade or so, the American Psychiatric Association (1952, 1968, 1980, 1987) publishes a *Diagnostic*

and Statistical Manual of Mental Disorders (DSM). The first DSM, published
in 1952, listed 60 types and subtypes of mental illness. Sixteen years later,
DSM II more than doubled the number of disorders. The number of disorders
grew to more than 200 with DSM III in 1980. The current guide, DSM III-R
(1987), includes tobacco dependence, developmental disorders and sexual
dysfunctions, school learning problems, and adolescent rebellion disorders.
DSM IV (in preparation) will add more disorders. Clearly the more of the
ordinary human problems in living that are labeled "mental illnesses," the
more people will be found who suffer from at least one of them – and, a
cynic might add, the more conditions that therapists can treat and for which
they can collect health-insurance payments.

From DSM II to DSM III, several conditions ceased to exist as officially
recognized mental disorders. Traditional neuroses no longer exist; their
numerous manifestations have been dropped or included in other DSM-III
classifications. As the neuroses were primarily a Freudian, psychodynamic
construction, rooted in alleged problems resulting from bad parenting, the
biological psychiatrists, now in control of the field, threw them out. The decision in 1973 by the American Psychiatric Association to remove "homosexuality" from its list of mental disorders lowered overnight by many millions
the total number of Americans considered mentally ill. However, the *International Classification of Diseases* (ICD-9, 1989) of the World Health Organization still includes homosexual behavior as a disease. The decision by the
National Association for Retarded Citizens to make a 70 IQ rather than an
80 IQ the cutoff point for defining mental retardation reduced by millions
the number of retarded Americans.

Clearly, most "mental disorders" are different from real organic illnesses.
In mental disorders there is ordinarily no physical marker that can be identified by objective tests and only the most vague beginning or ending is discernable. Most mental disorders are based solely on a judgment about
behavior. Wootton (1959) pointed out that the diagnosis of "mental illness"
nearly always requires a social judgment:

> . . . anti-social behavior is the precipitating factor that leads to mental treatment. But
> at the same time the fact of the illness is itself inferred from this behavior; indeed it is
> almost true to say that the illness is the behavior for which it is also the excuse. But
> any disease, the morbidity of which is established only by the social failure that it in-
> volves, must rank as fundamentally different from those with which the symptoms are
> independent of social norms. (p. 225)

While most "mental illnesses" are really learned patterns of disturbed behavior
for which psychotherapy is more helpful than organic treatment, it is only
necessary to look carefully at the prevalence data – nearly one in five
American adults exhibits disturbed behavior – to see the futility of relying
on individual intervention by individual therapists.

How Many Therapists Are There?

The public is regularly misinformed about the availablity of therapy. Each week Ann Landers, and other popular advisors, suggest counseling and therapy as the solution to individual problems described in letters from readers. Even as scientifically sophisticated a writer as Jane Brody (1981) can be misinformed, and therby misinform her readers, about the availability of help. In a *New York Times* article she stated that 34 million Americans are in psychotherapy. She was wrong. Probably no more than 1½ million are actually in therapy (see Albee, 1985) at any given time. To treat 34 million clients would require a 20-fold increase in the currently existing number of therapists. No foreseeable increase of this magnitude is in prospect.

How many therapists actually are available for the vast sea of troubled people? Kiesler and Sibulkin (1987, p. 812) have calculated the total number of (full-time equivalent) therapists in the United States to be about 45,000. This may be a conservative estimate but even if we add to this figure the unlicensed and unregulated personal counselors, yoga instructors, teachers of meditation, pastoral counselors, and school guidance personnel, we have only doubled or tripled the total number of licensed and unlicensed interventionists for people with personal problems. So one conventional argument for the futility of psychotherapy is the unbridgeable gap between need and available resources. Enormous sums of money spent on treating the few might be better spent on other interventions affecting more people. Self-help groups, for example, reach many times the number seen in individual therapy (see Silverman, 1978, and also the *Surgeon General's Workshop on Self Help and Public Health*, 1987, for optimistic examples of groups of people helping each other in support groups). But we must remind ourselves that even if there were twenty times as many psychotherapists there would be no reduction in the incidence of problems, a majority of which are caused by poverty, powerlessness, exploitation and social injustice (see Joffe and Albee, 1981).

Our American fixation on high technology individual medical treatment is as irrelevant and as tragic as our fixation on individual psychotherapy. It is simply not credible to suggest that "spare parts" of bodies (from "organ donors") and mechanical body organ devices (artificial hearts) are the most promising medical treatments of the future in a world in which millions die of the infectious diseases of childhood and the specter of mass starvation haunts much of humankind. Fifteen million of the world's children die each year of preventable conditions like infant diarrhea from polluted water, infectious diseases and starvation. Four hundred million women live in regions where the soil is deficient in iodine and as a result give birth to retarded children. The rate of epilepsy is high in the third world from too much lead and too little iron (Musarrat, 1988). Millions of children live with preventable handicaps — the underdeveloped, malnourished bodies and minds.

Part of the logic of this irrational American medical effort reflects the "industrial machine model" of the human body that, like other machines, is seen as an interacting mechanical system where parts are damaged or wear out and can be fixed or replaced. The prohibitive expense of individual high technology medicine that has developed in the Western world as a result of this industrial model has driven up the cost of health care (now 11% of our gross national product), enriched the health industry, provided the mass media with striking human interest stories and, in the process, misled the general public about the questionable value of one-to-one high-tech repair methods. In a similar way the human personality is often described as an interrelation of parts that can get out of balance and that can be corrected by therapy. The very high cost of these one-to-one interventions, both surgical and psychological, make them available only to (a) the affluent, (b) those who have health insurance, and (c) those who know about and accept the potential benefits of therapy. These constraints clearly limit the number of potential clients. Thirty-seven million Americans have no health insurance of any sort; most of those who do have union negotiated insurance have no (or very limited) mental health coverage (Sharfstein, 1988).

Psychotherapy Is a Luxury for the Affluent

It does not seem to matter whether or not mental health benefits are available to Class IV (blue collar) and Class V (no collar) people. They do not find therapy available, appropriate, or understandable. Auto workers with coverage for mental health benefits do not use them and the poor, like the migrant farm workers without benefits, are not even aware of them. Therapy is also unavailable to the growing army of the homeless. It is clear that psychotherapy is restricted largely to segments of the middle and upper classes while the most serious mental and emotional disorders are more prevalent among the very poor. The likelihood of migrant farm workers or homeless people receiving psychotherapy is about the same as the likelihood that they will receive artificial hearts or liver transplants: zero. The Task Panel on Migrant and Seasonal Farmworkers (1978) spelled out in chilling detail the horrors of the lives of agricultural migrant workers and their children — their health hazards, their powerlessness, low self-esteem, isolation, exploitation, poisoning by toxic pesticides . . . the list of risks is endless. Unlike hostages in the Middle East or MIA's in Southeast Asia, the names of the hundreds of thousands of these migrant worker hostages are unknown to the general public and their chances for rescue through any kind of therapy are nil.

Dörken and Cummings (1986) have argued that the poor will use mental health services including psychotherapy. They base their argument in large part on utilization rates in Hawaii. Hawaii is one of very few states with fairly extensive mental health service coverage in its Medicaid plan. It is also the only state with a universal health care program covering all employees and dependents for outpatient mental health visits. Referrals to a psychologist or psychiatrist must be made by a primary care physician, and so, not unexpectedly, psychiatrists provide more services than psychologists. It is interesting to note that the heavy users of basic health care are most often the ones referred by physicans for mental health care. It seems quite possible that those referred are the higher user chronic complainers and "character disorders," and that "the poor" in general do not seek mental health services directly on their own initiative. Only some of "the poor" get referred and they are a highly selective sample.

In an interview with a leading health care insurance expert and official for Blue Cross/Blue Shield, VandenBos (1983) elicited the following information. First, purchasers of group coverage for their employees do not typically ask for mental health coverage. Second, unions also do not ask for mental health coverage. Third, insurers worry about offering a benefit that will be attractive only to high risk or high user groups. Fourth, problems in defining appropriate "mental health services" make it difficult for insurers to predict utilization. For these and other reasons, currently emerging approaches to reimbursement for "psychiatric treatment" (see Sharfstein, 1988, for current thinking on this topic) are increasingly cool toward coverage of psychotherapy.

The training of psychotherapists makes them unsuited for most kinds of intervention except one-to-one psychotherapy with middle-class people like themselves. Therapists in training most often work in agencies that serve the less affluent; they learn that these clients are not valued by the high status professionals they emulate. On completion of their training they put such cases behind them or refer them to public mental health centers where the "therapists" are often poorly qualified and always underpaid. Most psychotherapists are drawn from the middle class and are familiar with middle-class problems. Middle-class people tend to be more conscience-laden and guilt-plagued than the poor. Such middle-class anxiety is often reduced by individual psychotherapy, and so the process is rewarding and reinforcing. Neurotic anxiety is less common among the poor who exhibit "reality anxiety." The real problems of poverty, unemployment, homelessness, exploitation, powerlessness, discrimination, poor housing, etc. are more urgent than interpersonal relationship problems or guilt over impulses.

The taxes and insurance deductions of the poor do, however, help support the psychotherapy of the affluent (Albee, 1977a). Senator Edward M. Kennedy (1975) pointed out this injustice. Kennedy sees new public programs of mental health care as "contain[ing] the apparent risk of subsidizing services to higher-income citizens directly from tax contributions of middle- and low-income Americans" (pp. 151–152).

Six Patients, Three Years, Little Change, Big Bucks

A television show in the late 1970s starring Bob Newhart as Dr. Hartley, a clinical psychologist, acquainted millions of viewers with a financially attractively, high status, and apparently undemanding career option. Dr. Hartley, a somewhat bumbling but well-meaning psychologist-therapist, saw the same small group of clients for three years. None of them got better, nor worse, but they (or their insurance) paid enough to allow him and his fashionable spouse to live in an obviously expensive high-rise apartment in an upper-middle class setting. Being a psychotherapist, it was clear, takes no more intellectual competence than being a real estate sales person, a stock broker, or a navigator of an airliner, and clearly has as high or higher social status.

In spite of the small number of therapists, there is no dearth of recruits to the field of therapy. And because of the importance of a protective professional guild to lobby for third party payments to cover or push for a whole range of interventions (including, recently, hospital privileges and psychotropic drug prescription privileges), the psychotherapists are quick to join state and national professional organizations (with ever increasing dues) that lobby to safeguard or advance their financial interests. Almost any bright student can get into a therapy training program. Failing to obtain admission to an accredited Ph.D. program, or to a Psy.D.-granting accredited professional school, need not end the quest. There are many other therapy programs with modest academic demands where, for a price, an aspiring therapist can obtain a degree. And a week of intensive drill (advertised regularly in the *APA Monitor*) is sufficient to master enough core knowledge of psychology to pass the national licensing examination. Psychology as it has existed traditionally – persons engaged in the scientific study of human behavior – is all but disappearing from view in the rising tide of psychotherapists.

Let us be clear that it is not sacrilegious, illegal or unconstitutional to choose a career as a psychotherapist in an affluent society. After facing the fact that doctoral level therapists serve primarily well-educated clients, that psychotherapy is rarely available to the poor, not much sought after by blue collar workers, and ineffective in rectifying social injustices, the choice of this "health profession" is no more blameworthy than the decision to become a dentist or a funeral director. Many people want or require the service and they or their insurance programs are willing to pay.

However, there is an ethical question worth pursuing about therapy. Rawls (1971) argues that in order to achieve social justice a society's efforts must be aimed at ensuring equality of opportunity. A just society must make every attempt to redress the social inequities that have led to disadvantage. This means more attention and effort in support of those in less favorable social positions. Limiting psychotherapy to the affluent does nothing to advance the cause of social justice and may actually dull sensitivity to injustice. But even if psychotherapy were available to all, the cause of social justice would not be advanced. Only with radical social changes leading to a just society will there be a reduction in the incidence of emotional problems.

The Value of Psychotherapy

Psychotherapy is a window on the damage done to children by uncaring, thoughtless, hostile or disturbed parents, and the damage done to everyone by a social system that encourages mindless competition and implicitly embraces the philosophy of social Darwinism. Psychotherapy often reveals the human effects of an economic system that produces jobs of incredible boredom and meaninglessness and that periodically throws out of work millions of people who want to work. One of four preschool children in the United States is poor and the rate is growing. For them, poverty leads to school failure which leads in turn to crime and delinquency. For their parents, it results – among other calamities – in parenting problems, child abuse and neglect (Schweinhart and Weikart, 1987). Therapy also reveals the devastating personal consequences on both the perpetrators and the victims of sexism, ageism, racism, ethnocentrism, homophobia, and exploitation of workers. While psychotherapy uncovers the individual damage inflicted by all of these social problems, treating the victims does nothing to correct the basic causes. Only when the findings of psychotherapists are translated into well-formulated preventive actions to correct or change the social and economic structure will it have made a significant contribution to prevention. But most therapists, like most professionals in other fields, have a major stake in defending the social order, not in attacking it.

When it is recognized clearly that even successful therapy does nothing to reduce the *incidence* of distress in the population, further questions may be raised as to its social value. (*Incidence* is a public health term that refers to the number of new cases occurring in a given time period.) The goal of primary prevention is to reduce the probability of future new cases and the social value of any intervention activity may arguably be related to its success in reducing (down the road) the rate of distress in the population. Both dentists and psychotherapists relieve individual pain and suffering. But fluoridation of the public water supply is preventing more cavities than dentists repair. There is no comparable massive prevention program to ensure more consistent loving and caring parenting so as to prevent future psychopathology.

Is psychotherapy a form of primary prevention because persons successfully treated for emotional problems become better parents, better spouses, and better citizens? The answer is no, though therapy may achieve all these desirable outcomes. For many years we have had successful individual treat-ment of gonorrhea with the result that persons cured do not pass on their infection to others. But there has been no reduction in the *incidence* of this disease in the society (see the United States Bureau of the Census, 1975, 1989). Early individual treatment is *secondary* prevention and has little or no effect on incidence. Early treatment often does reduce *prevalence*, the total number of cases in the population in a given time period. But early treatment resulting from early identification of both physical and mental problems may actually increase both measured incidence and prevalence. The identification of child abuse, or the borderline personality, as newly diagnosed conditions, has had this effect.

What Is To Be Done?

It is hard to see how the ongoing massive shift of psychology's focus toward the practice of psychotherapy can be arrested or altered very soon. In a society composed largely of lonely persons, and with the breakdown of the nuclear family and the decline of religion among much of the population, there is a widespread strong yearning for new guides and gurus. A craving for psycho-therapy, and its increasing social acceptability, may be preferable to other addictions like drugs and alcohol, or even to the acceptance of religious ideas. If it is true that the task of the therapist in treating neurotics is to make un-conscious material conscious, then the task of the preventionist in "treating" psychotherapists is to make their unconscious needs conscious. Therapists get gratification from their high social status, their generous income, and their satisfaction with seeing the positive results of their efforts in many of their clients. If therapists also face and accept the fact that they are having no ef-fect on incidence — that not being part of the solution defines them as being part of the problem — and choose anyway to continue, they may not merit our unqualified admiration, but at least we can respect them for their honesty.

Psychotherapy often is a form of reparenting. I have frequent discussions, and arguments, with a friend who is in full-time practice of psychotherapy. He deals largely with "borderline" cases, some of the most difficult and damaged people. He often has achieved real success with a client after three or four years of weekly therapy. They stop acting out and stop showing clear symp-toms of the negative consequences of early childhood damage. His case load averages 25 clients per week. Because of the stress and pain he experiences in reparenting his clients, who transfer onto him all their childhood anger and resentments, he becomes emotionally depleted, in danger of burnout. So he works four days a week and relaxes with his hobbies the rest of the time. If the average length of his intervention is three years then he has room in his practice for about eight new clients a year. He has taught me a great deal about the findings of the ego psychologists, about the devastating lifelong consequences of bad parenting, and about the reversibility through therapy of even extremely serious psychological distress. But his experience has also shown me graphically that society will never be able to deal with the very large number of persons with borderline personalities by concentrating its energy and resources on individual psychotherapy. While he may be helping a handful of people a year, many, many times that number of new borderlines is being created in our community by the bad parenting that can be traced to social marginality, economic powerlessness and social pathology.

It is interesting to observe the widespread denial of parental responsibility for the emotional disturbances of today's adolescents and young adults. Jack Hinckley has established the American Mental Health Fund that denies the role of parenting in mental disorders. The Fund has acquired the powerful support of the National Advertising Council to trumpet its message: "All mental illness is a medical illness." A similar group, the National Alliance for the Mentally Ill (NAMI) lobbies for more long treatment (organic type) and even involuntary hospitalization. Both groups enjoy the strong endorsement of prominent biological psychiatrists and political conservatives.

But it is hard to deny the evidence that bad childhood experiences (physical abuse, sexual abuse, neglect, emotional abandonment) have long-term damaging consequences. We also know that the worst parents were damaged themselves. British poet Philip Larkin (1974) sums it up:

> They fuck you up, your mum and dad.
>   They may not mean to, but they do
> They fill you with the faults they had
>   And add some extra, just for you.
>
> But they were fucked up in their turn
>   By fools in old-style hats and coats,
> Who half the time were soppy-stern
>   And half at one another's throats.
>
> Man hands on misery to man.
>   It deepens like a coastal shelf.
> Get out as early as you can.
>   And don't have any kids yourself.[1]

In a way, psychotherapy is comparable to some of the efforts of Lyndon Johnson's Great Society and its War on Poverty. The argument was advanced

---

[1]"This Be the Verse" from HIGH WINDOWS. Copyright © 1974 by Philip Larkin. Reprinted by permission of Farrar, Straus, and Giroux, Inc.

that if we gave remedial training to the socially disadvantaged, if we took children reared in poverty and degradation, in broken homes and pathological neighborhoods, and gave them remedial education we would help them achieve equality. Such help has been described as giving better running shoes to people, but still forcing them to play on an uneven playing field. The Great Society program failed because it attempted to change individuals through individual remediation. The programs of the War on Poverty were designed by therapy-oriented professionals, not by public health people. Goldenberg (1988) clearly identified the reason for their failure: the War on Poverty did far too little to end societal injustice and inequality so as to affect the self-esteem of all those millions damaged by prejudice and discrimination. The civil rights movement and the women's movement were much more effective because they aimed at societal change – true primary prevention. Similarly, psychotherapy may partially reduce the handicaps of a few of the emotionally damaged but this kind of war on emotional poverty cannot succeed because it does nothing to alter the social forces that keep producing more victims than are helped.

The Answer is Primary Prevention

If psychotherapy has such little social value, what should take its place? The obvious answer, validated in history, is primary prevention. Primary prevention is an approach to reducing the future incidence of a condition through proactive efforts aimed at groups, or even at a whole society. While most historical examples of primary prevention from the field of public health involve the reduction in new cases of disease, the concept is applicable to a wide range of conditions – crime and delinquency, child abuse, alcohol and drug abuse, suicide and murder, racism and sexism, homophobia, etc. Historically primary prevention efforts in the field of public health have reduced the incidence of several major plagues that have afflicted humankind. One of the most important recent successes is the complete elimination of smallpox, a plague that once afflicted millions and now is gone, probably forever.

Most mental disorders are not diseases but the traditional methods of primary prevention apply: (1) discovering and controlling the noxious agents (like bad parenting and the stresses of sexism, racism, exploitation, etc.); (2) strengthening the resistance of the susceptable (like empowerment, social coping skills, political action to improve self-esteem of the disadvantaged, and developing social support networks); and (3) preventing transmission (controlling child physical and sexual abuse, neglect, exploitation, and emotional damage). Primary prevention efforts, being proactive, generally require social and political action.

Critics of primary prevention argue that these efforts have not proven their value with demonstrable results. The only objective response to such critics is to suggest they read the literature of the field. Primary prevention efforts, described in some detail in the *Report of the Task Panel on Prevention* (1978) to the President's Commission on Mental Health, in the *Report of the Commission on Prevention* of the National Mental Health Association (1986), in Kessler and Goldston's (1986) *A Decade of Progress in Primary Prevention* and in the American Psychological Association's *Fourteen Ounces of Prevention* (see Price, Cowen, Lorian, and Ramos-McKay, 1989) are shown to be the most logical and promising approaches to reducing the incidence of psychopathology. But extending such efforts by psychologists and social workers would require a conceptual reorientation of the field, a change that would occur only with major and revolutionary social and political changes (see Joffe and Albee, 1981).

One social change, not improbable to occur, would be a decision by the federal government and third party insurers to exclude from payment the non-physician professionals engaging in interventions with persons with mental/emotional problems. While such a decision would be based on the erroneous belief that mental conditions are real diseases, and that diseases should be treated exclusively by physicians, such a curtailment of reimbursement would be advantageous to psychologists and social workers in the long run. Earlier I argued (Albee, 1975) that reimbursement for *all* professional interventions (including treatment by psychiatrists) with persons with neurotic and functional psychotic disorders should not be covered by third party payments because these persons are not suffering from real illnesses. I proposed limiting reimbursement only to those professionals treating organic conditions. This step, I thought, would put psychologists and most psychiatrists (as well as social workers and counselors) out of the financial reimbursement health system, keep competition fairly equal and limit the growth of the field. But I failed to anticipate the elimination of the neuroses (those Freudian inventions) by organized psychiatry's DSM-III, the sacking of psychodynamic professors in psychiatry, and the redefinition of most human problems as "medical diseases," caused by biochemical imbalances and genetic defects. Still more redefinitions of problems in living as diseases can be expected in successive revisions of psychiatric diagnostic systems. Unfortunately, psychologists and social workers accepted meekly the DSM-III (and DSM-III-R) diagnostic system. Instead of fighting it as scientifically dishonest and logically defective, they fell on their knees and begged to be included for reimbursement. (A few notable exceptions in psychology severely critized DSM-III: Garmezy [1978]; Zubin [1978]; and Schacht and Nathan [1977] are outstanding examples.) Abnormal psychology textbook writers, however, also yielded and publishers actually boast about up-to-date coverage of DSM-III-R. And psychologists are now lobbying hard for hospital privileges and for limited power to prescribe drugs for their "patients."

In addition to classifying most problems in living as illnesses, American psychiatry has joined forces with the reactionary citizens' groups described above to advance the position that "All mental illness is medical illness." This conservative message serves the dual purpose of raising more public funds for coverage of psychiatric drug treatment and reduction or elimination of support for social change as prevention. If all mental conditions are caused by organic, biochemical defects in the brain, then bad social environments are not to blame, parents and social exploiters are home free, NIMH can support only organic biological research, and the Establishment is not threatened. Whether we do it to ourselves, or have it done to us, psychotherapy has an uncertain future because of this rightward movement of American psychiatry and its citizen allies.

Psychologists whose careers are invested in helping people (through the medium of therapy) could join forces with the preventionists and social activists to fight for a social learning model of mental and emotional disturbances. Psychologists could turn to the study of social and economic origins of these disturbances and to strategies for developing a just society and a just world. It will happen eventually. Now is the time to begin.

References

American Psychiatric Association. (1952). *Mental disorders: Diagnostic and statistical manual.* Washington, D.C.: Author.

American Psychiatric Association. (1968). *Diagnostic and statistical manual of mental disorders* (second edition). Washington, D.C.: Author.

American Psychiatric Association. (1980). *Diagnostic and statistical manual of mental disorders* (third edition). Washington, D.C.: Author.

American Psychiatric Association. (1987). *Diagnostic and statistical manual of mental disorders* (third edition, revised). Washington, D.C.: Author.

American Psychological Association. (1988). *Fourteen ounces of prevention.* Washington, D.C.: Author.

Albee, G.W. (1975). To thine own self be true: Comments on insurance reimbursement. *American Psychologist, 30,* 1156–1158.

Albee, G.W. (1977a). Does including psychotherapy in health insurance represent a subsidy to the rich from the poor? *American Psychologist, 32,* 719–721.

Albee, G.W. (1977b). Problems in living are not sickness: Psychotherapy should not be included under national health insurance. *The Clinical Psychologist, 30,* 3–5, 6–8, 13.

Albee, G.W. (1985). The answer is prevention. *Psychology Today,* February, 60–64.

Brody, J. (1981). Guide through the maze of psychotherapies. *New York Times,* October 28, pp. C3, C8.

Dörkin, H., and Cummings, N.A. (1986). Impact of medical referral on outpatient psychological services. *Professional Psychology: Research and Practice, 17,* 431–436.

Eysenck, H. (1952). The effects of psychotherapy: An evaluation. *Journal of Consulting Psychology, 16,* 319–324.

Eysenck, H. (1964). The effects of psychotherapy. *International Journal of Psychiatry, 1,* 99–142.

Garmezy, N. (1978). Never mind the psychologists: Is it good for children? *Clinical Psychologist*, 31, 1–6.

Glasscote, R., Sanders, D., Forstenzer, H., and Foley, A. (Eds.). (1964). *The community mental health center: An analysis of existing models*. Washington, D.C.: American Psychiatric Association.

Goldenberg, I. (1988). The politics of timidity. In G.W. Albee, J.M. Joffe, and L.A. Dusenburg (Eds.), *Prevention, powerlessness, and politics. Readings on social change* (pp. 485–497). Newbury Park, California: SAGE Publications, Inc.

Henderson, J. (1975). Object relations and the new psychiatry: The illusion of primary prevention. *Bulletin of the Menninger Clinic*, 39, 233–245.

International classification of diseases, 9th revision. (1989). Clinical modification ICD-9-CM. Third Edition. Volume 1. *Diseases tabular list*. DHHS Publication No. (PHS) 89–1260, United States Department of Health and Human Services, Public Health Service, Health Care Financing Administration.

Joffe, J.M., and Albee, G.W. (Eds.). (1981). *Prevention through political action and social change*. Hanover, New Hampshire: The University Press of New England.

Joint Commission on Mental Illness and Health. (1960). *Action for mental health*. New York: Basic Books, Inc.

Kennedy, E.M. (1975). Commentary. In J. Marmor (Ed.), *Psychiatrists and their patients* (pp. 149–152). Washington, D.C.: Joint Information Service of the American Psychiatric Association and the National Association for Mental Health.

Kessler, M., and Goldston, S. (Eds.). (1986). *A decade of progress in primary prevention*. Newbury Park, California: SAGE Publications, Inc.

Kiesler, C.A., and Sibulkin, A.E. (1987). *Mental hospitalization. Myths and facts about a national crises*. Newbury Park, California: SAGE Publications, Inc.

Kramer, M. (1983). The continuing challenge: The rising prevalence of mental disorders, associated chronic diseases and disabling conditions. *American Journal of Social Psychiatry*, 3, 13–24.

Larkin, P. (1974). This be the verse. *High windows*. New York: Farrar, Straus, and Giroux.

Meehl, P.E. (1965). Discussions of Eysenck's "The effects of psychotherapy." *International Journal of Psychiatry*, 1, 156–157.

Musarrat, H. (1988, December). *Community mental health in Pakistan*. Paper presented at the 7th International Conference in Psychiatry, Karachi, Pakistan.

National Mental Health Association. (1986). *The prevention of mental-emotional disabilities. Report of the commission on prevention*. Alexandria, Virginia: Author.

Price, R.H., Cowen, E.L., Lorian, R.P., and Ramos-McKay, J. (1989). *Fourteen ounces of prevention*. Washington, D.C.: American Psychological Association.

Raimy, V. (1950). *Training in clinical psychology*. New York: Prentice Hall.

Rawls, J. (1971). *A theory of justice*. Cambridge, Massachusetts: Harvard University Press.

Regier, D.A., Myers, J.K., Kramer, M., Robins, L.N., Blazer, D.G., Hough, R.L., Eaton, W.W., and Locke, B.Z. (1984). The NIMH epidemiologic catchment area program. *Archives of General Psychiatry*, 41, 934–941.

Saxe, L. (1980). *The efficacy and cost-effectiveness of psychotherapy*. Office of Technology Assessment, Congress of the United States, Washington, D.C.: United States Government Printing Office.

Schacht, T.E., and Nathan, P.E. (1977). But is it good for the psychologists? Appraisal and status of DSM-III. *American Psychologist*, 32, 1017–1025.

Schofield, W. (1964). *Psychotherapy: The purchase of friendship*. Englewood Cliffs, New Jersey: Prentice Hall.

Schweinhart, L., and Weikart, D. (1987). Evidence of problem prevention by early childhood education. In K. Hurrelmann, F-X. Kaufmann, and F. Lösel (Eds), *Social intervention: Potential and constraints* (pp. 87–101). Berlin and New York: Walter de Gruyter.

Sharfstein, S. (1988). Financial incentives for alternatives to hospital care. *Proceedings of the Oklahoma Mental Health Research Institute 1988 Professional Symposium*, Volume 2, pp. 175–200. Oklahoma Department of Mental Health.

Silverman, P. (1978). *Mutual help groups: A guide for mental health workers*. DHEW Publication No. (ADM) 78–646. Washington, D.C.: United States Government Printing Office.

Strupp, H.H. (1986). Psychotherapy: Research, practice, and public policy (How to avoid dead ends). *American Psychologist*, 41, 120–130.

Surgeon General's Workshop on Self-help and Public Health (1987). Washington, D.C.: United States Department of Health and Human Services, Public Health Service.

Task Panel on Migrant and Seasonal Farmworkers. (1978, February). *Report to the President's commission on mental health*, Volume III, Appendix. Washington, D.C.: United States Government Printing Office.

Task Panel on Prevention. (1978). *Report to the President's commission on mental health*. Volume IV, Appendix. Washington, D.C.: United States Government Printing Office.

United States Bureau of the Census. (1975). *Historical statistics of the United States, Colonial times to 1970*. Bicentennial Edition, Part 2. Washington, D.C.

United States Bureau of the Census. (1989). *Statistical abstracts of the United States, 1989*. (109th Edition). Washington, D.C.

VandenBos, G.R. (1983). Health financing, service utilization, and national policy: A conversation with Stan Jones. *American Psychologist, 38*, 948–955.

VandenBos, G.R. (Ed.). (1986). Special Issue: Psychotherapy research. *American Psychologist, 41*, 111–214.

Wootton, B. (1959). *Social science and social pathology*. London: George Allen and Unwin.

Zubin, J. (1978). But is it good for science? *Clinical Psychologist, 31*, 1–7.

©1990 The Institute of Mind and Behavior, Inc.
The Journal of Mind and Behavior
Summer and Autumn 1990, Volume 11, Numbers 3 and 4
Pages 385 [139] – 406 [160]
ISSN 0271-0137
ISBN 0-930195-05-1

The Name Game: Toward a Sociology of Diagnosis

Phil Brown

Brown University and *Harvard Medical School*

Although diagnosis is integral to the theory and practice of psychiatry, social scientists have not developed a comprehensive approach to diagnosis. This paper presents a preliminary outline of the issues which a sociology of diagnosis should integrate. These include bias and social control in psychiatric diagnosis, diagnosis as part of a new extension of the biopsychiatric medical model, and flaws in contemporary diagnostic categorization. These issues are then viewed in terms of professional practice styles, diagnostic biases, psychiatry's professional dominance over the mental health field, and psychiatric hegemony over the clinical interaction with patients.

Diagnosis is integral to the theory and practice of psychiatry, yet it is loosely studied by social scientists. In this paper I lay out what I consider to be the main areas which a sociology of diagnosis should examine. The field is still new, and not all the components are well-developed. Some are more well-developed than others, for instance sex, race, and class bias, though they are not usually integrated with each other or with the other major areas of concern. There is also a small tradition of examining diagnosis in clinical interaction as a social construction. But we have not seen adequate attention to conceptual models which integrate medical sociology and sociology of science in order to understand the pivotal position which diagnosis plays in the larger professional project of biopsychiatry. Although much of the recent attention to diagnostic issues specifically addresses the DSM-III-R biopsychiatric project, it does not pay attention to other diagnostic currents. In this paper I discuss diagnosis historically, epistemologically, and sociologically, working to make links between the often disconnected components of the sociology of diagnosis.

Below I shall present an outline for a *sociology of diagnosis*. I view this as

David Cohen, William Gronfein, and Joel Kovel read an earlier draft of this paper and provided valuable comments and suggestions. Requests for reprints should be sent to Phil Brown, Ph.D., Department of Sociology, Brown University, Box 1916, Providence, Rhode Island 02912.

both an approach to the study of diagnosis, as well as an overall critique of modern psychiatry. The critical approach to psychiatry seen in the 1960s and 1970s has been fairly dissipated, owing to the general conservative trend in society, the success of organized psychiatry in promoting its new face, and the abandonment by many social scientists of their interest in this area. There are, however, signs of a renewal of interest in a critical perspective, stemming in large part from an interest in critiquing the new diagnostic project of psychiatry — a project blind to the entire past history of that profession.

In exploring the potential for a rich subject matter in the sociology of diagnosis, I can only mention briefly some of the key work already done. Many components of a sociology of diagnosis already exist in varying degrees of development. The task is to solidify those that are least developed, and to synthesize all the components into a new focus. Although I am concerned here with psychiatric diagnosis, I think that many of the issues can be extended to medical diagnosis. Indeed, a considerable body of work in medical sociology is concerned with lay-professional differences in disease and illness conception and experience, and with the social construction of disease (c.f. Freidson, 1970; Schneider and Conrad, 1983). That research directly touches on diagnostic issues, although they are not usually considered specifically as such.

I begin by discussing some historical examples of bias and social control in psychiatric diagnosis. I then situate current concern with diagnosis in the context of a new extension of the biopsychiatric medical model. That leads to a discussion of flaws in the theory and measurement of contemporary diagnostic categorization. These issues are then situated in specific phenomena of professional practice styles and their social biases. Following that, I examine psychiatry's professional dominance over the mental health field and its control over the clinical interaction with patients. Last, I take up the social gatekeeping functions of diagnosis by looking at diagnosis as an arena of struggle, and at the ahistorical nature of psychiatric diagnosis.

The Vagaries of Psychiatric Diagnosis

Benjamin Rush, a signer of the Declaration of the Independence and Physician General of the Continental Army, is considered the "founder" of American psychiatry. His cameo appears as a logo on the American Psychiatric Association's publications. In the period immediately following the American Revolution, Rush named an interesting diagnosis called "anarchia" (Szasz, 1970, pp. 138–149). Anarchia was the "form of insanity" in which people were unhappy with the new political structure of the United States (there were problems, such as black slavery and the restriction of the vote to white men who held landed property), and sought a more democratic society. Rather than deal with these opponents on their own political terms, Rush found it easier to transform their opinions into the symptoms of a mental disease.

Rush was also an innovator in treatment. He developed the "tranquilizer," a chair which held patients immobile by straps on their limbs and a cage over their head. He originated the "gyrator," a rotating board to which patients were strapped and then spun at high speeds. And when a patient presented the delusion of feeling fragile like glass, Rush figured out that the best thing to do was to pull a chair out from under them and then to show them glass pieces in order to demonstrate the wrongness of their belief (Szasz, 1970, pp. 138–149). Evidently, there was some connection between Rush's social control ideology of diagnosis and his social control practice of treatment.

Rush's psychologization via diagnosis was by no means new. The Catholic Church had a long medieval history of "diagnosing" nonconforming women as witches who were possessed by the devil and his legions. This was a complementary phenomenon to the then current religious/demoniacal perspective on social deviance. Indeed, a central element of Szasz' (1970) critique of institutional psychiatry is the latter's functional resemblance to the Inquisition. The Catholic Church's persecution for what it identified as deviance was torture and murder. There was a clear connection between labeling and social control practices: the purpose of both was to ensure fear, division, and supernaturalism in the working population, in order to maintain the feudal solidarity of exploiting nobles and authoritarian clergy.

In 1843 Dr. Samuel Cartwright identified the disease of "drapetomania," which occurred only in black slaves and which resulted in a curious form of pathology — the victims had a compulsion to run away. Blacks also were the only people to contract "dyaesthesia Aethiopica," which caused such pathology as "pay[ing] no attention to property" (Thomas and Sillen, 1972, p. 2). The function of these diagnostic practices was to provide support for a social order based on slavery.

In the early 20th century, psychiatrists developed a new use for the diagnosis of "psychopathic." Originally used to label a variety of male deviants such as vagabonds, criminals, and revolutionaries, the diagnosis was used by Progressive Era psychiatrists to label sexually active women. Lunbeck (1987) provides a fascinating account from her research in the archives of the Boston Psychopathic Hospital covering the years 1912–1921. Typically, women committed to the hospital for "hypersexual behavior" were working class women living on their own who had chosen to forego or delay marriage, or who were widowed or divorced. Psychiatry's response to the new sexual morality of the time was to target it as a mental disease. Sexual freedom was but one manifestation of these new women's autonomy in the world of work, pleasure, and social and familial relations. However, the women were out of character with traditional norms, and (male) psychiatrists could only see them as having a mental disease.

Psychiatrists classified sexually active women along with prostitutes, blaming them equally for enticing men into illicit sex; this diagnosis let men off the hook. The psychiatrists found further evidence of derangement in that "immoral" women would not accept money for sex. The doctors followed the general social values that proclaimed sex as a commodity: a moral woman saved her virtue as her best asset; an immoral one could only give it up for pay — otherwise she was crazy. Psychiatrists had earlier tried out the diagnosis of "feeblemindedness," but the patients scored too high on IQ tests. Some were intelligent enough to openly debate with their caretakers the sexual double standard. Hospital psychiatrists in turn warned them not to read or discuss those other social issues, since education was bad for women (Lunbeck, 1987).[1]

In the turbulent 1960s, Bettleheim (1969) told the United States Congress of his findings: student antiwar protesters who charged the University of Chicago with complicity in the war machine had no serious political agenda; they were acting out an unresolved Oedipal conflict by attacking the university as a surrogate father. Bettelheim's appellation worked well to pathologize essentially rational political protest.

The Logic of A Sociology of Diagnosis

The few examples above are manifestations of the application of psychiatry for social control, and from our current vantage point they seem very crude. I emphasize them, however, precisely because in their own time they were part of very ordinary worldviews. There are certainly other forms of social control, especially today, which are far less overt. Indeed, critiques of the "psy complex" (Castel, Castel, and Lovell, 1982) argue that it involves social control at very routine levels of socialization, labeling of behavior, and prescriptions for medical/psychiatric intervention.

The entire history of the sociological study of mental health, as well as the tradition of radical critiques of the mental health field, have revolved around this common theme of psychiatry's role in social control. What has not always been clear is that *diagnosis* has been a central component of this social control. *Giving the name* has been the starting point for social labelers. The power to give the name has been a core element in the social control nature of the mental health professionals and institutions.

In one sense the critique of diagnosis *is* the critique of psychiatry, because

[1]This was the same prescription given to Charlotte Perkins Gilman in the last decade of the 19th century, and in fact we usually associate this with the psychiatric approach to upper class women.

diagnosis is the *language of psychiatry*, which by extension defines the practice of psychiatry. Diagnosis locates the parameters of normality and abnormality, demarcates the professional and institutional boundaries of the mental health system, and authorizes psychiatry to label and deal with people on behalf of society at large (or, more appropriately, certain sectors of society). It is the legal basis for provision of benefits, and often for involuntary commitment.[2] Especially in the guise of DSM-III-R (American Psychiatric Association, 1987), psychiatric diagnosis is the social representation of psychiatric knowledge, as well as the psychiatric profession's presentation of self. Diagnosis, Blaxter (1978) notes, is "a museum of past and present concepts of the nature of disease" (p. 12).

Diagnosis thus cannot be studied on its own: it is integral to the whole of psychiatry. We are compelled to question what I term the *diagnostic project* of psychiatry in the context of the entirety of psychiatric knowledge and practice. This means, in particular, putting it in the context of all the errors and maltreatments of organized psychiatry — overreliance on drugs, abusive treatment such as psychosurgery, conscious and unconscious social control, replication and support of racism, sexism, and class bias. Put simply, if modern diagnosis is the *culmination* of psychiatry — which DSM-III proponents certainly claim it to be — then what are we to make of the history of psychiatry leading up to this modern phenomenon? I think the answer is that diagnosis reaps the sad legacy of the mental health system and mental health professions.

This is not to be read as a simplistic antipsychiatry which sees all mental health services as social control. Many people and facilities sincerely strive to help patients. However, as I discuss below, they do so mainly *without* reference to the official diagnostic framework, and often enough do so with knowing or unknowing circumvention of and opposition to official diagnosis (Brown, 1987).

Diagnosis and the Biomedical Model

The increasing faith in DSM (hereafter used in place of the cumbersome DSM-III-R) is central to the new biopsychiatry. We are in a period of "remedicalization" of psychiatry. I say "remedicalization" because the prior medicalization process was challenged by attention to social factors and the role of the mental health system in social change. The newer biopsychiatry has taken aim at the proponents of a social context, offering an assortment of new work in molecular biological studies of psychosis, with a new armamen-

---

[2]Committment, however, requires varying degrees of *behavioral* characteristics, such as actual or imminent violence to self or others, or in more broad-based statutes, inability to care for oneself. These characteristics cannot be read directly from diagnoses, although some diagnoses imply a greater likelihood of those characteristics.

tarium of laboratory tests and brain imaging. Apparently the proponents hope that such "hard" data will legitimate their biopsychiatry more than have descriptive neo-Kraepelinian categories and observations of the effects of psychoactive drugs. But the new molecular biological approach only offers simple correlations between biochemical states and accepted diagnostic categories. Further, it accounts for only a small fraction of categories of the official nosology.

Let me give an example of the attitude of this new biopsychiatry. In 1987 I attended the founding conference of the Commonwealth Research Center, a major research center funded by the Massachusetts Department of Mental Health. Most invited speakers were fully locked into the molecular biological levels of psychiatry, eager to show the biochemical bases of mental illness. A small minority of speakers represented a social context, though clearly from within the medical model. One was Bruce Dohrenwend, probably the most respected psychiatric epidemiologist in the United States; he has worked closely with many leaders of biopsychiatry, and has developed rating scales widely used by biopsychiatrically oriented people. The other was Courtney Harding, a psychologist who has been a principal investigator of the Vermont Longitudinal Study (Harding, Brooks, Ashikaga, Strauss, and Breier, 1987). This is a remarkable study which shows that diagnosed schizophrenics have a higher rate of recovery than previously expected, and that psychosocial rehabilitation prior to discharge plays a major role in reducing future symptoms. Despite the fact that both these respected scholars have always worked alongside psychiatrists, and adhered to a medical model (albeit with a strong social component), most conference speakers and participants sharply challenged them for arguing that social factors were significant determinants of mental illness. It was simply astounding − the biopsychiatrists went against the grain of well-established research findings about social factors, and stridently challenged these two speakers. There was no apparent need for it − the biopsychiatrists already dominated the conference. Yet, clearly, they perceived a need to demonstrate the worth of their perspective and to guard against future usurpation of their dominance.

Organized biopsychiatry has embarked on what it self-consciously styles a "neo-Kraepelinian" project. Quite literally, its adherents seek a return to Emil Kraepelin because he was such a remarkable labeler and classifier. They desire the neo-Kraepelinian model because it is hyper-empirical, easily measurable and computable. This approach states that it disregards etiology and dismisses conflicting theoretical standpoints (Andreasen, 1984; Blashfield, 1984). Early diagnostic schema of physical illness were also accumulated without reference to etiology, but when etiological knowledge later accumulated, doctors typically tried to apply it. We certainly do not expect doctors today to return to an atheoretical, descriptive framework simply to avoid controversy. Yet this is what the current diagnostic project in psychiatry is purportedly all about. Further, despite their claims, the neo-Kraepelinians do not disregard etiology so much as history, whether personal or social. They would most likely be satisfied with some form of genetic and biochemical etiology, which is in fact what they aim for. The neo-Kraepelinians simply do not want to deal with any form of *social* etiology.

In addition, the growth of drug treatment as the intervention of choice has cemented the centrality of diagnosis. Interest in formal diagnosis was rekindled in the 1950s as a result of the introduction of psychoactive drugs (Guimon, 1989). Since medication requires a match between disease and treatment, exact diagnosis became increasingly important. Unfortunately, the advent of widespread drug prescription often led to an uncritical reliance on medication, while at the same time diminishing the importance of social and institutional contexts in generating and maintaining what we call mental disorders. In fact, unlike medicine where diagnosis typically leads the doctor to prescribe a medication with known effect, psychiatry often reverses this logic by making a diagnosis based on the patient's *response* to medication.

The forefront of social psychiatry during World War II and immediately after presented a vibrant criticism of biological reductionist thinking. Jones (1953) and later Wing and Brown (1970) noted the significance of "institutionalism" caused by hospitals rather than biological processes. This did not imply that *all* symptoms were socially and institutionally caused, but rather that *many* were. Sociological studies in the 1950s and 1960s heightened this awareness (Belknap, 1956; Caudill, 1958; Goffman, 1961; Stanton and Schwartz, 1954). Community mental health approaches grew up in this environment, leading to emphasis on non-institutional treatment and to attention to social factors.

Pseudoscience

Such changes in orientation created disagreement within psychiatry. As we know, all science is full of controversy, and claims makers are always attempting to win colleagues and the rest of society to their perspective. What becomes accepted as science is often the result of successful social organizing and claims-making (Latour, 1987). In large part the biopsychiatry project is a way of securing unity in a disunified profession. The purpose of this unity is largely to secure professional dominance over the mental health field, since psychology and social work have grown to be important mental health disciplines in the last several decades. Unity within psychiatry also solidifies the psychiatric claim that it is a "hard" medicine worthy of third party reimbursement.

The leaders of the diagnostic project claim that they are being atheoretical. While it is true that they are emphasizing symptom clusters and avoiding traditional arguments, such as those between organic and psychoanalytic perspectives, they cannot be atheoretical. As Faust and Miner (1986) point out, even the most descriptive observations in psychiatry are based on criteria of normality which are at bottom value judgements, e.g., "aggressive behavior" by five year-olds, cut-off points for IQ measurements of mental retardation. Faust and Miner, following recent work in the social studies of science, argue that facts are largely defined by prior theoretical or organizing constructs. To insist on only facts, in fact, obstructs scientific development. Natural science, upon which psychiatry unsuccessfully attempts to measure itself, typically hypothesizes abstract concepts which go beyond observable entities. But there is no way to bracket the prior organizing configuration. That configuration may just be very subtle, even unnoticeable.

Everything is based on some theory, and the theory in this case is a biopsychiatric one. The neo-Kraepelinians actually put forth a claim to a neo-Kraepelinian theory, while at the same time denying the existence of *any* theory. They thus put forth a theory in the guise of a non-theory, and at the same time command others to avoid theoretical models. The claim to be atheoretical is really a technical means to avoid a political question, namely, who should have the power to define and implement psychiatric knowledge and practice?

According to biopsychiatric nosologists, the symptom clusters and categorical entities which form the basis for DSM-III and DSM-III-R have been scientifically detected. Mirowsky and Ross (1989) describe some fundamental problems in the diagnostic project. In the absence of "gold standards" to prove disease (e.g., demonstrable lesions), psychiatry uses concepts of latent biological classes as evidence for the validity of its diagnostic system. As Mirowsky and Ross note, however, "The problem is that the categorical biological state may not cause the symptoms on which a diagnosis is based" (p. 16).

Factor analytic studies by DSM-III developers came up with symptom clusters which do not correspond to DSM groupings, although DSM diagnostic groups have distinct profiles of mean scores on the factors. This can be understood in two ways. First, each diagnostic category can be seen as a latent class, with still unknown pathophysiologic entities (this is the belief of the DSM-III developers). Second, "We can regard the factors as separable attributes of people and the diagnostic categories as subjective constellations of those attributes" (Mirowsky and Ross, 1989, p. 17). Just as stellar constellations are mythical creations of human perception, so too, Mirowsky and Ross tell us, the diagnostic groupings are "mental overlays grouping elements that seem to form something distinct, but which may have no real connection with each other" (p. 17).

In addition to these conceptual errors, the diagnostic project contains measurement flaws. By collapsing continuous metric scales into categorical assessments, certainty is increased at the expense of reliability. Mirowsky and Ross point out that if cut-points were used on bathroom scales to categorize light and heavy, almost everyone would be classified correctly, but without any reliability of measurement.

Psychiatry seeks to achieve predictive power in a situation where certainty is low. This phenomenon is common to positivist approaches to the social world — uncertainty is viewed as an interloper to be overcome rather than as a basic feature which may provide problems that cannot be surmounted. DSM proponents claim they have achieved a high degree of interrater reliability (Klerman, 1983). A careful review by Kutchins and Kirk (1986) of a number of field trials of DSM reliability, however, demonstrates otherwise. Even using their own standard of good agreement on diagnosis (Cohen's kappa of 0.7 or higher), DSM originators only reached that level on 31 kappas, while falling below that mark on 49. Further, no major diagnostic category attained that level of agreement.

The psychiatric literature is full of DSM reliability studies on countless numbers of diagnoses on all the axes. Yet hardly any research addresses validity. Anyone can achieve interrater reliability by teaching all people the "wrong" material, and getting them to all agree on it. Chang and Bidder (1985, p. 202) put the problem this way:

> At the current stage of psychiatric knowledge, grouping patients according to selected properties rather than in terms of their total phenomenology is analogous to classifying a car by observing any four of the following eight properties: wheels, motors, headlights, radio, seats, body, windshield wipers, and exhaust systems. While an object with four of these properties might well be a car, it might also be an airplane, a helicopter, a derrick, or a tunnel driller.

Put otherwise, witch trials showed a much higher degree of interrater reliability than any DSM category (Kovel, 1988), yet we would not impute any validity to those social diagnoses.

Validity requires that the variable or item be highly correlated with a known measure, such as clinical diagnosis in medical records. Biopsychiatry is satisfied to take as construct validity the fact that DSM-III and DSM-III-R have been widely accepted by courts, prisons, third party payers, and medical schools. Actually this is merely successful social hegemony, yet the neo-Kraepelinains mistakenly take it as evidence of scientific breakthrough (Kovel, 1988). Of course, from a social constructivist approach to science, such successful social hegemony is in fact a scientific breakthrough. This is because when a society's leading institutions accept the beliefs, practices, and implications of a scientific model, a form of scientific knowledge has been "created."

By criticizing the existing attempts at "objective" measurement in psychiatry, I do not mean to imply that these can be sufficiently refined to the point that they offer a very valid picture. Indeed, my point is that psychiatry is approaching the problem incorrectly by examining patients and their symptoms as discrete phenomena without context. More so than other medical fields, psychiatry faces a large gap between *signs* noticed by the doctor and *symptoms* reported by the patient. To a large degree, the attribution of mental illness is made not on the basis of characteristics of the patient in isolation, but on the interaction between patient and provider (Rosenberg, 1984). Given what we know of the disparity between medical and lay perspectives of illness, and given the many communication problems in medical interaction, we would expect psychiatry to be particularly prone to attaining distorted information. Thus, methodological and measurement refinements will not be likely to increase the validity of psychiatric diagnosis. We can understand this better by examining professional practice styles and psychiatry's social biases.

Professional Practice Styles

Not only is validation generally lacking, but when researchers study validity the results are startling — validity is very low. For a good example, let us examine the well-known data on the diagnostic differences between the United States and the United Kingdom (Kendell, Cooper, Gourlay, Copeland, Sharpe, and Gurland, 1971). Professionals were surprised to learn that depression occurred far more often in the United Kingdom than in the United States, and that schizophrenia occurred more frequently in the United States than in the United Kingdom. In researching this problem, it was found that the differences were due to practice styles and their underlying belief systems. American practitioners were simply more likely to read certain psychotic symptoms as signs of schizophrenia when they should have done otherwise. DSM-III leaders point to their diagnostic project as a way to avoid such biases (and hence to improve validity), through the use of clear checklists and decision-trees. Yet Lipton and Simon (1985) restudied the same hospital (Manhattan State) years later, examining patient charts, and found the same level of erroneous diagnosis. In particular, clinicians picked up on a single symptom (i.e., hallucinations) which is often associated with schizophrenia, yet failed to examine corroborating symptoms. In fact, hallucinations are seen in affective disorders as well, and more details are required to make the differential diagnosis.

In other research, Rubinson, Asnis, and Friedman (1988) surveyed mental health professionals and found serious misconceptions about the diagnosis of major depression. The most common errors were erroneous beliefs that this diagnosis required vegetative signs and a distinct quality of mood, and that it could not be made if the condition was chronic. Respondents answered incorrectly on these items 48%, 41%, and 37%, respectively.

There are not enough such studies — largely because they are threatening, or at least perceived as of doubtful value — so we cannot tell how common such errors are. But there is good reason to believe that idiosyncratic use of DSM is widespread. My own field work in the psychiatric walk-in clinic of a free-standing community mental health center provides ample evidence that clinicians resisted official diagnostic classification in order to make their own work easier, to help patients, and to criticize the official nomenclature and its underlying theory (Brown, 1987). The staff used humor and sarcasm, and invented alternative diagnoses. They minimized and normalized certain behaviors by giving mild diagnoses to protect people from employers and others. They evaded formal diagnosis when possible, in order to cover their own potential errors or to protect patients from outside agencies. Clinicians also downplayed formal, accurate diagnosis when patients came from non-psychiatric agencies (homeless shelters, welfare department, prison pre-release) since they did not want to be doing the "dirty work" for those agencies (Brown, 1989).

In examining more closely one component of the diagnostic process, the Mental Status Exam (MSE), I found other curious features. The MSE was employed in a highly variable manner in patient interviews and discussions with supervisors, and this variation was not consistent with research, teaching, and theoretical models of the MSE. In addition, clinicians and patients often found the MSE to be awkward and embarrassing. As a result there was much humor, as well as clinician disclaimers (e.g., "Some of these questions may sound silly") [Brown and Drugovich, 1989].

Arising from these observations, it makes sense to think of diagnoses as involving both *diagnostic technique* and *diagnostic work*. *Diagnostic technique* involves the formalization of classification, including the specific tasks, techniques, interviews, and chart recording necessary to make the formalized classification. These elements are mostly discrete, measurable phenomena which can be taught in specific training programs. However, the discrete and measurable aspects of these elements are only *potential*, and their actual practice varies greatly across clinicians and institutions.

Diagnostic work consists of the process by which clinicians concretely proceed with their evaluation and therapeutic tasks. Many clinicians — especially young ones in training — employ short-cuts and individual practice styles. This stems in part from their awareness that their senior colleagues do not completely accept the given standardization and formalization. Most clinicians have a basic distrust of the attempt to force fit scientifically repeatable measurements into a framework which is much too "soft" for such measurement. The use of short-cuts and individual styles also comes from a desire to feel more "experienced," like the elder practitioners. Diagnostic work is thus embedded in routine work, and clinicians' desire to be more advanced makes them less accepting of the rigors of routine "scut-work" of diagnostic technique.

Looking at surveys of psychiatrists' opinions on DSM-III, we see that even those who agreed that DSM contributed positively to psychiatric training and practice nevertheless believed that it emphasized signs and symptoms at the expense of overall understanding. In one survey (Kutchins and Kirk, 1988), 35% of psychiatrists sampled said they would stop using DSM if not required to use it. Clinical psychologists are more critical; 90% said their chief application was for insurance purposes (Kutchins and Kirk, 1988). A survey of social workers found that 81% saw DSM as very important for insurance purposes. Their top four categories of usefulness – insurance, agency, Medicaid, and legal requirements – all had nothing intrinsically to do with clinical practice (Kutchins and Kirk, 1988). Another survey found that psychologists prefer social-interpersonal, nondiagnostic, and behavioral analysis rather than DSM. Nearly one-half rejected the notion that a universal nosology was valuable (Smith and Kraft, 1983).

We see, then, a significant ambivalence in that clinicians both laud and criticize the official nomenclature. This stems from the diverse social functions and mixed agendas of diagnosis. Mental health institutions, government agencies, clinicians, professional groups, and third party payers all have different needs for the diagnostic project. Generally these needs are incompatible, and prone to generate conflict.

Professional practice styles regarding diagnosis are not necessarily helpful to patients. Some of the above examples about clinician avoidance of DSM classifications – such as aiding reimbursement or defending against stigma and bias – are in the patient's interest. Yet much diagnostic behavior is part and parcel of traditional professionalism. This involves professionals' social biases, professional dominance in the mental health field, and control over the clinical interaction.

Professionals' Social Biases

Neo-Kraepelinians and their allies believe that past biases were due to lack of objective criteria, and thus new "objective diagnostic criteria" will eradicate the potential for biases (Maxmen, 1985, p. 45). This grand claim is evidence of a striking problematic which drives the biopsychiatric nosologists – employing a technical means to obtain a social end. The situation is impossible on two counts. First, as I have already pointed out, professional practice styles vary across providers and institutions – even on the ostensibly less value-laden matter of DSM classifications of schizophrenia versus affective disorder. Post-DSM-III studies have shown that misdiagnosis remains common. Clinicians often simply do not follow the codified diagnostic schema, and even when they attempt to do so, they make many errors. In addition, ongoing struggles betwen biopsychiatric, psychoanalytic, behaviorist, and community approaches lead clinicians to come up with varying diagnoses.

Second, race, sex, and class bias – which have long been central features of psychiatric diagnosis – are much more value-laden, and will undoubtedly be even harder to eradicate with technical classification. These biases are part of the overall culture, and invariably will show up in major social institutions. This is especially the case in the mental health field, since it has so much latitude for interpretation.

Sexism in diagnosis has been shown to reflect continual social attitudes, as well as historically changing patterns (Chesler, 1972; Smith and David, 1975). Continual social attitudes are usually seen in sex differences in definitions of mental health and illness. In Broverman, Broverman, Clarkson, Rosenkrantz, and Vogel's (1970) classic study, mental health professionals responded to an open-ended question on the nature of mental health for men, women, and humans in general. The mentally healthy woman was defined by her similarity to overall stereotypes of female passivity; the mentally healthy man by his similarity to acceptable male dominance; the human in general was the same as the man.

It is in the historically changing patterns that we observe drastic evidence of diagnostic sexism. I have already mentioned Lunbeck's (1987) analysis of female psychopathy. In the late 19th century, neurasthenia was widely abused as a disease category designed to keep middle and upper class women from active participation in social life. Hysteria has been another widely disputed diagnosis, now discredited, although many observers believe that the "borderline" diagnosis today serves some of the same functions.

Researchers continue to find differentials in diagnosis by sex. Women are more likely to be diagnosed with depression, phobias, and histrionic personality disorders, while men are more disposed to paranoid personality disorders and antisocial personality disorders. It is unclear to what extent these are real differences attributable to social factors, the result of professional bias, or a combination of both. What is clear is that these differences provoke considerable criticism of official diagnostic approaches, and demand our attention.

Racism in diagnosis has also been widely studied. As with sexism, we can look at both continual ideology and historically specific diagnoses. Beginning in slavery, racism led psychiatrists to conceptualize blacks as belonging to a separate race which was inferior in neurological, physiological, and emotional capacity. In the 19th and early 20th centuries such eminent mental health professionals as G. Stanley Hall, William McDougall, and William Alanson White pursued this "scientific racism" which viewed blacks as a race still in a childlike social development (Thomas and Sillen, 1972, pp. 1–22).

In terms of specific diagnostic practices, perhaps the best known early epidemiological example is the exaggeration of black insanity according to the 1840 census. This data, reported as true in the *American Journal of Insanity*, claimed that blacks had higher rates of madness in free states — as high as one in 14. The data were clearly fabricated, since insane blacks were reported in counties where no blacks at all lived. Yet the data were widely used for such significant political action as President John Calhoun's 1844 extension of slavery to Texas. Despite clear disproof of this data, psychiatrists in the Reconstruction era continued to cite it as evidence of the beneficial aspects of slavery (Thomas and Sillen, 1972, pp. 16–20).

From the 19th century well into the 20th, psychiatry maintained that blacks were rarely depressed. The explanations usually centered around the idea of a happy-go-lucky personality or the notion that blacks have less to lose in terms of prestige, esteem, possessions, and relationships (Thomas and Sillen, 1972, p. 128–129). Higher black rates of schizophrenia and paranoid personality disorders, combined with lower black rates of affective disorders, were often explained in terms of innate racial differences. Critics of traditional diagnosis have argued that the prevailing diagnostic categories are largely a result of professional bias. As with sex biases, there is undoubtedly a combination of bias and real difference.

To the extent that differentials are caused by professional ideology, sex and race biases have not been altered in the post-DSM-III era. Loring and Powell (1988) were interested in whether sex and race of psychiatrist and client affected diagnosis. They used an analogue study providing two real cases, and varying four categories of race and sex and a fifth category of no information. Loring and Powell found that psychiatrists were more likely to concur on the diagnosis of case studies when no information on the client's race and sex was available. When such information was available, psychiatrists tended to come up with the correct diagnosis when the client's race and sex were the same as their own. Male psychiatrists were more likely to find depression in women clients; women were unlikely to apply that category at all. Black psychiatrists gave white males the least serious diagnoses. All psychiatrists tended to give blacks the more serious diagnoses. These findings suggest that people view more seriously the abnormality or rule-breaking of those who are different from them. In a similar vein, Rosenfield (1982) found that people were more likely to be committed to mental hospitals for behaviors incongruent with their sex roles. From evidence so far, then, DSM-III has not succeeded in its promise to eradicate diagnostic bias.

Let me offer one conceptual caution. That there are diagnostic biases does not, however, mitigate the fact that there may well be class, sex, and race differences in actual mental health status. In particular, Hollingshead and Redlich (1958) showed that the class differences in mental illness are to some extent "real," and attributable to varying stresses and living conditions in the social world. Likewise, women may have higher rates of depression as a result of their social roles which lead them to be more attuned to emotional life. And blacks may have higher rates of antisocial behavior due to living in a world hostile to them. A culturally sensitive mental health system would have to deal both with social differentials in diagnosis and diagnostic bias. Further, a research effort in the sociology of diagnosis faces a major challenge in partialling out these two phenomena.

Professional Dominance

The ascendancy of the diagnostic project reflects the elite stature of research over clinical practice. Developments within and without the mental health professions have combined to make research on diagnostic categories a valued endeavor. Diagnostic researchers also see themselves as "correcting" the errors of clinical impressionism. This is related to psychiatric defensiveness against the growth of non-medical mental health professions. A strict diagnostic schema, particularly one seeking to incorporate medical evidence, allows psychiatrists to reassert their dominance over the other professions. Diagnosis has, of course, previously been affected by the degree of professional power. Temerlin's (1968) famous experiment showed how clinicians were prone to follow the suggestion effects of experts. Psychiatrists' suggestions were most likely to be followed, leading to a more or less severe diagnosis depending upon the expert's overt cues.

This is but one example of the certainty which psychiatry holds up to safeguard its professional position. We see another case of unwarranted certainty in Rosenhan's (1973) oft-cited study, which showed that psychiatrists diagnosed and admitted to hospitals healthy "pseudopatients" who presented themselves with no other evidence than that they heard voices.

This certitude is planted in young psychiatric residents during the professional socialization of the training process. Blum and Rosenberg (1968) concluded from their study of residents that journeymen held apprentices to a higher standard of purity than would later be necessary. The purpose was to convince the residents that there is a clear set of skills which must be mastered in order to progress. Light (1980) also observed resident training, and found that diagnostic instruction was a central part of overall socialization which sought to provide certainty to a disunified profession which holds multiple needs and goals.

Control of the Clinical Interaction

The same professional desire for certainty which permeates professional hierarchies also dominates the clinical encounter. DSM-based diagnosis represents a *power-linguistic approach* to categorization, in which patient subjectivity is sacrificed to clinical objectivity. As Kovel (1988) points out, DSM allows for an "objectifying gaze" rather than an intersubjective dialogue. Although mental disorders are parts of a system of social relations, DSM makes diagnosis in the abstract by separating persons from their social world. At the same time, relying on diagnosis provides detachment. Detachment is taught as a positive form of achieving objective understanding, and is also a desired goal for clinicians who feel overburdened by their work.

Although diagnosis is so crucial to the official approach to mental illness, it is treated in a curiously secretive fashion. Psychiatrists are somewhat reluctant to inform patients and families of the diagnosis, especially for schizophrenia. A survey of 221 psychiatrists (Green and Gantt, 1987) found that 75% would always tell the patient of manic-depressive illness, 73% of unipolar depression, and 31% of schizophrenia. If the category "usually inform" is added, the figure is 91% for the two affective disorders and 58% for schizophrenia. Among the clinicians I studied, two-thirds would share the diagnosis with the patient, but only 5% would bring it up on their own. This secrecy and aversion to disclosure clearly cements professional control of the interaction.

Apart from any of the other constraints I have already addressed, the status and knowledge differentials between patient and professional are enough to produce disparate viewpoints among doctors and patients concerning the meaningfulness of certain data and how it should be used. Even if there is a generally consensual approach between client and professional, the process of decoding and interpreting information is dynamic and interactive. Certain bits of information are sought or offered, leading to decisions to ask for other bits. Opinions, attitudes, emotions, and styles are in play at each step of this process, for the diagnosis carries with it a large number of implications: future treatment, future limitations, reimbursement, stigma, potential reconstruction of identity as a chronic patient. Further, the process by which the diagnosis is arrived at contains the kernel — or even the template — of the continuing therapeutic relationship in terms of authority relations, mutual participation, comfortableness, directedness, and satisfaction. As Glaser and Strauss (1965, p. 18) argue, "From a sociological perspective, the important thing about any diagnosis, whether correctly established or not, is that it involves questions of definition."

The *goals* of diagnosis are more important for the clinician than the patient. The clinician is bound by financial, bureaucratic, and professional pressures which demand official diagnosis. As well, the clinician wishes the certainty and control which is obtainable from naming the problem. To some degree, the patient also wants the control which comes with the name. A diagnosis seems to remove the mystery of the problem by giving it a name upon which hinge future considerations of treatment, cure, personal and social implication of the problem, and social acceptance of one's diminished abilities. Yet for patients, diagnosis is less important than a broad understanding of their problems and what can be done for them.

Patients, like clinicians, use cues as a way of recognizing the disorder. Three types of cues — symptomatological, behavioral, and communicative — disturb the taken-for-granted sense of order. This is to some degree complementary to doctors' diagnostic actions: for both parties, the naming of a diagnosis helps people in "making sense of problematic experience," since "something unknown, potentially dangerous, and worrying becomes assimilated into a familiar order" (Locker, 1981, pp. 47–50).

Twenty years ago, Levinson, Merrifield, and Berg (1967) examined the same clinic where I conducted research. They found that an ideal, objective "diagnostic model" was in fact less common than a "suitability model" that selected psychotherapy clients. Despite changes in the mandate of the clinic, twenty years later suitability remains a powerful characteristic of patient selection. Suitable candidates typically are verbal and articulate middle-class persons who staff view as "healthy neurotics." Thus the "objective" gaze of DSM is short-circuited by a more subjective approach which carries its own biases.

Thus what purports to be a *diagnostic* process is in fact a *disposition* process, since the same diagnosis can lead to different dispositions. Adjustment reactions of various types and dysthymic disorder (what pre-DSM-III nomenclautre called "depressive neurosis") are often diagnosed for persons who are not very troubled, functioning well on their own, and who are able to discuss and interpret their problems. But a middle-class college or graduate student is more likely than a working-class person or welfare recipient to be offered therapy, despite similarities in diagnosis.

One woman in her early 20s, mother of 5- and 8-year-old children, came to the clinic I studied. An AFDC (welfare) recipient with a clerical work background, she felt in a rut with trying to find work. She felt she was getting little empathy and support form others though she put herself out a lot for people. One such person struck her and broke several vertebrae. She also retained many unexamined emotions about her mother being raped in their house eight years ago. This patient was able to present herself quite clearly and was articulate about many things in her history. She took an active role in asking sensible questions about the clinic, such as whether she would see the same clinician each time and whether she would have to repeat her story over again. She engaged very much with the clinician, and responded fully to questions. But in crucial ways, her vocabulary differed from the staff's. This client came looking for help, but was not savvy enough to say she was looking for "therapy"; this was one example of the limitations of her "treatment vocabulary." Similarly, her "vocabulary of discomfort" (Bart, 1968) was not congruent with the clinicians' vocabulary. She said too much about concrete life experiences, rather than making abstract connections. She also said she was "lonely," but not "depressed." Staff in fact took this literally, and believed the woman needed what they term "supportive therapy," i.e., periodic contact with a social worker who would encourage her to make certain social contacts. Interestingly, one of those recommended contacts would be her minister, to whom she had spoken about her problems, and who she claimed had been of minimal help. One other noncongruent discomfort vocabulary item was that she expressed guilt about her mother's rape, but did not use the term, "guilt." Compared to most working class women who came to the clinic, particularly those who like her had been teen mothers, this patient was extremely articulate and insightful. One might think that she would be an interesting challenge to take on as a psychotherapy candidate. But a query to the clinician about this elicited no answer.

From the standpoint of Balint's (1957) concept of "organizing" the illness, the psychiatrist in this case did not interpret the client's problems broadly enough so as to "organize" it as requiring therapy. If anything, the intake clinician merely listened, without interpreting. In other cases, clinicians can provide excessive interpretation which minimizes the client's problems by recasting them as inner conflicts without any reference to social surroundings. An excellent analysis is found in Scheff's (1968) analysis of a training session, found both on a phonograph recording and in a written transcript. A woman presented herself for therapy because her alcoholic husband abused her verbally and prevented her from working outside the home. The psychiatrist was hostile to her, and reframed her problem as a personal shortcoming. Only when she accepted this new "organized" illness did he offer her treatment.

Thus either with the objective DSM gaze or the subjective suitability gaze, diagnostic reasoning is the central form by which many clients judge their patients and reframe their problems and needs. Diagnosis, then, serves a gatekeeping function, in which individual practice styles and local cultures of appropriate care are manifested. I next turn to some large social gatekeeping functions.

Diagnosis as an Arena of Struggle

A sociology of diagnosis can also point to the importance of diagnosis as an arena of struggle. Diagnosis is often the location in the psychiatric world where both lay and professional critics fight over the roles and functions of diagnoses. These struggles are ample proof that scientific discoveries are not the result of an ongoing "march of science" as much as of political battles.

Bayer's (1981) study of the psychiatric profession's response to homosexuality presents a classic example of diagnosis as an arena of struggle. Without any change in the internal "science" of psychiatry, the American Psychiatric Association dropped homosexuality as a mental disorder, based on widespread opposition from the gay rights movement and from people sympathetic to that movement's demands concerning diagnosis. Feminists, too, have taken up struggles in this arena. Proposed DSM-III-R revision discussions included "paraphilic coercive disorder" which many felt would let child sexual abusers off the hook by calling them mentally ill rather than criminal. Women's groups fought this, and the proposed diagnosis was dropped. Feminist pressure also led the APA to change "masochistic personality disorder" to "self-defeating personality disorder" (this labels the victim of wife battering, rather than the batterer), and "premenstrual syndrome" was changed to "periluteal phase dysphoric disorder" (Kaplan, 1983).

Diagnostic struggles are sometimes directed toward the inclusion of new categories. Post-traumatic stress disorder, for example, was added to DSM-III through the concerted action of Vietnam Veterans Against the War and sympathetic mental health professionals. Supporters faced opposition from the Veterans' Administration and the American Psychiatric Association, and were able to overcome this by successful mobilization of mental health professionals, veterans groups, and by media attention (Scott, 1989).

Conclusion: The Ahistorical Nature of Diagnosis

Biopsychiatric neo-Kraepelinians lay claim to a project far grander than merely a comprehensive, objective diagnostic schema. Their goal is to lead the transformation of the mental health system. This is largely defined negatively — opposing the labeling/societal reaction perspective and the anti-institutionalist attitudes that have played such a large role. These new leaders seek to strip psychiatry of any social context. They wish to place psychiatry in a technocratic framework rather than an interpretive, humanistic one. But even if the professional project goes beyond diagnosis, the diagnostic project is at the core of a larger goal. One reason for the centrality of diagnosis is that diagnosis plays a coordinating role in laying out the terms of medico-psychiatric discourse. Professional leaders have taken the diagnostic terminology of DSM and reified it into the essential statement and rationale of biopsychiatry. Another reason is that the significant social powers to whom organized psychiatry asks for support view the diagnostic schema as the proper codification of psychiatry. Third-party payers, both private and governmental, as well as state and federal bureaucrats who run mental health agencies, have established a diagnostic determinism. Quite literally, the mental health of a client only becomes "official" when the proper DSM code is affixed.

Psychiatry is ahistorical in many ways, especially in ignoring the history of its own traditions and errors. It is striking that there has been so little criticism of DSM. As we would expect, more criticism comes from social workers and psychologists, since they lose out to psychiatry's professional dominance. Within psychiatry there is very little criticism. Criticism is stifled by a general impression, fostered by DSM leaders, that the "old way" was merely a simplistic psychoanalysis or a radical antipsychiatry. DSM proponents argue that their system avoids the social expansionism of previous times. Earlier expansionism was marked during the rich funding of the 1950s and 1960s. In that period, many large-scale epidemiological studies employed diagnosis as a major vehicle for their work, which resulted in greater social, professional, and economic attention to mental illness. Yet there is a new expansionism today, again in the self-interest of psychiatry. We see expansionism now in general research areas of rich funding and prestige, such as AIDS, aging, and homelessness. Also, some new diagnoses have the same expansionist quality, e.g., "post-luteal phase disorder," "post-traumatic stress disorder."

Psychiatry's ahistoricity is illuminated by these new categories. Despite the inclusion of new categories which have clear social contexts, psychiatry ignores its own history and the history of society. In particular, psychiatry does not ask why certain diagnostic categories appear and disappear over time. Quite simply, psychiatry cannot explain why hysteria has declined, or why narcissistic problems and codependency have grown. These are essentially sociopolitical phenomena which are not comprehensible within the medical framework of diagnosis. Because psychiatry cannot comprehend diagnosis as a socio-political phenomena, alterations to the existing traditional diagnosis models will not lead to a greater understanding of mental disorder. For that reason, a sociology of diagnosis should be further developed in order to offer a more comprehensive perspective.

References

American Psychiatric Association. (1987). *Diagnostic and statistical manual of mental disorders* (third edition, revised). Washington, D.C.: American Psychiatric Association.

Andreasen, N.C. (1984). *The broken brain: The biological revolution in psychiatry.* New York: Harper & Row.

Balint, M. (1957). *The doctor, his patient, and the illness.* New York: International Universities Press.

Bart, P. (1968). Social structure and vocabularies of discomfort. *Journal of Health and Social Behavior, 9,* 188–193.

Bayer, R. (1981). *Homosexuality and American psychiatry: The politics of diagnosis.* New York: Basic.

Belknap, I. (1956). *Human problems of a state mental hospital.* Detroit: Wayne State University Press.

Bettleheim, B. (1969). Student revolt: The hard core [Testimony presented to the House Special Subcommittee on Education, March 20, 1969]. *Vital Speeches of the Day, 15,* 405–410.

Blashfield, R.K. (1984). *The classification of psychopathology: Neo-Kraepelinian and quantitative approaches*. New York: Plenum.

Blaxter, M. (1978). Diagnosis as a category and process: The case of alcoholism. *Social Science and Medicine, 12*, 9–17.

Blum, A.F., and Rosenberg, L. (1968). Some problems involved in professionalizing social interaction: The case of psychotherapeutic training. *Journal of Health and Social Behavior, 9*, 72–85.

Broverman, I.K., Broverman, D.M., Clarkson, F.E., Rosenkrantz, P.S., and Vogel, S.R. (1970). Sex-role stereotypes and clinical judgments of mental health. *Journal of Consulting and Clinical Psychology, 34*, 1–7.

Brown, P. (1987). Diagnostic conflict and contradiction in psychiatry. *Journal of Health and Social Behavior, 28*, 37–50.

Brown, P. (1989). Psychiatric dirty work revisited: Conflicts in servicing non-psychiatric agencies. *Journal of Contemporary Ethnography, 2*, 182–201.

Brown, P., and Drugovich, M. (1989, August 12). Some of these questions may sound silly: Empirical standardization versus clinical application of the Mental Status Examination. *Paper presented at the Annual Meeting of the American Sociological Association*. San Francisco, California.

Castel, R., Castel, F., and Lovell, A. (1982). *The psychiatric society*. New York: Columbia University Press.

Caudill, W. (1958). *The psychiatric hospital as a small society*. Cambridge, Massachusetts: Harvard University Press.

Chang, M.M., and Bidder, G. (1985). Noncomparability of research results that are related to psychiatric diagnosis. *Comprehensive Psychiatry, 26*, 195–207.

Chesler, P. (1972). *Women and madness*. New York: Doubleday.

Faust, D., and Miner, R.A. (1986). The empiricist and his new clothes. *American Journal of Psychiatry, 143*, 962–967.

Freidson, E. (1970). *Profession of medicine*. New York: Dodd, Mead.

Glaser, B.G., and Strauss, A.L. (1965). *Awareness of dying*. Chicago: Aldine.

Goffman, E. (1961). *Asylums*. Garden City: Doubleday.

Guimon, J. (1989). The biases of psychiatric diagnosis. *British Journal of Psychiatry, 36*, 366–373.

Green, R.S., and Gantt, A.B. (1987). Telling patients and families the psychiatric diagnosis: A survey of psychiatrists. *Hospital and Community Psychiatry, 38*, 33–37.

Harding, C.M., Brooks, G.W., Ashikaga, T., Strauss, J.S., and Breier, A. (1987). The Vermont longitudinal study of persons with severe mental illness, I: Methodology, study sample, and overall status 32 years later. *American Journal of Psychiatry, 144*, 718–726.

Hollingshead, A.B., and Redlich, F.C. (1958). *Social class and mental illness*. New York: Wiley.

Jones, M. (1953). *The therapeutic community*. New York: Basic.

Kaplan, M. (1983). A woman's view of DSM-III. *American Psychologist, 38*, 786–792.

Kendell, R.E. (1983). DSM-III: A major advance in psychiatric nosology. In R.L. Spitzer, J.B.W. Williams, and A.E. Skodol (Eds.), *International perspectives on DSM-III* (pp. 55–68). Washington, D.C.: American Psychiatric Press.

Kendell, R.E., Cooper, J.E., Gourlay, A.J., Copeland, J.R.M., Sharpe, L., and Gurland, B.J. (1971). Diagnostic criteria of American and British psychiatrists. *Archives of General Psychiatry, 25*, 123–130.

Klerman, G.L. (1983). The significance of DSM-III in American psychiatry. In R.L. Spitzer, J.B.W. Williams, and A.E. Skodol (Eds.), *International perspectives on DSM-III* (pp. 3–25). Washington, D.C.: American Psychiatric Press.

Kovel, J. (1988). A critique of DSM-III. *Research in Law, Deviance, and Social Control, 9*, 127–146.

Kutchins, H., and Kirk, S.A. (1986). The reliability of DSM-III: A critical review. *Social Work Research and Abstracts, Winter*, 3–12.

Kutchins, H., and Kirk, S.A. (1988). The business of diagnosis: DSM-III and clinical social work. *Social Work, 33*, 215–220.

Latour, B. (1987). *Science in action: How to follow scientists and engineers through society*. Cambridge, Massachusetts: Harvard University Press.

Levinson, D.J., Merrifield, J., and Berg, K. (1967). Becoming a patient. *Archives of General Psychiatry, 17*, 385–406.

Light, D. (1980). *Becoming psychiatrists: The professional transformation of self*. New York: Norton.

Lipton, A., and Simon, F. (1985). Psychiatric diagnosis in a state hospital: Manhattan State revisited. *Hospital and Community Psychiatry, 36,* 368–373.

Locker, D. (1981). *Symptoms and illness: The cognitive organization of disorder.* London: Tavistock.

Loring, M., and Powell, B. (1988). Gender, race, and DSM-III: A study of the objectivity of psychiatric diagnostic behavior. *Journal of Health and Social Behavior, 29,* 1–22.

Lunbeck, E. (1987). A new generation of women: Progressive psychiatrists and the hypersexual female. *Feminist Studies, 13,* 513–543.

Maxmen, J.S. (1985). *The new psychiatry.* New York: Morrow.

Mirowsky, J., and Ross, C.E. (1989). Psychiatric diagnosis as reified measurement. *Journal of Health and Social Behavior, 30,* 11–25.

Rosenberg, M. (1984). A symbolic-interactionist view of psychosis. *Journal of Health and Social Behavior, 25,* 289–302.

Rosenfield, S. (1982). Sex roles and societal reactions to mental illness: The labeling of "deviant" deviance. *Journal of Health and Social Behavior, 23,* 18–24.

Rosenhan, D.L. (1973). On being sane in insane places. *Science, 179,* 250–258.

Rubinson, E., Asnis, G.M., and Friedman, J.M. (1988). Knowledge of the diagnostic criteria for major depression: A survey of mental health professionals. *Journal of Nervous and Mental Disease, 176,* 480–484.

Scheff, T.J. (1968). Negotiating reality: Notes on power in the assessment of responsibility. *Social Problems, 16,* 3–17.

Schneider, J.W., and Conrad, P. (1983). *Having epilepsy: The experience and control of illness.* Philadelphia: Temple University Press.

Scott, W.J. (1989, August 6). PTSD in DSM-III. A case study in the politics of readjustment from combat. *Paper presented at the Annual Meeting of the Society for the Study of Social Problems.* San Francisco, California.

Sharma, S.L. (1970). A historical background for the development of nosology in psychiatry and psychology. *American Psychologist, 23,* 248–253.

Smith, D., and Kraft, W.A. (1983). DSM-III: Do psychologists really want an alternative? *American Psychologist, 38,* 777–785.

Smith, D.E., and David, S.J. (Eds.). (1975). *Women look at psychiatry.* Vancouver, British Columbia: Press Gang Publishers.

Stanton, A., and Schwartz, M. (1954). *The mental hospital.* New York: Basic.

Szasz, T.S. (1970). *The manufacture of madness: A comparative study of the Inquisition and the mental health movement.* New York: Delta.

Temerlin, M.K. (1968). Suggestion effects in psychiatric diagnosis. *Journal of Nervous and Mental Diseases, 147,* 349–353.

Thomas, A., and Sillen, S. (1972). *Racism and psychiatry.* New York: Brunner/Mazel.

Wing, J.K., and Brown, G.W. (1970). *Institutionalism and schizophrenia.* London: Cambridge University Press.

©1990 The Institute of Mind and Behavior, Inc.
The Journal of Mind and Behavior
Summer and Autumn 1990, Volume 11, Numbers 3 and 4
Pages 407 [161] – 424 [178]
ISSN 0271-0137
ISBN 0-930195-05-1

Subjective Boundaries and Combinations in Psychiatric Diagnoses

John Mirowsky

University of Illinois at Urbana-Champaign

This distinctions embodied in official psychiatric diagnoses represent arbitrary and subjective views of patients' problems. Historically, individual psychiatrists were free to superimpose their own distinctions and categories. In recent decades, a uniform set of concepts has been negotiated, promoted, and enforced. The uniform diagnoses improve descriptive communication and meet administrative needs. However, they remain arbitrary. This essay argues that a descriptive theory of psychiatric problems should distinguish the objective pattern of correlation among the thoughts, feelings, and behaviors in question from the subjective view of them embodied in diagnoses. A map of correlations among psychiatric symptoms reveals a graded circular spectrum, analogous to a color wheel. The psychiatric types are *not* empirical islands in correlational space. They are subjective points of reference on a circular continuum. Problems that appear to be of one type shade into those that appear to be of another. Salient locations on the circle correspond to the following labels, in the following order: schizophrenia, alcoholism, autonomic arousal, sleep problems, emotional distress, fear and panic, paranoia, and back to schizophrenia.

The boundaries of psychiatric diagnoses are arbitrary, somewhat like lines of longitude and latitude superimposed on the earth's globe; even more like Munsell chips of just-noticeably-different colors superimposed on the visual continua of hue, value, and chroma. As I will show, the analogy between psychiatric problems and perceived colors is particularly apt. The questions one can ask about distinctions among mental illnesses parallel those about distinctions among colors. How many distinct colors are there? How many distinct mental illnesses? Where is the boundary between red and yellow? Where is the boundary between schizophrenia and depression? Are red and

Data presented in this paper were collected by Richard L. Hough and Dianne Timbers as part of the Life Change and Illness Research Project, supported by grants from the National Institute of Mental Health (NIMH-CER RO1-MH16108), the Hogg Foundation for Mental Health, and the University of Texas at El Paso. Requests for reprints should be sent to John Mirowsky, Ph.D., Department of Sociology, University of Illinois, 326 Lincoln Hall, 702 South Wright Street, Urbana, Illinois 61801.

pink the same color? Are depression and dysthymia the same problem? The theory of color also illustrates the kind of thinking that can lead psychiatric assessment out of its morass of distinctions. The neo-Kraepelineans are trying to pave the ground with reified diagnoses, yielding predictable results (Mirowsky and Ross, 1989a, 1989b). The subject matter continually shifts beneath the misplaced concreteness. A lighter step, guided by reference posts, may provide a surer means of traversing the ground.

What basis is there for saying that the boundaries of psychiatric diagnoses are arbitrary? Most of the evidence comes from the creators and proponents of diagnostic schemes. The task of negotiating and promulgating diagnostic standards was not brief or easy, and it is not finished. This essay begins with a brief history of the current official psychiatric diagnoses, describes the degree and sources of variability and uncertainty in the official scheme, maps the correlations among the symptoms on which diagnoses are based, discusses the relationship of diagnostic overlays to symptom patterns, and recommends a theory of psychiatric diagnosis that distinguishes objective patterns of symptoms from diagnostic overlays.

Origins and Validity of Contemporary Psychiatric Diagnoses

Chaotic Beginnings

The crisp "syndromes" described in diagnostic manuals are not distinct and characteristic collections of symptoms and signs that immediately impress themselves on the minds of clinical observers. They are official classifications laboriously negotiated over decades, promulgated by the American Psychiatric Association and the National Institute of Mental Health, and enforced through control of grants and reimbursements. Before the push to institute official standards in the late 1970s, there was little agreement on concepts, definitions, and diagnostic criteria. Rates of psychiatric rejection at World War II induction centers ranged from 0.5% to 50.6%, and the specific diagnoses selected at different sites were "bizarrely at odds (Robins, 1985, p. 919). The natural variety of diagnostic ideas and practices gave no hint of distinct, empirical syndromes with universal inter-observer validity. There were tantalizing broad similarities in the distinctions made, but nothing to suggest that the boundaries between one mental illness and another, or between mental illness and wellness, could be found in the observations themselves.

A Glimpse at Patterns

The late 1960s and early 1970s produced a wave of serious attempts to shape psychiatric diagnoses by reference to empirical syndromes. The results of those studies led psychiatric nosologists and epidemiologists to abandon objective patterns of correlation as a basis for discovering or evaluating diagnostic constructs. The studies of that era used exploratory factor analysis to search for syndromes. A factor is a set of symptoms and signs with two things in common: they covary among themselves more than with other symptoms and signs, and their profiles of correlations with other symptoms, signs, traits, statuses, etc. are similar. A syndrome is one of two things: either a distinct *combination* of symptoms known to result from a single cause, or a set of symptoms that occur together so commonly that they appear to constitute a distinct clinical picture. The first definition of a syndrome could not be applied because there was little knowledge of, and even less agreement about, the causes of psychiatric symptoms. Researchers turned to the second definition of a syndrome, which is very close to that of a factor.

A number of large studies collected uniform information on the symptoms of patients in psychiatric treatment. Factor analyses of the data revealed problems that clustered empirically, but did not correspond one-to-one with clinical diagnoses. For example, one group of researchers found that symptom patterns could be summarized in the following factors: inappropriate or bizarre appearance or behavior, belligerence and negativism, agitation and excitement, retardation and emotional withdrawal, speech disorganization, suspicion or a sense of persecution, hallucinations and delusions, grandiosity, depression and anxiety, tendency to suicide or self-mutilation, somatic concerns, social isolation, disorientation and memory problems, antisocial impulses or acts, drug abuse, and alcohol abuse (Endicott and Spitzer, 1972; Spitzer, Endicott, Fleiss, and Cohen, 1970; Spitzer, Fleiss, Endicott, and Cohen, 1967). On the whole these factors did not, and still do not, correspond to the diagnostic categories in fashion.

The factor analytic studies showed that clinical psychiatric categories are not empirical syndromes in one sense: they do not constitute distinct factors. In fact, the symptoms treated as attributes of each diagnostic category are drawn from a number of factors that often have little or no correlation with each other, and that often correlate equally well with a number of different diagnoses. The researchers might have tailored new diagnostic categories to reflect the empirical syndromes (that is, a diagnosis of bizarre appearance and behavior, of belligence and negativism, of agitation and excitement, etc). Instead they chose to save the traditional clinical categories by reinterpreting the results. The researchers showed that patients grouped by clinical diagnosis have distince profiles of average scores on the factors. For example, patients diagnosed as depressed *and* those diagnosed as paranoid schizophrenic have higher than average scores than others on indexes of agitation, anxiety, social isolation, thoughts of suicide, and depressed mood. The two diagnostic groups are distinguished from each other by higher than average scores among those diagnosed as paranoid schizophrenic on indexes of suspicion, belligerence, grandiosity, and bizarre behavior. By treating the clinical categories as *causes* of the symptom factors, the researchers presented each distinct factor profile as a syndrome in the first sense given above – as a distinct *combination* of symptoms known to result from a single cause.

There is a fallacy in interpreting the distinct factor profiles as evidence that the clinical categories are empirical syndromes. The fallacy is obvious to anyone not committed to psychiatric culture and thus not inclined to reify its categories. *Patients' symptoms are not caused by the categories through which their doctors perceive and organize symptoms* (except for the secondary problems resulting from labeling). Only someone who believes a psychiatric category is as real as a microorganism could see its factor profile as a distinct combination of symptoms resulting from a single cause. Anyone else would see the psychiatric category as an arbitrary subjective combination of factors. With 16 factors, treated for simplicity as present or absent, there are 65,536 possible clinical categories with distinct profiles. Each of the phantom categories not in use has just as much validity, by the test of having a distinct factor profile, as the relatively small number fashionable at any one time. The diagnostic categories exist in the subjective and interpretive culture of psychiatry, and not in the objective pattern of correlation among mental, emotional, and behavioral problems.

Marshaling Consensus

The growing realization that clinical diagnoses do not correspond to symptom factors led clinical researchers to abandon factor analysis as a means of validating or shaping diagnostic practice. Factor analysis was temporarily banished to community studies of so-called screening scales, and finally displaced altogether by approaches more congenial to psychiatric preconception. To do this successfully, it was necessary to hone and unify that preconception. The evolving strategy was to demonstrate "procedural validation" (Robins, 1985; Robins, Helzer, Ratcliff, and Seyfried, 1982) by building professional consensus and measuring it as inter-rater reliability. Several major research centers developed their own systems of diagnostic categories and criteria for use in their own clinical research (Weissman, Myers, and Ross, 1986). Committees of the American Psychiatric Association developed somewhat looser descriptions and criteria for clinical use (American Psychiatric Association, 1980). The National Institute of Mental Health contracted to develop a diagnostic protocol for use in a large, multi-city survey called the Epidemiologic Catchment Area (ECA) study. NIMH wanted the ECA protocol to reflect the existing systems. An NIMH committee reviewed the four major research instruments in use at the time, and brought together the researchers to hash out differences in definitions and criteria. Of the four research instruments considered, only one had been developed and validated using factor analysis. It was immediately eliminated from any further consideration because "its scales were based on internal consistency rather than approximating traditional clinical syndromes" (Robins, 1986, p. 415).

Clearly, the researchers and NIMH scientists realized they could not count on the objective patterns of correlation among symptoms to approximate traditional clinical syndromes. How, then, could they develop an instrument that would be accepted as valid by researchers and clinicians? The answer was to use inter-rater reliability as the measure of validity (Mirowsky and Ross, 1989a, 1989b). Inter-rater reliability measures the extent of agreement between two judges. Inter-rater reliability is notoriously low in psychiatric diagnosis, but it can be increased dramatically through the use of standardized interview schedules and rote diagnostic rules. Developers of ECA's *Diagnostic Interview Schedule* (DIS) labored to demonstrate that firm guidance and oversight can coax psychiatrists into a higher level of diagnostic agreement, and that a similar level of agreement can be induced between psychiatrists and lay interviewers operating under the same constraints (Robins, 1985; Robins et al., 1982).

The ingenuity of the "procedural validation" is that it sidesteps any reference to empirical correlation between symptoms, let alone deeper forms of validation. It is only necessary to get the judges to consider the same information and follow the same decision rules. The pieces of information do not have to be related, and the rules do not have to reflect anything more than the ability and willingness of the judges to use them. Take the medieval diagnosis of witchcraft as an example. Several highly respected inquisitors agree that witches may be known by three or more of the following signs: talking to animals, foul breath, avoiding churches and men of the cloth, walking on moonlit nights, and dancing alone. To validate the diagnostic category and criteria, we only need show that any pair of trained inquisitors using these signs and the three-or-more rule will agree on who is or is not a witch more frequently than expected by chance. The more the inquisitors follow these guidelines, the more they will find themselves in agreement, which will bolster professional use of the diagnostic system and public confidence in the profession's determinations.

Sharp Distinctions Along Fuzzy Boundaries
Between Uncertain Locations

Variability in the Clinic

Despite official psychiatry's strenuous efforts to promote uniformity, clinical diagnosis remains highly variable. Clinical studies show that the large majority of diagnostic categories have inadequate inter-rater reliability, with agree-ment less than 70% of that possible above random chance (Kutchins and Kirk, 1986). In all likelihood, agreement is even lower among psychiatrists not working at a research center and not having their diagnoses reviewed and compared. A study of actual diagnostic practice at a community mental health center found that the psychiatrists frequently criticized the official diagnostic system as rigid, inapplicable, or beside the point (Brown, 1987). Commonly, a specific diagnosis was chosen for its administrative effect from a list of diagnoses that seemed to fit about equally well. Clinical social workers who use official psychiatric diagnoses say they do so primarily for insurance pur-poses (Kutchins and Kirk, 1988). Most find the psychiatric diagnoses of little or no value for understanding and predicting clients' behavior or for plan-ning treatment. Most feel the diagnoses overlay medical labels on psycho-social problems, and particularly do not help in understanding marital and family problems. However, the great majority contend that the official diag-noses establish a common language to communicate about mental disorders. On the whole, clinicians seem to treat the official diagnoses as administrative pigeon holes and linguistic tags that do little to explain the nature and cause of problems, and that rarely provide an apt description of a patient's symp-toms and problems.

Variability in Research

Unlike clinicians, epidemiologists ask standard questions, record answers in a standard format, and use computers to make diagnoses according to highly explicit rules. As a consequence, epidemiologists achieve higher inter-rater reliability than clinicians. Evaluations of the diagnostic systems used by epidemiologists underscore the fact that the distinctions being made are not inherent in the pattern of observed symptoms, but rather exist in the minds that formulate the categories. First, each set of diagnostic rules is different from the others. Using the same data from the same set of patients, the four most commonly used sets of rules often disagree. Overall diagnostic agree-ment between systems is about 70% of the agreement possible above that due to chance (Robins, Helzer, Croughan, and Ratcliff, 1981). (The percent of agreement above chance is measured using the $\varkappa$ coefficient discussed by Kutchins and Kirk [1986].) Between NIMH's rules used in the ECA studies and the APA's clinical rules, agreement on who is depressed or schizophrenic is only about 65% of the agreement possible above that due to chance. Second, the more leeway psychiatrists are allowed in interviewing and judging, the lower the agreement between their diagnoses and those of a standardized pro-tocol, dropping to 19% for schizophrenia and from 25% to 50% for depres-sion (Anthony, Folstein, Romanoski, VonKorff, Nestadt, Chahal, Merchant,

Brown, Shapiro, Kramer, and Gruenberg, 1985; Helzer, Robins, McEvoy, Spitznagel, Stoltzman, Farmer, and Brockington, 1985). Every psychiatrist knows and recognizes depression and schizophrenia, yet diagnostic agreement among psychiatrists is remarkably low and consequently difficult to codify.

Overlapping Circles

The inherent fuzziness of psychiatric problems produces very high correlations between diagnoses. For example, the distinction between depression and schizophrenia is the most basic. Nevertheless, the odds of qualifying for a diagnosis of schizophrenia are 28.5 times greater among those who qualify for a diagnosis of major depression than among those who do not (Boyd, Burke, Gruenberg, Holzer, Rae, George, Karno, Stolzman, McEnvoy, and Nestadt, 1984). Odds ratios work both ways, so the opposite is also true: the odds of qualifying for a diagnosis of major depression are 28.5 times greater among those who qualify for a diagnoses of schizophrenia than among those who do not. In fact, qualifying for any one NIMH–ECA diagnosis increases the odds of qualifying for every other one. The multiples range from a low of 1.6 for alcoholism and somatization to a high of 89.1 for schizophrenia and mania, with the average of being 10.3 (geometric mean). (To put these values in perspective, the odds of qualifying for a diagnosis of schizophrenia are 3.4 times greater among those with a family history of mental disorder compared to those without [Link, Dohrenwend, and Skodol, 1986], and they are 7.8 times greater among those in the bottom 25% of socioeconomic status compared to those in the top 25% [Holzer, Shea, Swanson, Leaf, Myers, George, Weissman, and Bednarsky, 1986]). The odds of getting lung cancer are 14.0 times greater for those who smoke than for those who do not [Mausner and Bahn, 1974]). Clearly, the superimposed psychiatric categories overlap a great deal.

Several things account for the remarkably large odds ratios between diagnoses. One way or another, they all reflect the fact that the boundaries between disorders are superimposed, and not found in the phenomena themselves. First, a number of the most important causes or risk factors affect several different disorders. The most notable is low social status, which increases the odds of just about every disorder (e.g., Holzer et al., 1986). Also, a family history of one type of disorder increases the risk of developing other types (Boyd et al., 1984). Second, problems tend to cascade from one type to another, as when alcoholism results in depression and hallucinations, or when delusions lead to antisocial behavior (e.g., Kendell, 1988). Third, almost all psychiatric cases have in common the symptoms and signs of demoralization, which include dread, anxiety, sadness, feelings of helplessness and hopelessness, and poor self-esteem (Dohrenwend, Shrout, Egri, and Mendelson, 1980).

Rare or distinctive problems are accompanied by these common ones (Boyd et al., 1984). Fourth, the ideal types represented by diagnostic rules often share defining features with other types. For example, withdrawal is considered an attribute of both schizophrenia and depression, and delusions of grandeur are considered attributes of both schizophrenia and mania. Shared attributes increase the correlations among diagnoses.

In Between, Just Short of, and Left Over

The inherent fuzziness of psychiatric problems generates diagnostic categories defined as in between, just short of, or left over from other categories (American Psychiatric Association, 1980; Srole and Fischer, 1980). Categories defined as in between others cover the blend of primary categories, like naming orange the hue blending red and yellow. Schizoaffective disorder blends schizophrenia and depression. Paranoid schizophrenia blends paranoia and schizophrenia. Categories defined as just short of others cover variations in intensity, like calling pink the color red in hue but light and low in saturation. Dysthymia is just short of major depression. Cyclothymia is just short of major bipolar depression. Schizophreniform personality is just short of schizophreniform disorder, which is just short of schizophrenia. Finally, there are diagnoses for cases that cannot be classified with any degree of certainty as in between or just short of anything specific. They are designated "unspecified" if the case does not provide sufficient information for making a judgment, "residual" if the case does not fit any of the defined subcategories in a larger class, and "atypical" if a case does not quite meet the minimum criteria for one major class and instead blends aspects of others. These are the beige, taupe, heather and tweed of the diagnostic order.

A Circular Spectrum: Correlations from a Community Survey

A map of the correlations among symptoms provides the best illustration of why psychiatric categories are so blurry. The reason is that the problems on which diagnoses are based do not divide themselves neatly into distinct syndromes. Problems classified as one type mix with and shade into problems classified as another type. A map of the correlations also shows why there seem to be different types of problems, despite the difficulty of drawing clear boundaries between them. The reason is that the broadest psychiatric concepts represent salient loci on a circular gradient of problems, much like red, yellow and blue on a color wheel.

Mapping the 4,095 Correlations Among 91 Symptoms

Modern psychometric techniques can map the location and clusters of symptoms in correlational space. By definition, the correlation between two symptoms increases to the extent that the presence of one multiplies the odds of the presence of the other. The higher the correlation between two symptoms, and the more similar their profiles of correlation with other symptoms, the closer they are in correlational space.

To map correlations, a computer program begins by giving each symptom a random location. Then it measures the distance between all the pairs of locations and compares the distances to the respective correlations. If two symptoms are farther apart than their correlation says they should be, the program moves them closer together. If the symptoms are too close, the program moves them farther apart. The program keeps shuffling the points around until the fit of the distances to the correlations stops improving (Kruskal and Wish, 1978).

Figure 1 shows a map of 4,095 correlations among 91 of the most important psychiatric symptoms. Complete descriptions of them are in Table 1. The symptoms were chosen from standard research indexes and diagnostic questionnaires (Spitzer and Endicott, 1978; Wheaton, 1985). These are the symptoms on which psychiatric diagnosis is based. They represent the problems of the overwhelming majority of all patients seen and diagnosed by psychiatrists.

For most of the symptoms, individuals were asked how often they had it or how often it happened in the last 12 months. Seven of the symptoms are the interviewers' observations of behavior during the interview. Most people do not have, or rarely have, most of the symptoms. However, everyone has some of them, and every symptom is experienced frequently by at least some people.

The data come from a community survey of 463 people living in El Paso, Texas, and Juarez, Mexico, called the Life Stress and Illness Project (Burnam, Timbers, and Hough, 1984; Hough, Fairbank, and Garcia, 1976). This survey has, to our knowledge, the most complete list of symptoms of all forms of psychological problems of any community study. The respondents were selected by careful random-sampling. They represent the typical range of people living in El Paso and Juarez. Most people in the community have symptoms that range in severity from mild to moderate, although some have severe problems. Very few are psychiatric patients or have ever been psychiatric patients. All were interviewed in their homes, in English or Spanish depending on the person's preference. (One of the original purposes of the study was to find out if the pattern of correlations among symptoms depends on the subjects' language and culture. In these data, it does not. The patterns are essentially the same for the Mexicans as for the Anglos.)

In order to show the relationship of diagnostic concepts to the pattern of correlations, symptoms are classified into five main categories: depression, anxiety, schizophrenia, paranoia, and alcoholism. The assignment of symp-

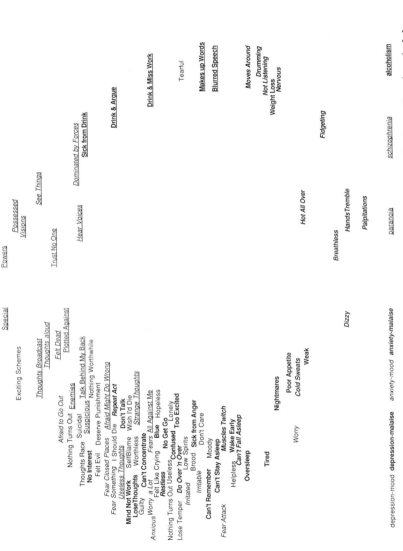

Figure 1. Map of the correlations of 91 psychiatric symptoms. See Table 1 for the wording of each item. Data from the Life Stress and Illness Research Project (Hough, Fairbank, and Garcia, 1976). This graph is reprinted with permission from *Social Causes of Psychological Distress* (Mirowsky and Ross, 1989c, pp. 42 and 43) [Copyright ©1989 by Aldine de Gruyter.]

Table 1

List of Symptoms Mapped in Figure 1, Categorized by Psychiatric Diagnosis

---

Schizophrenia

Dominated by forces: felt that your mind was dominated by forces beyond your control

Hear voices: heard voices without knowing where they came from

See things: seen things or animals or people around you that others did not see

Visions: had visions or seen things other people say they cannot see

Possessed: felt that you were possessed by a spirit or devil

Special powers: felt you had special powers

Felt dead: felt that you did not exist at all, that you were dead, dissolved

Thoughts aloud: seemed to hear your thoughts spoken aloud — almost as if someone standing nearby could hear them

Thoughts broadcast: felt that your unspoken thoughts were being broadcast or transmitted, so that everyone knew what you were thinking

Afraid might do wrong: felt afraid that you might do something seriously wrong against your own will

Strange thoughts: had unusual thoughts that kept bothering you

Useless thoughts: had useless thoughts that kept running through your mind

Paranoia

Trust no one: felt it was safer to trust no one

Plotted against: believed you were being plotted against

Talk behind back: felt that people were saying all kinds of things about you behind your back

Enemies: felt you had enemies who really wished to do you harm

Suspicious: been very suspicious, didn't trust anybody

All against me: been sure that everyone was against you

Depression-mood

Nothing worthwile: wondered if anything was worthwhile anymore

Suicidal: thought about taking your own life

Nothing turns out: felt that nothing turned out for you the way you wanted it to

Deserve punishment: felt you deserved to be punished

Should die: felt that others would be better off if you were dead

Felt evil: felt that you have done something evil or wrong

Wish I'd die: wished you were dead

Worthless: felt very bad or worthless

Self blame: blamed yourself for something that went wrong

Hopeless: felt completely hopeless about everything

Lonely: felt lonely

Felt like crying: felt like crying

Guilty; felt guilty about things you did or did not do

Useless: felt useless

Lose temper: lost your temper

Low spirits: been in low spirits

Brood: brooded over unpleasant thoughts or feelings

Don't care: just didn't care what happened to you

Moody: been moody and unhappy

Helpless: felt completely helpless

Tearful: the respondent cried or was tearful

(Manic)

Exciting schemes: had times when exciting new ideas and schemes occurred to you one after another

Thoughts race: became so excited that your thoughts raced ahead faster than you could speak them

Table 1 continued

List of Symptoms Mapped in Figure 1, Categorized by Psychiatric Diagnosis

Depression-malaise

Don't talk: became very quiet and didn't talk to anyone
No interest: shown no interest in anything or anybody
Can't concentrate: had trouble concentrating or keeping your mind on what you were doing
Lose thoughts: kept loosing your train of thought
Mind not work: felt that your mind did not work as well as it used to
Blue: had periods of feeling blue or depressed that interfered with your daily activity
No get go: had periods of days or weeks when you couldn't take care of things because you couldn't "get going"
Confused: felt confused; had trouble thinking
Sick from anger: got angry and afterward felt uncomfortable, like getting headaches, stomach pains, cold sweats and things like that
Can't remember: began having trouble remembering things
Can't stay asleep: had trouble staying asleep
Wake early: had trouble with waking up early and not being able to fall asleep again
Oversleep: had trouble with oversleeping; that is, sleeping past the time you wanted to get up
Tired: troubled by feeling tired all the time
Nightmares: been bothered by nightmares
Poor appitite: had poor appetite
Weak: felt weak all over
Weight loss: experienced any weight loss of 10 lbs. (5 kg) or more over the past year, without going on special diets

(Manic)
Too excited: felt so great (excited, talkative or active) that it was difficult to concentrate

Anxiety-mood

Worry a lot: worried a lot about little things
Anxious: felt anxious about something or someone
Irritated: got easily irritated
Worry: I am a person who is the worrying type

(Panic)
Afraid to go out: felt afraid to leave the house because you were afraid something might happen to it
Fear closed places: been afraid to be in closed places
Fear something: feared something terrible would happen to you
Fears: had special fears that kept bothering you
Fear attack: feared being robbed, attacked, or physically injured

Anxiety-malaise

(Autonomic)
Muscles twitch: had trouble with your muscles twitching or jumping
Can't fall asleep: had trouble falling asleep
Cold sweats: had cold sweats
Dizzy: had dizziness
Breathless: had shortness of breath when you were not exercising or working hard
Hands tremble: had your hands tremble
Palpitations: had your heart beating hard when you were not exercising or working hard
Hot all over: suddenly feel hot all over

Table 1 continued

List of Symptoms Mapped in Figure 1, Categorized by Psychiatric Diagnosis

Anxiety-malaise continued

(Behavioral)

Restless: had periods of such great restlessness that you could not sit in a chair for very long
Fidgeting: the respondent kept fidgeting and squirming
Nervous: the respondent appeared nervous and fidgety
Not listening: the content of the respondent's answers often have little or nothing to do with the questions asked
Drumming: the respondent drums on surfaces with fingers or taps on floor
Moves around: the respondent kept getting up and moving around restlessly

(Obsessive)

Repeat act: had to repeat an act over and over again though it is hard to explain to others why you did it
Do over 'n over: found yourself doing the same things over and over again to be sure they were right

Alcoholism

Blurred speech: the respondent's speech was blurred
Makes up words: the respondent makes up new words
Drink and miss work: missed work or been late to work because of drinking
Drink and argue: had arguments with your family because of your drinking
Sick from drink: had trouble with your health because of drinking

---

toms to categories follows standard research and diagnostic practice (American Psychiatric Association, 1980; Wheaton, 1985). Symptoms of depression and anxiety are further subdivided into mood (feelings) and malaise (bodily states).

Reading the Map

The map shows a circular gradient of correlation. There are salient loci that suggest some of the standard psychiatric distinctions, such as paranoia, schizophrenia, and alcoholism. The psychiatric types are *not* empirical islands in correlational space. They are subjective points of reference on the circular continuum. Proglems that appear to be of one type shade into those that appear to be of another.

Viewers of the map are likely to share some rough, common perceptions of the primary loci and major distinctions. Each viewer also is likely to have a unique sense of the number and location of primary loci, and of the boundaries between them. The distinctions in Table 2 represent the author's reading of the map.

The map of symptom correlations illustrates the relationship of objective patterns to official diagnostic constructs and to individual differences in the perception of disorders. The symptoms representing the core of a specific official diagnosis, such as schizophrenia, concentrate in a particular region

Table 2

Author's View of Salient Loci on the Map of Symptom Correlations (Figure 1)

Primary Type	Clock Location	Clock Range
Schizophrenia	12:00	11:00 - 1:00
Alcoholism	2:45	2:00 - 3:00
Autonomic arousal	5:30	4:00 - 7:00
Sleep problems	8:00	7:30 - 8:30
Emotional distress	9:00	8:30 - 9:30
Fear and panic	10:00	9:30 - 10:30
Paranoia	10:45	10:30 - 11:00
Schizophrenia	12:00	11:00 - 1:00

of the circular spectrum. However, they also blend into adjacent regions, and some appear far from the main concentration. A researcher interpreting the pattern of correlations tends to see a number of distinct salient locations. The individual's distinctions roughly correspond to official psychiatric constructs because of two things: the concentration of apparently similar symptoms near specific loci, and trained predisposition to subdivide the spectrum along traditional lines. On the other hand, an individual researcher's distinctions would rarely coincide exactly with official ones, or with those of another researcher. Because the symptoms do not form isolated islands in the correlational space, the number of salient loci and the boundaries between them can vary considerably from observer to observer. This explains why the traditional diagnoses can seem to have inter-observer validity despite low diagnostic concordance and despite drifting fashions in diagnostic rules.

Designing Better Concepts and Measures

The traditional categorical form of thinking inherited by psychiatry from medicine provides the poorest possible means of representing mental, emotional, and behavioral problems. Each diagnosis is an arbitrary subjective combination of problems from multicible loci in correlational space. Developing, promoting, and enforcing the use of official combinations does not make them any less arbitrary. It creates an illusion of objectivity and concreteness. The illusion may suit the institutional needs of insurance companies, government agencies, and the medical profession. The danger is that it discourages the development of non-diagnostic concepts and measures that are more efficient, flexible, and exact for scientific and clinical purposes.

Contemporary psychiatric epidemiology illustrates some of the problems with diagnostic concepts and measures. The ECA studies estimate the prevalence and socio-demographic patterns of various diagnoses in the population.

What does it mean to say that X% of the population has a combination of problems from multiple locations in correlational space that fits the arbitrary but official definition of a traditional psychiatric concept? Any desired prevalence can be estimated by adjusting the decision rules over a wide range of equally plausible and acceptable ones. How is it possible to predict the risk factors for membership in a class that is a just-noticeably-different subjective combination of problems from disparate locations in correlational space? The only consistently detectable risk factors must be ones that increase all kinds of problems regardless of their location in the space (factors such as low income, low education, and a family history of problems). Arbitrary prevalence and obscured patterns of risk are a poor scientific yield.

The circular spectrum suggests concepts and measures that avoid problems created by overlapping, arbitrary, and reified diagnoses. Rather than categorize individuals, researchers and clinicians can assess each person's severity of problems of various types. Each type of problem is a salient location on the spectrum. A type of problem is represented by an index composed of items in or near the location that appear similar and distinctive. The types are subjective, but their locations are not. The correlation between types of problems represents the proximity of their central locations, which is partly objective (based on symptom locations) and partly subjective (based on how one divides the spectrum). Severity is the frequency or duration of problems in a location. Severity is represented by the average frequency or duration of problems of a particular type.

An individual's profile of index scores can be thought of in several ways. One way is as arrows pointing from the center of the circle toward the salient locations represented by each type. The length of each arrow reflects the severity of its type of symptom. Another way is as gradations of saturation or shading that vary from one location to another on the rim of the circle.

Risk factors can be represented in the correlational space, too. One way is to draw a small symbol at each symptom's location, varying the symbol according to the symptom's correlation with a risk factor. For example, the symbols for Mars and Venus can represent symptoms more common among men and women respectively. Alternately, the correlation between a risk factor and different types of symptoms can be represented as arrows of varying length pointing from the center toward the location of each type.

Thinking of psychiatric problems as locations on the spectrum of problems eliminates the confusion introduced by subjective categorical distinctions and combinations. Although some researchers and clinicians may prefer graphic representations, many will prefer index scores. The important thing is to break the constraints of categorical diagnostic *concepts*. Doing so has three main advantages. First, it eliminates the confusion between types of problems and types of people. It does this by not categorizing people. Second, it explicitly distinguishes the objective pattern of correlations among problems from the subjective division of problems into noticeably different types. Third, it encourages us to wonder why the pattern is as it is, and why we see it as we do.

The third advantage brings us back to color theory as a model for developing a theory of psychiatric disorder. Color theory has three parts: a physical theory of energy waves that include visible light, a biological theory of the anatomy and physiology of human vision, and a psychophysical theory of color phenomena. The three main parts of the theory developed together over a period of centuries. The links among the components are particularly revealing. For example, violet and purple appear similar, but they are at opposite ends of the physical spectrum. The similarity is purely in our visual system. Likewise, the fact that all colors can be mixed from three primary colors (plus black) is built into our visual system. It reflects the fact that our color receptors have maximum sensitivity at three distinct wavelengths of light. Much of the power of color theory comes from distinguishing and linking the physical, biological, and subjective.

In building a theory of psychiatric problems, we need to distinguish various components. One is the pattern of correlation among problems. Another is the set of systems that produce the pattern of correlations. Locations in the correlational space may represent organic structures such as the adrenal glands, biochemical processes such as the synaptic release and uptake of norepinepherine, behavioral systems such as learned helplessness, or cultural systems such as sex roles. Another element is the way people with what we call psychiatric problems perceive and experience their thoughts, feelings, and behaviors. The final element is the way that friends, family, the community, and professionals think about and respond to problems. In the final analysis, a problem is only a problem because someone says it is. Who? On what basis? For what reason? A good theory of psychiatric problems must distinguish the thoughts, feelings, and behaviors addressed by psychiatry from the psychiatric view of them.

References

American Psychiatric Association. (1980). *Diagnostic and statistical manual of mental disorders* (third edition). Washington, D.C.: American Psychiatric Association.

Anthony, J.D., Folstein, M., Romanoski, A.J., VonKorff, M.R., Nestadt, G.R., Chahal, R., Merchant, A., Brown, C.H., Shapiro, S., Kramer, M., and Gruenberg, E.M. (1985). Comparison of the lay Diagnostic Interview Schedule and a standardized psychiatric diagnosis: Experience in eastern Baltimore. *Archives of General Psychiatry, 42*, 667-675.

Boyd, J.H., Burke, J.D., Gruenberg, E., Holzer, C.E., Rae, D.S., George, L.K., Karno, M., Stolzman, R., McEnvoy, L., and Nestadt, G. (1984). Exclusion criteria of DSM-III: A study of co-occurrence of hierarchy-free syndromes. *Archives of General Psychiatry, 41*, 983-989.

Brown, P. (1987). Diagnostic conflict and contradiction in psychiatry. *Journal of Health and Social Behavior, 28*, 37-50.

Burnam, M.A., Timbers, D.M., and Hough, R.L. (1984). Two measures of psychological distress among Mexican Americans, Mexicans, and Anglos. *Journal of Health and Social Behavior, 25,* 24–33.

Dohrenwend, B.P., Shrout, P.E., Egri, G.G., and Mendelson, F.S. (1980). Nonspecific psychological distress and other dimensions of psychopathology. *Archives of General Psychiatry, 37,* 1229–1236.

Endicott, J., and Spitzer, R.L. (1972). What! Another rating scale? The Psychiatric Evaluation Form. *The Journal of Nervous and Mental Disease, 154,* 88–104.

Helzer, J.E., Robins, L.N., McEvoy, L.T., Spitznagel, E.L., Stoltzman, R.Z., Farmer, A., and Brockington, I.F. (1985). A comparison of clinical and Diagnostic Interview Schedule diagnosis: Physician reexamination of lay-interviewed cases in the general population. *Archives of General Psychiatry, 42,* 657–666.

Holzer, C.E. III, Shea, B.M., Swanson, J.W., Leaf, P.J., Myers, J.K., George, L., Weissman, M.M., and Bednarski, P. (1986). The increased risk for specific psychiatric disorders among persons of low socioeconomic status: Evidence from the Epidemiological Catchment Area surveys. *American Journal of Social Psychiatry, 6,* 259–271.

Hough, R.L., Fairbank, D.T., and Garcia, A.M. (1976). Problems in the ratio meaasurement of life stress. *Journal of Health and Social Behavior, 17,* 70–82.

Kendell, R.E. (1988). What is a case? Food for thought for epidemiologists. *Archives of General Psychiatry, 45,* 374–376.

Kruskal, J.B., and Wish, M. (1978). *Multidimensional scaling.* Beverly Hills: Sage.

Kutchins, H., and Kirk, S.A. (1986). The reliability of DSM-III: A critical review. *Social Work Research and Abstracts, Winter,* 3–12.

Kutchins, H., and Kirk, S.A. (1988). The business of diagnosis: DSM-III and clinical social work. *Social Work, 33,* 215–220.

Link, B.G., Dohrenwend, B.P., and Skodol, A.E. (1986). Socio-economic status and schizophrenia: Noisome occupational characteristics as a risk factor. *American Sociological Review, 51,* 242–258.

Mausner, J.S., and Bahn, A.K. (1974). *Epidemiology: An introductory text.* Philadelphia: W.B. Saunders.

Mirowsky, J., and Ross, C.E. (1989a). Psychiatric diagnosis as reified measurement. *Journal of Health and Social Behavior, 30,* 11–25.

Mirowsky, J., and Ross, C.E. (1989b). Rejoinder – assessing the type and severity of psychological problems: An alternative to diagnosis. *Journal of Health and Social Behavior, 30,* 38–40.

Mirowsky, J., and Ross, C.E. (1989c). *Social causes of psychological distress.* New York: Aldine-de-Gruyter.

Robins, L.N. (1985). Epidemiology: Reflections on testing the validity of psychiatric interviews. *Archives of General Psychiatry, 42,* 918–924.

Robins, L.N. (1986). The development and characteristics of the NIMH Diagnostic Interview Schedule. In M.M. Weissman, J.K. Myers, and C.E. Ross (Eds.), *Community surveys of psychiatric disorders* (pp. 402–427). New Brunswick, New Jersey: Rutgers University Press.

Robins, L.N., Helzer, J.E., Croughan, J., and Ratcliff, W. (1981). National Institute of Mental Health Diagnostic Interview Schedule. *Archives of General Psychiatry, 38,* 381–389.

Robins, L.N., Helzer, J.E., Ratcliff, K.S., and Seyfried, W. (1982). Validity of the Diagnostic Interview Schedule, version II: DSM-III diagnoses. *Psychological Medicine, 12,* 855–870.

Spitzer, R., and Endicott, J. (1978). *Schedule for affective disroders and schizophrenia.* New York: Biometric Division, Evaluation Section, New York Psychiatric Institute.

Spitzer, R.L., Endicott, J., Fleiss, J.L., and Cohen, J. (1970). The Psychiatric Status Schedule: A technique for evaluating psychopathology and impairment of role functioning. *Archives of General Psychiatry, 23,* 41–55.

Spitzer, R.L., Fleiss, J.L., Endicott, J., and Cohen, J. (1967). Mental Status Schedule: Properties of factor-analytically derived scales. *Archives of General Psychiatry, 16,* 479–493.

Srole, L., and Fisher, A.K. (1980). To the editor. *Archives of General Psychiatry, 37,* 1424–1426.

Weissman, M.M., Myers, J.K., and Ross, C.E. (1986). *Community surveys of psychiatric disorders.* New Brunswick, New Jersey: Rutgers University Press.

Wheaton, B. (1985). Personal resources and mental health: Can there be too much of a good thing? In J.R. Greenley (Ed.), *Research in community and mental health* (pp. 139–184). Greenwich, Connecticut: JAI.

©1990 The Institute of Mind and Behavior, Inc.
The Journal of Mind and Behavior
Summer and Autumn 1990, Volume 11, Numbers 3 and 4
Pages 425 [179] – 464 [218]
ISSN 0271-0137
ISBN 0-930195-05-1

Brain Damage, Dementia and Persistent Cognitive Dysfunction Associated With Neuroleptic Drugs: Evidence, Etiology, Implications

Peter R. Breggin

Center for the Study of Psychiatry and George Mason University

Several million people are treated with neuroleptic medications (major tranquilizers or antipsychotics) in North America each year. A large percentage of these patients develop a chronic neurologic disorder — tardive dyskinesia — characterized by abnormal movements of the voluntary muscles. Most cases are permanent and there is no known treatment. Evidence has been accumulating that the neuroleptics also cause damage to the highest centers of the brain, producing chronic mental dysfunction, tardive dementia and tardive psychosis. These drug effects may be considered a mental equivalent of tardive dyskinesia. Relevant data are derived from human autopsies, brain imaging (CT, MRI and PET scans), neuropsychological tests, and clinical research. That the neuroleptics can damage higher brain centers is confirmed by their known neurotoxicity and neurophysiological impact, animal autopsies, and a comparison to diseases that mimic neuroleptic effects, such as Huntington's chorea and lethargic encephalitis. Patients and the public should be informed of the danger of both tardive dyskinesia and tardive dementia. The mental health professions should severely limit the use of neuroleptics and develop safer and better alternatives to these dangerous substances.

The neuroleptics, also known as major tranquilizers or antipsychotics, are among the most widely used drugs in psychiatry. In the United States and Canada alone, millions of adults and children receive these medications in general hospitals, private and public mental hospitals, board and care homes, institutions for the developmentally disabled, nursing homes, prisons, clinics and private practice. While the medications are most often advocated for patients diagnosed as schizophrenic or manic, they are in fact widely used as a method of social control. In many institutions, most of the inmates will be receiving them (Breggin, 1983).

Wade Hudson, Research Associate at the Center for the Study of Psychiatry (1988–89), was involved in the final stages of research for this project, which would not have been completed without his help. Requests for reprints should be sent to Peter R. Breggin, M.D., Center for the Study of Psychiatry, 4628 Chestnut Street, Bethesda, Maryland 20814.

It is now widely recognized that the neuroleptics frequently produce a largely irreversible neurological disease, tardive dyskinesia, in a significant number of patients. New evidence is accumulating that the same drugs can also cause persistent damage or dysfunction to the highest centers of the brain, resulting in irreversible intellectual and emotional impairments, including tardive dementia and tardive psychosis. These effects may be viewed as the mental equivalent to tardive dyskinesia.

Although concerns about neuroleptic-induced damage to the highest centers of the brain have been voiced for more than a decade (Marsden, 1976), it was not until 1983 that the subject was analyzed in depth (Breggin, 1983, pp. 110–146). Since then, a considerable amount of relevant evidence has been published. In the first part of this article, I will review evidence of cognitive deficits, dementia and atrophy in neuroleptic-treated patients. In the second part I will explore the etiology.

The term dementia will be used as defined in the *Diagnostic and Statistical Manual of Mental Disorders* (third edition, revised, American Psychiatric Association [APA], 1987) [DSM-III-R]: "The essential feature of Dementia is impairment in short- and long-term memory, associated with impairment in abstract thinking, impaired judgment, other disturbances of higher cortical function, or personality change" (p. 103). The DSM-III-R states "As in all Organic Mental Syndromes, an underlying causative organic factor is always assumed" (p. 103). Acute drug-induced disorders that can cause brain damage and impair mental function, such as neuroleptic malignant syndrome or toxic psychoses, will not be considered in this article which deals with more gradually evolving persistent brain damage and dysfunction associated with chronic exposure to neuroleptics.

Reliance upon the neuroleptics for the treatment of acute schizophrenia is almost universal in psychiatry and most psychiatrists use them as the first line of treatment in these cases (see any recent textbook of psychiatry, for example, Nicholi, 1988; or Talbott, Hales, and Yudofsky, 1988). Occasional criticism of their use has been made (Breggin, 1983; Cohen and Cohen, 1986; Mosher and Burti, 1989). I have documented that the neuroleptics have no specific ameliorative effect on any mental disorder and that they are nonspecific brain-disabling agents that perform a chemical lobotomy, in part through disruption of dopamine neurotransmission in the limbic and frontal lobe pathways (Breggin, 1983). The drugs do not cure a disorder but instead flatten the emotions, produce disinterest or apathy, and enforce docility. In a controlled study, Mosher and Burti (1989) demonstrated that almost all patients undergoing their first schizophrenic episode can be treated more successfully without neuroleptics than with them.

Terms like schizophrenia and schizophreniform, based on DSM-III or DSM-III-R, are used largely without reservation in most of the studies reviewed, and I have adopted this language for convenience in communicating. Several fundamental assumptions behind this classification – including the disease model – create a bias toward believing that a supposedly medical disease, schizophrenia, has caused the physical disorders found in the brains of these patients. This built-in bias should not distract us from properly evaluating the etiology of the damage. In my own opinion, schizophrenia is neither genetic nor physical in origin (Breggin, in press). The lay term, madness, is more appropriate to this psychosocial phenomenon. I have suggested alternative explanations elsewhere (Breggin, 1980d, in press).

Evidence from Studies of Drug-Treated Patients

Background: Tardive Dyskinesia

In a large percentage of patients the neuroleptic medications produce a neurologic disorder called tardive dyskinesia [TD]. The disease, characterized by abnormal involuntary movements, can manifest itself after a few weeks or months. More commonly it develops after six months to two years or more of treatment. In the majority of cases it is irreversible and there is no effective treatment. If it is detected early and the medications are discontinued, an estimated 20–50% of patients may greatly improve or recover (APA, 1980). However, a recent report indicated that among patients with persistent TD, followed for a period of 5 years, 82% showed no overall significant change, 11% improved, and 7% became worse (Bergen, Eyland, Campbell, Jenkings, Kellehear, Richards, and Beumont, 1989).

TD often begins with uncontrolled movements of the face, including the tongue, lips, mouth and cheeks; but it can start with almost any group of muscles. The most common early sign is a quivering or curling of the tongue. Tongue protrusions and chewing movements are also common, and can become serious enough to harm teeth. The hands and feet, arms and legs, neck, back and torso can be involved. The movements displayed are highly variable, and include writhing contortions, tics, spasms, and tremors. The person's gait can be badly impaired. More subtle functions can be affected and are easily overlooked: respiration (involving the diaphragm), swallowing (involving the pharyngeal and esophageal musculature), the gag relflex, and speech (Yassa and Jones, 1985). The movements disappear during sleep. They sometimes can be partially suppressed by willpower and frequently are made worse by anxiety. They can vary from time to time.

Many cases of TD appear to be relatively mild, often limited to movements of the tongue, mouth, jaw, face, or eyelids. Nonetheless, they are disfiguring and often embarrassing. A rare case is totally disabling and patients have been known to commit suicide (Yassa and Jones, 1985).

There is increasing awareness of two related variants of TD, tardive dystonia and tardive akathisia. Tardive dystonia involves "sustained involuntary twisting movements, generally slow, which may affect the limbs, trunk, neck, or face" (Burke, Fahn, Jankovic, Marsden, Lang, Gollomp, and Ilson, 1982, p. 1335). It can produce cramp-like, painful spasms that temporarily prevent the individual from carrying out normal activities. Tardive akathisia involves a feeling of inner tension or anxiety that drives the individual into restless activity, such as pacing (Jeste, Wisniewski, and Wyatt, 1986).

Recognition of TD's existence became widespread in 1973 with the publication of reports by George Crane and by the American College of Neuropsycopharmacology–Food and Drug Administration Task Force. In the same year, the *Physician's Desk Reference* (*PDR*, see Thorazine) began to include persistent dyskinesias among neuroleptic side-effects and reports began to flood the psychiatric literature.

In 1980 the APA produced a detailed analysis of the disease in its *Task Force Report: Tardive Dyskinesia*. It made clear that TD is a serious, usually irreversible, untreatable, and highly prevalent disease resulting from therapy with the neuroleptics. The *Task Force* estimated the prevalence rate for TD in routine treatment (several months to two years) as *at least* 10–20% for *more than minimal disease*. For older and chronically exposed patients, the rate was at least 40% for more than minimal disease. A recent study of elderly nursing home patients found that 41% developed tardive dyskinesia over a period of only twenty-four months and that none fully recovered (Yassa, Nastase, Camille, and Belzile, 1988). While long-term studies have found a spontaneous dyskinesia prevalence of 1–5% in the elderly, none of the non-drug treated controls developed spontaneous dyskinesias during the two years.

As high as the *Task Force* rates are, a number of studies indicate that the rates may in fact be still higher, especially in older and long-term patients for whom the prevalence may exceed 50% (see APA, 1980, Table 9, p. 50; reviewed in Breggin, 1983). Furthermore, there is general agreement in the literature that for unknown reasons the overall rates of tardive dyskinesia have been increasing in recent years (Jeste and Wyatt, 1980, p. 27); this suggests that the *Task Force* figures have been eclipsed by increasing rates.

As an exception to the usually higher prevalence estimates, Jeste and Wyatt (1982) estimated a prevalence rate of only 13%; but they obtained this lower estimate by two most unusual manipulations of the data. First, they excluded all minimal and mild cases, and included only moderate and severe ones (pp. 22–23), even though most studies indicate that the great majority cases are in fact minimal or mild (APA, 1980, p. 45). Thus they excluded most cases from consideration. Second, the authors assumed that one-fourth of the remaining cases did not have drug-induced dyskinesias (p. 32), even though they themselves cite studies indicating that the pre-drug era rate of dyskinesias was as low as 0.5% (p. 16). Without their severe pruning of the data, the prevalence rates derived from Jeste and Wyatt's data would surpass 25% by a considerable amount. On the other hand, even a rate of 13% for a moderate to severe treatment-induced neurological disease constitutes an iatrogenic disaster.

Children are susceptible to a particularly virulent form of TD with truncal involvement that can interfere with posture and locomotion (Breggin, 1983; Gualtieri and Barnhill, 1988; Gualtieri, Quade, Hicks, Mayo, and Schroeder, 1984; Gualtieri, Schroeder, Hicks, and Quade, 1986).

In 1985 the Food and Drug Administration (FDA) took the unusual step of setting specifically worded requirements for a warning in association with all neuroleptic advertising ("Neuroleptics," 1985). In a wholly unprecedented move, in the same year the APA sent out a warning letter about the dangers of tardive dyskinesia to its entire membership.

Various authors have noted that cases of dyskinesia were reported among psychiatric patients prior to the neuroleptic era. However, the APA's *Task Force on Tardive Dyskinesia* (1980, pp. 47–48), as well as Jeste and Wyatt (1982, pp. 15–20), and others have concluded that the particular syndrome of TD is a product of the drug era. TD is recognized as a disease produced by neuroleptics in all contemporary textbooks of psychiatry (e.g., Nicholi, 1988; Talbott, Hales, and Yudofsky, 1988).

It is difficult to determine the total number of TD cases. Van Putten (see Lund, 1989) recently estimated 400,000–1,000,000 cases in the United States. My own estimate is higher, ranging in the several millions (Breggin, 1983). It is no exaggeration to call tardive dyskinesia a widespread epidemic and possibly the worst medically-induced castastrophe in history.

Neuroleptic-Induced Persistent or Permanent Damage to the Highest Centers of the Brain

Evidence is accumulating that there are higher-brain and mental function equivalents to TD in the form of damage in the limbic system and frontal lobes, with associated persistent mental dysfunction.

Brain Atrophy and Associated Mental Deficits from Brain Imaging Studies

In one of the earliest studies attempting to measure cerebral atrophy in neuroleptic-treated schizophrenic patients, Sabuncu, Sabacin, Saygill, Kumral, and Ornek (1977) used pneumoencephalography (PEG) to show enlarged ventricles. Other PEG studies have demonstrated similar findings, but we shall focus on the newer and more sophisticated brain imaging techniques.

Many studies involving computerized axial tomography (CT scans) of schizophrenic patients, nearly all of them neuroleptic-treated, have found enlarged lateral ventricles and sometimes enlarged sulci, indicating shrinkage or atrophy of the brain. The ventricles tend to expand in proportion to tissue shrinkage within the confines of the skull. The sulci deepen or enlarge when there is shrinkage of the cerebral cortex. Enlargement of the lateral ventricles is the most common finding in CT studies of drug-treated schizophrenic patients.

Johnstone and his colleagues (Johnstone, Crow, Frith, Husband, and Kreel, 1976; Johnstone, Crow, Frith, Stevens, Kreel, and Husband, 1978) were among the first researchers to show increased ventricular size on CT scan of schizophrenic patients. They also found mental impairment on the *Withers and Hinton Test* and the *Inglis Paired Association Learning Test*. Weinberger, Cannon-Spoor, Potkin, and Wyatt (1980) and Weinberger, Torrey, Neophytides, and Wyatt (1979) found increased ventricular size in schizophrenic patients, nearly all of whom had been treated with drugs. Jeste, Wagner, Weinberger, Reith, and Wyatt (1980) found no difference on a CT scan between a TD group and a matched control group of neuroleptic-treated patients without TD. Both groups were chronic inmates (mean duration 33.5 years) with many years of neuroleptic therapy. Famuyiwa, Eccleston, Donaldson, and Garside (1979) found cerebral atrophy on CT scan in schizophrenic patients with and without TD, and also found an increased rate of dementia compared to controls, especially among TD patients. On the *Withers and Hinton* and the *Inglis Paired Association Learning Test* they found increased mental dysfunction. Golden, Moses, Zelazowski, Graber, Zatz, Horvath, and Berger (1980) found brain atrophy on CT scan in neuroleptic-treated schizophrenics and correlated it with mental dysfunction on the *Luria-Nebraska* battery.

DeMeyer, Gilmore, DeMeyer, Hendrie, Edwards, and Franco (1984) found that third ventricle size was correlated with both length of illness and length of neuroleptic treatment. In a second study, DeMeyer, Gilmore, Hendrie, DeMeyer, and Franco (1984) reviewed the CT literature on measurements of brain tissue density rather than ventricular size, and found several studies which demonstrated a loss of density in drug-treated schizophrenics. In their own research they found a loss of density among neuroleptic-treated schizophrenic patients compared to unmedicated hospital controls, as well as a direct correlation with mental impairment as measured by psychological tests.

Lawson, Waldman, and Weinberger (1988) studied twenty-seven schizophrenic patients with the CT and with neuropsychological batteries, including the *WAIS* and *Halstead-Reitan*. They found enlarged ventricles or cortical atrophy in twelve of the patients. Their study revealed a significant correlation between cognitive impairment on the psychological batteries and brain damage. The patients with cerebral abnormalities averaged more than nine years in duration of illness with long-term exposure to neuroleptics and other psychotropic drugs. As in other studies, no correlation was found between the damage and the degree of schizophrenic pathology. Also in 1988, Shelton, Karson, Doran, Pitkar, Bigelow, and Weinberger found prefrontal atrophy in schizophrenics.

Thus far nearly all studies demonstrating cerebral atrophy involved patients heavily treated with neuroleptics, and sometimes with electroshock and other brain-disabling regimens (see Breggin, 1979, for a review of brain damage from electroshock). Two studies that have evaluated relatively young and relatively untreated patients have found enlarged ventricles, and several others have not.

Weinberger, DeLisi, Perman, Targum, and Wyatt (1982) reported enlarged ventricles in seven of thirty-five (20%) of "first-episode schizophreniform disorders." Of these seven with abnormalities, five had scans within two weeks of their initial exposure to neuroleptic drugs, the other two within four weeks. The study found a similar rate of ventricular enlargement in chronic schizophrenic patients (four of seventeen or 23.5%). Twelve patients in their experimental group had already been given CT scans "because of a suspicion of 'organicity.' " This could raise questions about the composition of the group, but only one of twelve had enlarged ventricles. There was no correlation between ventricular enlargement and duration of treatment or illness. The investigators labelled their CT criteria as "suggestive of CNS abnormality."

Schulz, Koller, Kishore, Hamer, Gehl, and Friedel (1983) studied 15 teenage patients, including twelve schizophrenic and three schizophreniform. The patients had been ill for less than two years. Of the fifteen patients, eight were found to have enlarged ventricles. Ten of the patients had never received neuroleptics, and six of these had enlarged ventricles. As in Weinberger et al. (1982), there was no correlation between length of treatment or illness and CT abnormalities.

The above two studies are frequently cited as conclusive evidence that enlarged ventricles are found in untreated patients and that therefore the abnormalities are not due to medication. Anticipating more extensive discussion ahead, three points can be made.

First, other studies of young schizophrenics do not find abnormal CT findings. Tanaka, Hazama, Kawahara, and Kobayashi (1981) found no ventricular enlargement or cortical atrophy in thirty-two patients ages 21–40, while they did find abnormalities in patients aged 41–60. Benes, Sunderland, Jones, LeMay, Cohen, and Lipinski (1982) found no abnormalities in a group with a mean duration of illness of 1.1 years. Jernigan, Zatz, Moses, and Cardellino (1982) found no abnormalities in a group that ranged from age 23 to 58. Iacono, Smith, Moreau, Beiser, Fleming, Lin, and Flak (1988) studied 85 individuals experiencing a first psychotic episode. They ranged in age from 15 to 40 years.

There was no enlargement of lateral ventricles and no succal expansion, and therefore no confirmation of the findings of Weinberger et al. (1982) and Schulz et al. (1983). The authors did find an unexplained enlargement of the third ventricle in their patients which they did not feel they could attribute to schizophrenia. Second, the total numbers of patients in the two studies are small, with only ten patients who were never exposed to neuroleptics (Schulz et al., 1983). Third, a disorder associated with ventricular enlargement and cerebral atrophy, sometimes leading toward dementia, is likely to be progressive. Weinberger et al.'s (1982) finding of similar rates in first-episode schizophreniform patients and chronic schizophrenics would seem unlikely. More frequently, studies have found increasing rates among patients exposed to a longer duration of treatment and illness. All of the patients in Weinberger et al. (1982) and one-fifth of the patients in Schulz et al. (1983) were schizophreniform. This diagnosis means the patients had one acute episode of six months or less duration without deterioration and without recurrence. It seems especially improbable that CNS pathology involving enlarged ventricles would cause this short-lived disorder with good outcome.

A study by Nyback, Weisel, Berggren, and Hindmarsh (1982) is occasionally cited as indicating that relatively young and untreated patients suffer from enlarged ventricles and brain atrophy. The abstract for the paper described the subjects as "relatively young patients with acute psychoses" (p. 403). However, it turns out that "relatively young" meant under the age of forty-five, typically with multiple hospitalizations. Similarly, "acute psychosis" did not indicate a first episode, but merely that the patients were actually psychotic at the time of the study.

Recently, magnetic resonance imaging (MRI) has begun to replace the CT scan for determining brain tissue density. A 1988 MRI study by Kelsoe, Cadet, Pickar, and Weinberger confirms the general findings on many CT studies. So does an unpublished study by Andreasen and her colleages (cited in Andreasen, 1988). In the eight studies reviewed by Kelsoe et al. (1988), a few showed no abnormalities, and the majority showed a variety of somewhat inconsistent abnormalities. However, the weight of the studies leans toward a finding of atrophy in the brains of neuroleptic-treated schizophrenic patients. Surprisingly few studies have attempted to correlate CT scan findings with the presence of TD. Bartels and Themelis (1983) found abnormalities in the basal ganglia of TD patients; but overall the results have been mixed and inconclusive (see Goetz and van Kammen, 1986).

Recently the positron emission tomography (PET scan) has been used to measure the metabolic rate and blood flow of various parts of the brain. This instrument can detect dysfunction before it necessarily manifests as gross pathology. From the earliest studies, there has been a somewhat consistent finding of hypoactivity in the frontal lobes and frontal cortex of neuroleptic-treated schizophrenics (Buchsbaum, Ingvar, Kessler, Waters, Cappelletti, van Kammen, King, Johnson, Manning, Flynn, Mann, Bunney, and Sokoloff, 1982; Farkas, Wolf, Jaeger, Brodie, Christman, and Fowler, 1984; Wolkin, Angrist, Wolf, Brodie, Wolkin, Jaeger, Cancro, and Rotrosen, 1988 [reviewed in Andreasen, 1988]; Wolkin, Jaeger, Brodie, Wolf, Fowler, Rotrosen, Gomez-Mont, and Cancro, 1985). However, not all reports confirm the finding of frontal hypoactivity (Gur, Resnick, Alavi, Gur, Caroff, Dann, Silver, Saykin, Chawluk, Kushner, and Reivich, 1987; Gur, Resnick, Gur, Alavi, Caroff, Kushner, and Reivich, 1987). There has been no consistent correlation with atrophy on CT scans. In each study, the patients had long histories of neuroleptic treatment prior to being removed temporarily for the PET scans.

The PET has been used to study specific parts of the brain in which the neuroleptics are known to produce dysfunction by blockade of the dopamine neurotransmitter system, including the basal ganglia (see ahead). A variety of studies show that the basal ganglia of neuroleptic-treated patients can develop dopamine related abnormalities (Farde, Wiesel, Halldin, and Sedvall, 1988).

PET studies of untreated schizophrenic patients have been contradictory (reviewed by Andreasen, 1988). One PET study involving unmedicated patients found no frontal hypoactivity (Sheppard, Gruzelier, Manchanda, Hirsch, Wise, Frackowiak, and Jones, 1983). It included a dozen patients, six who had never received any neuroleptics, and four who had received between 1 and 4 single doses. Neither PET, MRI nor CT scan studies are as yet conclusive concerning the existence of brain abnormalities prior to neuroleptic treatment. One CT scan project was specifically developed for the purpose of evaluating lifetime intake of neuroleptics. Lyon, Wilson, Golden, Graber, Coffman, and Bloch (1981) found a correlation between lifetime intake and shrinkage of the posterior but not anterior quadrants of the brain. The study has a relatively small sample of sixteen patients; but as a preliminary study, it points the way toward a much neglected area of research.

In summary, mounting radiological evidence from PET, MRI and CT scans confirms the presence of chronic brain dysfunction (PET scans) and brain atrophy (MRI and CT scans) in neuroleptic-treated schizophrenic patients. The total number of relevant CT scan studies is estimated to be over 90 (Kelsoe, Cadet, Pickar, and Weinberger, 1988), most of which show damage. Other studies implicate the total lifetime amount of neuroleptic intake (DeMeyer, Gilmore, DeMeyer et al., 1984; Lyon et al., 1981), but that is not a frequently replicated finding. There is some indication that early in their disorder and their treatment, patients tend not to display CT scan abnormalities; and that later in the disorder and treatment, the abnormalities become more frequent. There is insufficient data to determine whether or not cerebral atrophy or other abnormalities are consistently found in TD, although some researchers have found electroencephalographic evidence that the cerebral cortex is afflicted (Koshino, Hiramatsu, Isaki, and Yamaguchi, 1986).

In published series, the percentage of drug-treated schizophrenic patients with atrophy on CT scan varies from zero to over 50%. It is premature to establish a prevalence rate for any particular group of patients, but the reported rates are substantial, typically in a range of 10–40%. Independently, Andreasen (1988) recently reviewed the literature and found a very similar range of 6–40%, using the criterion of two standard deviations larger than the control mean. Andreasen noted that higher rates were reported with increasing severity and length of illness. This would also correlate with length and intensity of treatment with neuroleptics.

A number of the CT scan studies we have reviewed found a correlation between atrophy and persistent cognitive deficits or frank dementia (DeMeyer, Gilmore, Hendrie et al., 1984; Famuyiwa et al., 1979; Golden et al., 1980; Johnstone et al., 1976; Lawson et al., 1988). This material is reviewed next.

Clinical studies and neuropsychological tests for persistent cognitive deficits and tardive dyskinesia. Evidence for mental deterioration in association with neuroleptic therapy has been mounting. An earlier review (Breggin, 1983) disclosed that many patients with TD are also suffering from severe mental deterioration (e.g., Edwards, 1970; Hunter, Earl, and Thornicroft, 1964; Rosenbaum, 1979). Often the data had to be culled from charts and footnotes because most of the studies relegated this correlation to obscurity within the article. Other studies concluded, without evidence, that the brain damage must have pre-dated the TD.

Ivnik (1979) observed that many TD patients at the Mayo Clinic were demented and decided to investigate the problem by studying one case in detail using a battery of neuropsychological tests before and after termination of neuroleptic therapy. Ivnik took the position that the dementia observed frequently among TD patients at the Mayo Clinic was not permanent — this one case tended to clear up partially upon discontinuation of the drug. However, partial clearing without complete recovery is expected in dementia after the causative agent has been removed. The patient remained severely and permanently mentally impaired on psychological tests.

A national research project evaluated brain dysfunction caused by polydrug abuse, including street drugs (for a more detailed analysis, see Breggin, 1983). Using the *Halstead-Reitan*, the study unexpectedly uncovered a significant correlation between generalized brain dysfunction and total lifetime psychiatric drug consumption in schizophrenics (Grant, Adams, Carlin, Rennick, Judd, Schooff, and Reed, 1978; Grant, Adams, Carlin, Rennick, Lewis, and Schooff, 1978). More than one quarter of the neuroleptic-treated patients had persistent brain dysfunction. The statistical analysis related the chronic brain dysfunction more to the lifetime neuroleptic intake than to the schizophrenia: "Neuropsychological abnormality was associated with greater antipsychotic drug experience" (Grant, Adams, Carlin, Rennick, Lewis, and Schooff, 1978, p. 1069). Indeed, schizophrenic patients who abused street drugs rather than taking neuroleptics showed no correlation between schizophrenia and increased brain dysfunction. None of the patients had been exposed to neuroleptics for more than five years.

In an unpublished version of the paper presented at a professional meeting (Grant, Adams, Carlin, Rennick, Judd, and Schooff, 1978), the authors underscored the connection between tardive dyskinesia and cognitive deficits, and warned in their concluding sentence, "It is also clear that the antipsychotic drugs must continue to be scrutinized for the possibility that their extensive consumption might cause general cerebral dysfunction" (p. 31). The version published in *Archives of General Psychiatry* (Grant, Adams, Carlin, Rennick, Lewis, and Schooff, 1978) warned of the possibility of long-term cognitive deficits associated with neuroleptic use, but in somewhat less threatening language. However, the danger was wholly expurgated from the *American Journal of Psychiatry* version (Grant, Adams, Carlin, Rennick, Judd, Schooff, and Reed, 1978). The misleading correlation with schizophrenia was highlighted, and the more important relationship with extent of psychiatric drug use was buried out of sight in the statistical analysis. The several warnings about cognitive deficits from neuroleptic use were edited out. This appears to have been part of a successful attempt to keep vital information from reaching the profession and the public. I have never seen the studies cited in a discussion of brain damage and dysfunction from neuroleptics.

More recently, a clinical study of hospitalized drug-treated patients found many suffering from mental deterioration typical of a chronic organic brain syndrome (Wilson, Garbutt, Lanier, Moylan, Nelson, and Prange, 1983). The mental abnormalities correlated positively with TD symptoms measured on the AIMS. In addition, length of neuroleptic treatment correlated with three measures of dementia – unstable mood, loud speech and euphoria. The authors stated: "It is our hypothesis that certain of the behavioral changes observed in schizophrenic patients over time represent a behavioral equivalent of tardive dyskinesia, which we will call tardive dysmentia" (p. 188). However, these symptoms are typically part of a more encompassing organic brain syndrome, including the cognitive deficits found in many studies, and the term tardive dementia would seem more appropriate. The tendency in the literature, perhaps in search of a euphemism, has been to use the term tardive dysmentia even when a fullblown dementing syndrome is being described.

In addition the *Schizophrenia Bulletin* has published several articles with commentaries discussing neuroleptic-induced "tardive dysmentia" (Goldberg, 1985; Jones, 1985; Mukherjee, 1984; Mukherjee and Bilder, 1985; Myslobodsky, 1986).

Jones distinguished between two types of permanent brain damage from such drugs — one producing apathy and the other euphoria. Goldberg pursued a similar line of reasoning and reviewed the literature.

We have already noted that many CT scan studies of brain atrophy have reported additional findings of cognitive loss on neuropsychological testing. However, the correlation is not wholly consistent (Goetz and van Kammen, 1986). Zec and Weinberger (1986) reviewed the subject at length. Using the *Withers and Hinton Test*, Johnstone's initial positive correlation between CT scan abnormalities and mental dysfunction was not confirmed by some later studies. However, the *Luria-Nebraska* and *Halstead-Reitan* batteries, considered among the most sensitive for detecting brain damage and dysfunction, do tend to indicate a relationship between ventricular enlargement and neuropsychological deficits. Overall, the trend is definitely toward a correlation between CT scan indices of atrophy and neuropsychological indices for persistent cognitive dysfunction and dementia.

Several studies in addition to Wilson et al. (1983) have reported an association between TD symptoms and generalized mental dysfunction. Itil, Reisberg, Huque, and Mehta (1981) found a clinical profile of severe organicity in TD patients. Waddington and Youssef (1986) found a correlation between TD and intellectual impairment, as well as blunted affect and poverty of speech, but attributed it to the underlying schizophrenia. Struve and Willner (1983) found a loss of abstract reasoning in TD patients compared to neuroleptic treated controls without TD. In a study of patients with affective disorder and TD, Wolf, Ryan, and Mosnaim (1982) found evidence of dementia: "relatively intact IQ scores but significant impairment in performing tasks of immediate memory and new learning abilities are similar to the findings of investigations of patients with Huntington's chorea" (p. 477). DeWolfe, Ryan, and Wolf (1988) found a strong correlation between cognitive deficits, including memory impairment, and facial tardive dyskinesia. They suggested that the degree of deficit was related to total lifetime intake of neuroleptics in patients with facial dyskinesias.

Wade, Taylor, Kasprisin, Rosenberg, and Fiducia (1987) pointed out that Huntington's and Parkinson's diseases might provide a model for tardive dyskinesia, including the development of cognitive impairments (see ahead, as well as Koshino et al., 1986; and Breggin, 1983, for similar discussions). They studied 54 manic or schizophrenic patients with tardive dyskinesia. Using a vareity of tests that had demonstrated cognitive deficits in patients with Parkinson's and Huntington's diseases, they found similar cognitive impairments in the tardive dyskinesia cases. Individuals with more severe TD had more severe cognitive losses. They concluded that the tardive dyskinesia was one expression of a larger "chronic neuroleptic-induced neurotoxic process" (p. 395).

Reports by Gualtieri and his colleagues (Gualtieri and Barnhill, 1988; Gualtieri, Quade, Hicks, Mayo, and Schroeder, 1984; Gualtieri, Schroeder, Hicks, and Quade, 1986) indicated that many institutionalized children and young adults go through a period of worsening of their psychiatric symptoms after withdrawal from neuroleptics. This occurs in developmentally disabled patients in whom there is no complicating schizophrenic process. The researchers attribute the withdrawal problems to a drug-induced dementing process. Some patients stabilize or improve if kept medication free, but others seemed permanently worsened by the medications, and like adult cases, require increased medication to control their drug-induced symptoms. Gualtieri and Barnhill (1988) discuss the various explanations and conclude that the most likely hypothesis is that the neuroleptics impair higher mental function. They point out that "In virtually every clinical survey that has addressed the question, it is found that TD patients, compared to non-TD patients, have more in the way of dementia" (p. 149). They believe that the dementia results from damage to the basal ganglia that is also found in TD (see below). Gualtieri and Barnhill declare that "neuroleptic treatment is considered by enlightened practitioners in the field to be an extraordinary intervention" (p. 137) requiring serious justification. In summary, a convincing body of literature indicates that patients treated long-term with neuroleptics develop persistent cognitive deficits and dementia.

There is another source of clinical evidence for damage to higher brain centers in patients suffering from TD: clinical reports of denial or anosognosia among TD patients. A review of the literature disclosed that most tardive dyskinesia patients do not complain about their symptoms and will even refuse to admit their existence when confronted with them (Alexopoulos, 1979; Breggin, 1983; DeVeaugh-Geiss, 1979; Smith, Kuchorski, Oswald, and Waterman, 1979; Wojcik, Gelenberg, LaBrie, Mieske, 1980). Myslobodsky, Tomer, Holden, Kempler, and Sigol (1985) found that 88% of the TD patients "showed complete lack of concern or anosognosia with regard to their involuntary movement" (p. 156). The study also found some indication for cognitive deficits in these patients. Myslobodsky (1986) reported "emotional indifference or frank anosognosia of abnormal movements" (p. 1) in 95% of TD patients. He concluded that the most probable cause was "some form of cognitive decline associated with dementia disorder, probably owing to some neuroleptic-induced deficiency within the dopaminergic circuitry" (p. 4). As Myslobodsky suggests, the denial of obvious symptoms of brain dysfunction can be a telltale sign of chronic damage to the highest centers of the brain. It is found, for example, in severe brain disease caused by alcoholism (Wernicke's encephalopathy) or syphillis.

Overall, there is increasing evidence that long-term use of neuroleptics produces or is strongly associated with persistent cognitive deficits and dementia in a significant but as yet undetermined percentage of patients, and that tardive dyskinesia patients are especially afflicted, perhaps in the majority of cases.

Tardive psychosis. Some reports have indicated that some neuroleptic-treated patients develop drug-induced tardive psychoses that can become more severe than their original psychiatric disorders (Chouinard and Jones, 1980; Chouinard and Jones, 1982; Chouinard, Jones, and Annable, 1978; Csernansky and Hollister, 1982; also see news reports by Jancin, 1979 and "Supersensitivity Psychosis," 1983). Tragically, patients can require lifetime medication for a disorder that could have had a much shorter natural history.

The authors of two studies (Chouinard and Jones, 1980; Csernansky and Hollister, 1982) believe that the exacerbation of psychotic symptoms after removal from the drugs is due to brain damage from the drugs. They have labelled the disease tardive psychosis to underscore its parallel with TD. It can be irreversible and, like TD, can require ever-increasing drug doses to suppress the drug-induced symptoms.

At present, tardive psychosis is considered a controversial clinical entity, and the number of studies is insufficient to determine a prevalence. Although Chouinard and Jones (reported in "Supersensitivity Psychosis," 1983) have found a prevalence of 30–40%, Hunt, Singh, and Simpson (1988) reviewed the charts of 265 patients and located 12 probable and no definite cases of tardive psychosis.

Tardive psychosis overlaps clinically with the more established entity of tardive dementia. Studies by Gualtieri and his colleagues (1984, 1986) indicate that their patients suffer from a mixture of increased dysphoria, psychotic symptomatology, and dementia.

Clinicians have become increasingly aware of the difficulty of removing patients from neuroleptics, in part because of what appears to be tardive psychosis. Withdrawal from the drugs also can produce transient or persistent dyskinesias, dysphoria, and autonomic imbalances, resulting in nausea and weight loss. These reactions to neuroleptic withdrawal have led to debate over classifying these medications as addictive (Breggin, 1989a, 1989b).

Direct examination of the brain. There are surprisingly few autopsy reports following chronic neuroleptic therapy and they have been somewhat inconclusive (reviewed in the following: Bracha and Kleinman, 1986; Breggin, 1983, pp. 103–105; Brown, Colter, Corsellis, Crow, Frith, Jagoe, Johnstone, and Marsh, 1986; Jeste, Iager, and Wyatt, 1986; Rupniak et al., 1983). However, several studies have demonstrated the expected pathological changes from neuroleptic treatment: cellular loss or degeneration in the basal ganglia. The term basal ganglia will be used to indicate the striatum (caudate, putamen and globus pallidus), plus the substantia nigra — areas known to be strongly affected by the neuroleptics (see below).

There is autopsy evidence that the neuroleptics can damage the basal ganglia, areas potentially critical in the production of both TD and tardive dementia. As early as 1959, Roizin, True, and Knight reported postmortem degeneration in the basal ganglia of a few neuroleptic-treated patients and correlated these findings with related neurologic dysfunctions caused by the drugs. Forrest, Forrest, and Roizin (1963) reported an autopsy evaluation of one case of long-term neuroleptic treatment which demonstrated neuronal loss in the cerebral cortex and degenerative changes in the substantia nigra. The most striking alterations were in the putamen of the basal ganglia. The patient had also been given shock treatment.

Gross and Kaltenbach (1968) found evidence from three autopsies of irreparable damage to the caudate nucleus. They suggested that neuroleptic treatment may cause reversible tissue lesions and lead to irreparable damage of the caudate nucleus. Christensen, Moller, and Faurbye (1970) found a considerably higher degree of cell degeneration in the substantia nigra, as well as other pathological findings, in patients with TD compared to their controls. Jellinger (1977) reviewed the literature, and in his own research he found "damage to large neurons in the caudate nuclei with increased satellitosis and slight glial reaction in 46%" (p. 38) of patients subjected to chronic neuroleptic therapy. The percentage of patients with pathological changes was higher among those suffering from tardive dyskinesia (57% versus 37.5%). The afflicted areas were among those most directly affected by neuroleptics.

Brown et al. (1986) performed postmortem examinations on 41 schizophrenic patients. They found that, compared to controls, the patients' brains were lighter in weight (by 6%) and displayed ventricular enlargement associated with temporal lobe atrophy. The authors believed that their findings substantiate the atrophy found on CT scans. They stated "There were no significant effects of insulin, phenothiazine treatment, or electroconvulsive therapy on the results reported herein" (p. 38) but gave no supporting data. The conclusion contradicts evidence indicating cell death and degeneration from insulin treatment (see Breggin, 1979, p. 137; Kalinowsky and Hippius, 1969, pp. 288–289), as well as from shock therapy (Breggin, 1979, pp. 38–62). According to a table in Brown et al. (1986, p. 38), 23% had shock treatment, 28% had insulin therapy, and 41% had neuroleptic treatment. A note indicated that the frequency of shock treatment might be under-estimated. How many patients had combined treatment was not indicated.

Since the patients had a mean length of illness of 31 years and had died in the hospital, many during the era before de-institutionalization, most or all were probably long-term inmates who would have been subjected to numerous other stresses that might have caused brain damage, including head trauma and undetected disease. It would appear that nearly all the patients were subjected to so many damaging stresses that it would be impossible to attribute the findings to schizophrenia or to rule out other causes, including treatment (see Marsden, 1976, for similar observations on brain damage found among chronic inmates). Finally, as Brown et al.'s (1986) review chart indicated, the only modern postmortem study of *drug-free schizophrenics* (Wildi, Linder, and Costoulas, 1967) found no brain atrophy.

Hunter, Blackwood, Smith, and Cumings (1968) concluded that they could find no pathology in three postmortem studies of neuroleptic-treated patients. However, all three individuals did have pathological changes in the substantia nigra which were interpreted as normal due to aging in two cases and dismissed as of unknown etiology in the other case. All three subjects were elderly, complicating the interpretation of the findings. Arai, Amano, Iseki, Yokoi, Saito, Takekawa, and Misugi (1987) found neuronal degeneration in the cerebellar dentate nucleus, rather than the basal ganglia, in four cases of oral TD.

Although inconclusive, postmortem findings tend to confirm the effects expected from neuroleptic treatment: deterioration in the basal ganglia and substantia nigra, plus more generalized pathology. Animal research also strongly suggests permanent brain damage from neuroleptic treatment (see below).

In a recent review of structural changes in the brain associated with TD, Krishnan, Ellinwood, and Rayasam (1988) concluded "In summary, neuropathological, CT, and MRI studies reveal neuroanatomical and physicochemical changes in the brain of TD patients, but the exact nature and significance of these changes remain an enigma" (p. 173). However, while the specific changes associated with TD do remain something of a puzzle, the finding of pathological changes of various kinds associated with neuroleptic therapy in general seems increasingly well-established, and many of the studies do localize the findings in the basal ganglia, where the greatest impact can be anticipated.

Summary of Evidence from Human Studies

Substantial evidence confirms the presence of persistent cognitive deficits, brain dysfunction, dementia and brain damage – especially atrophy– among neuroleptic-treated patients. The most consistent and convincing body of evidence has been produced by the new brain imaging techniques (CT, MRI and PET scans). A range of 10-40% of patients afflicted with brain damage is most consistently reported. The rates seem to increase with duration of treatment and the age of patient.

Numerous clinical and neuropsychological studies have reported persistent cognitive dysfunction, tardive psychosis and tardive dementia among neuroleptic-treated schizophrenic patients. Tardive dementia is becoming an increasingly recognized syndrome. There is some postmortem evidence of basal ganglia deterioration, as well as generalized neuropathology. Brain atrophy has also been found in at least one recent postmortem study of these patients, although few studies exist. Various kinds of pathology have also been found in association with TD, sometimes localized in the basal ganglia.

Overall, the evidence presented from brain imaging, clinical evaluations, neuropsychological testing, and human postmortems indicates that the neuroleptics are the probable cause of the cognitive dysfunction and brain damage found in many patients. Our analysis continues with further evidence pertaining to etiology and a discussion of the implications of these findings for the mental health professions.

Neuroleptics as the Cause

As reviewed in the preceding section, data from human studies indicate that the neuroleptics are the cause of damage to the higher brain and to the mind reported in various research studies. This section will explore a more definitive answer to the question "Is neuroleptic medication or schizophrenia the cause of persistent mental dysfunction and brain damage found in many neuroleptic-treated patients?"

The Lessons of Lethargic Encephalitis and Subcortical Dementia

The neuroleptic drug effect as clinically observed closely mimics the effects of lethargic encephalitis (encephalitis lethargica or von Economo's disease) as reported during and after World War I. Both the neuroleptics and the viral disease produce mental apathy and indifference, plus various acute dyskinesias, including Parkinson's syndrome, dystonias and tremors. The encephalitis epidemic, which afflicted tens of thousands, was well-known to neurologists and psychiatrists in the 1950s, including Delay and Deniker in France, who were among the first to use the neuroleptics for psychiatric purposes. In a 1970 retrospective, Deniker observed:

> It was found that neuroleptics could experimentally reproduce almost all symptoms of lethargic encephalitis. In fact, it would be possible to cause true encephalitis epidemics with the new drugs. Symptoms progressed from reversible somnolence to all types of dyskinesia and hyperkinesia, and finally to parkinsonism. The symptoms seemed reversible on interruption of the medication. (p. 160)

While the symptoms initially seemed reversible, Deniker realized that they were turning out to be permanent in some cases:

> Furthermore, it might have been feared that these drugs, whose action compares with that of encephalitis and parkinsonism, might eventually induce irreversible secondary neurological syndromes. Such effects cannot be denied: it has been known for some years that permanent dyskinsias may occur. . . . (p. 163)

The parallel between lethargic encephalitis and neuroleptic toxicity was remarkable in several respects. Both groups of patients initially displayed apathy or disinterest, followed by the onset of various dyskinesias; and then in both groups of patients, after a delay, the dyskinesias sometimes became permanent. In regard to lethargic encephalitis, many patients seemed to recover, only to relapse into devastating neurological disorders years later. Many cases of Parkinson's disease were traced, years later, to an earlier exposure of lethargic encephalitis. While Parkinson's disease was the most common "tardive" or delayed motor disorder associated with lethargic encephalitis, other dyskinesias more similar to drug-induced TD (see below) were also known to develop.

There was a still more menacing potential parallel between the viral disease and the drug-induced disease. Many of the post-encephalitic patients, after an apparent recovery, later went on to develop severe psychoses and dementia (Abrahamson, 1935; Matheson Commission, 1939). Thus, the completion of the parallel between lethargic encephalitis and neuroleptic effects awaited the discovery that in addition to TD, tardive psychosis and tardive dementia could follow the exposure to neuroleptics.

The parallel between the medication effects and the viral encephalopathic effects was not proof that the medications would also produce mental deterioration; but it sounded a warning that similar mechanisms and hence similar adverse outcomes were possible. This concern was raised early by Paulson (1959), who wrote:

> The sequelae of encephalitis include many muscular, psychic and autonomic responses; and most of the neurologic complications from the penhothiazines are within the range of post-encephalitic parkinsonism. (p. 800)

Paulson remarked that no "permanent lesions" had yet been discovered to correspond with the "muscular, psychic and autonomic responses"; but his concern was justified.

The same year, Brill (1959) also commented on the similarity between lethargic encephalitis and the neuroleptics "which, in full doses, can reproduce many of the most outstanding features of the chronic encephalitic syndrome. . ." (p. 1166). Brill pointed out that both the viral disease and the drug reaction produce similar neurological and mental effects, including "the rousable stupor of acute encephalitis." Apparently unimpressed with initial reports of persistent dyskinesias, Brill believed that the neuroleptic effects were "controllable, reversible, and nonprogressive." A few years later, Hunter et al. (1964) again noted the parallel between the epidemic viral disease and the drug effect, and suggested that the neuroleptics cause a chemically induced encephalitis.

Given the clinical similarity between the impact of lethargic encephalitis and that of the neuroleptics, we may wonder about similarities in brain pathology produced by each. Brill (1959) summarized the autopsy findings of patients suffering from lethargic encephalitis (see also Abrahamson, 1935; Brodal, 1969). Cell loss was marked in the basal ganglia and especially the substantia nigra, where the damage, according to Brill, "is outstanding and may be seen by inspection, even in gross freshly cut specimens" (p. 1165).

The hardest hit areas in lethargic encephalitis, the cells of the basal ganglia and the substantia nigra, are also the areas most affected by the neuroleptic medications in the production of TD. The substantia nigra and the basal ganglia (the caudate and putamen) constitute the nigra-striatal pathway. This pathway contains dopamine neurons whose function seems irreversibly affected by neuroleptics in the development of TD (see below). As reviewed earlier, these regions are sometimes found damaged in autopsies of neuroleptic-treated patients, as well as in neuroleptic-treated animals (see ahead).

We have already seen that lethargic encephalitis sometimes caused dementia as well as dyskinesias. A number of other diseases which cause dyskinesias also tend to produce dementia. Huntington's chorea, whose dyskinesias somewhat mimic TD, typically results in severe mental deterioration. The most characteristic pathology is found in the basal ganglia (caudate and putamen), with less severe loss of tissue in the frontal and temporal lobes (Adams and Victor, 1985). Postmortem findings in Huntington's disease resemble those found in postmortem studies of some neuroleptic-treated patients, but are more severe (Brown et al., 1986). Based on a review of pertinent literature and their own electroencephalographic studies, Koshino et al. (1986) come to the same conclusion as we do:

> The EEG similarities of TD and Huntington's chorea were discussed, and a suggestion was made that not only the basal ganglion, but also the cerebral cortex, could be involved in development of TD. (p. 34)

Parkinson's disease, which affects motor control, is also frequently associated with a gradually developing loss of mental faculties, sometimes leading to dementia. Like neuroleptic treatment, Parkinson's disease often produces a blunting or slowing of emotional responsiveness. The characteristic lesions of Parkinson's disease are found in the substantia nigra (Adams and Victor, 1985).

The association of mental deterioration with diseases of the basal ganglia and substantia nigra led to the concept of subcortical dementia (Huber and Paulson, 1985). According to this formulation, a type of dementia can arise from damage to the basal ganglia and surrounding structures rather than to the cerebral cortex. Patients with subcortical dementia are very similar to those with cortical dementia, except that they tend to be more depressed and apathetic, without as much evidence of impairment to higher cortical functions, such as speech. Patients with subcortical dementia display a slowing of mental operations and progressive memory impairment. Although Huber and Paulson do not make the connection, we will suggest that subcortical dementia is one more probable mechansim for the production of persistent mental dysfunction and deterioration by the neuroleptics, although there are other probable mechanisms as well (see below).

An important lesson may be learned from lethargic encephalitis, as well as from subcortical dementia in other diseases, such as Huntington's and Parkinson's diseases. Long-term pharmacological alteration in dopamine neurotransmission in the basal ganglia and substantia nigra has the potential risk of producing not only movement disorders but serious and potentially irreversible cognitive dysfunction, including dementia. These observations are extremely relevant in deciding whether the neuroleptics can cause persistent mental dysfunction and brain damage in medicated patients.

Neuroleptic Neurotoxicity

Deniker (1970, 1971) indicates that he and Delay were well aware of the neurotoxicity of the first neuroleptics. Many references in the literature also refer to the "neurotoxicity" of the drugs (e.g., DiMascio and Shader, 1970; Famuyiwa et al., 1979; van Sweden, 1984). In routine treatment, most patients demonstrate one or another manifestation of neurotoxicity, including Parkinson's syndrome, dystonia, akathisia and tremors. The disinterest, apathy and lethargy that develop more or less in proportion to dosage can also be attributed to toxic reactions (Breggin, 1983).

Occasional severe reactions to the drugs, such as neuroleptic malignant syndrome, closely mimic the described acute phase of the once-feared lethargic encephalitis. The neuroleptic malignant syndrome includes signs of severe central nervous system intoxication with extreme dyskinesias, hypertonicity of muscles, impaired consciousness, hypertension, and instability of the autonomic nervous system (Guze and Baxter, 1985; Levenson, 1985). It is fatal 10–20% of the time. The occurrence of such an extremely toxic reaction in even a small percentage of patients – an estimated 1–2% or less – again suggests the damaging potential of these drugs.

The adverse effects of neuroleptics on many biochemical processes in the brain, including protein synthesis, mitochondrial activity and membrane structure, and most enzymes are described in a substantial body of work (Matsubara and Hagihara, 1968; Teller and Denber, 1970). Various neurotransmitter systems are affected, including dopamine, gamma-aminobutyric acid (GABA) and acetylcholine (APA, 1980, pp. 75–79). Protein synthesis is maximally inhibited in the basal ganglia (Sellinger and Azcurra, 1970), a finding consistent with evidence from many sources demonstrating the impact of neuroleptics on that region of the brain (see below). Although attention will be focused on blockade of dopaminergic neurons, it should not be forgotten that the neuroleptics disrupt many processes in the brain. We should anticipate that many untoward effects of these drugs will escape our attention due to the complexity of their effects and the difficulty of detecting them with our present methods. The generalized neurotoxic impact of the neuroleptics provides another warning about potential dangers to the functioning of the brain and mind.

Neuroleptics, Tardive Dyskinesia, and Dopamine Neurons

TD is produced partly as a result of neuroleptic-induced chronic inhibition of dopaminergic neurons in area A9 of the substantia nigra. These A9 neurons project to the striatal nuclei (caudate and putamen) where they stimulate the release of dopamine. Following neuroleptic blockade of A9 neurons, post-synaptic dopamine receptor targets in the striatum undergo a compensatory increase in both the numbers of dopamine receptors and their sensitivity. This dopamine receptor supersensitivity or hyper-reactivity in the striatum produces TD (Chiodo and Bunney, 1983; Jenner and Marsden, 1983; Jeste, Iager, and Wyatt, 1986). Of recent interest, neuroleptic blockade of dopamine receptors in the putamen has been demonstrated on PET scan (Farde, Wiesel, Halldin, and Sedvall, 1988).

The dopamine model for TD indicates why the initial impact of the neuroleptics mimics Parkinson's disease (motor slowing), while the delayed effects (hyperkinesias) of the drugs mimic Huntington's chorea. The characteristic lesions of Parkinson's disease are found in the substantia nigra (Adams and Victor, 1985). The substantia nigra is the site of the dopamine neurons whose function is rapidly inhibited by the neuroleptics. The characteristic lesions of Huntington's chorea are found in the striatum [caudate and putamen] (Adams and Victor, 1985). The striatum is where the delayed supersensitivity of TD results from chronic neuroleptic inhibition. This emphasizes a point we have already noted: neuroleptic effects parallel neurological diseases which produce both motor impairment and severe cognitive dysfunction.

The neuroleptic threat to the highest mental centers becomes apparent when it is realized that dopaminergic neurons susceptible to similar neuroleptic inhibition are found in the highest centers of the brain, including the mesolimbic system and cortex, which regulate emotional and mental activities. The bodies of these neurons originate in the ventral midbrain tegmentum (A10) and project axons to limbic and cortical structures, including the nucleus accumbens, septal nuclei, amgydala, and frontal and cingulate cortex, where they stimulate the release of dopamine (Adams and Victor, 1985; Chiodo and Bunney, 1983; White and Wang, 1983).

Marsden (1976) was one of the few to point to the danger of irreversible neuroleptic-induced damage — similar to tardive dyskinesia — in the highest centers of the brain. He observed in a letter to *Lancet*, "If long-term neuroleptic therapy can cause an apparently permanent change in striatal dopamine-receptor action, then one must assume that the same can occur in the meso-limbic cortical dopamine receptors" (p. 1079).

Animal research has confirmed that supersensitivity of dopamine receptors develops in the meso-limbic and cerebral cortical areas, much as it does in the striatum (Chiodo and Bunney, 1983; White and Wang, 1983) and that it can become chronic after termination of neuroleptic treatment (Jenner and Marsden, 1983; Rupniak, Jenner, and Marsden, 1983).

While tardive dyskinesia is difficult to reproduce in animals, Gunne and Haggstrom (1985) have been able to create both acute and irreversible dyskinesias in monkeys and rats. With persistent dyskinesias, they demonstrated evidence of irreversible biochemical changes in the basal ganglia and related areas (substantia nigra, medial globus pallidus, and nucleus subthalamicus). The changes were thought to reflect suppression of the dopamine system with a corresponding hyper-reactivity or supersensitivity. The authors found that a limbic component of the dopamine systems was involved.

Many researchers have remarked on the relationship between inhibition of the meso-limbic and cortical dopamine system and the clinical production of blunting or apathy (White and Wang, 1983; reviewed in Breggin, 1983). Lehmann (1975), who introduced the neuroleptics into North America in 1954, offered this straightforward observation:

> Neuroleptic drugs are characterized by their effects on the ascending reticular activating formation, which result in reduced reactivity to external and internal stimuli and in decreased spontaneous activity. Furthermore, their effects on the limbic system lead to blunting of emotional arousal. . . . (p. 28)

That the neuroleptics currently suppress the activity of neurons in area A10, with their projections to higher brain centers, is confirmed clinically by the disinterest, indifference or apathy which the neuroleptics produce in routine clinical usage. As previously analyzed in detail (Breggin, 1983), this impact closely parallels the clinical effect of surgical disruption of the limbic system fibers by lobotomy and newer forms of psychosurgery. It is no exaggeration to label the impact of the neuroleptics a chemical lobotomy.

In summary, dopamine neurons play a major role in the functioning of basal ganglia, limbic and cerebral cortical regions, and are critical in the highest mental life of the individual. Evidence from human and animal research confirms that neuroleptics suppress dopamine neurotransmitter systems. The impact of the neuroleptics on the mind can be explained by inhibition of these neuronal systems. Finally, animal experimentation reveals that chronic neuroleptic treatment affects the limbic-cortical system much as it does the striatum, with the production of a persistent reactive supersensitivity of the dopamine receptors. From such observations, we can expect a limbic and cortical equivalent of tardive dyskinesia, capable of causing persistent cognitive deficits, tardive dementia and brain atrophy in neuroleptic-treated patients.

In addition, some dopamine neurons in the substantia nigra (A9) project to the cortex rather than to the striatum. These neurons are blockaded by the neuroleptics, and dysfunction in these cortical projections can be expected to have a negative impact on the highest mental functions. Furthermore, it has been known for some time that the striatum itself is not a purely motor area and that it is involved with higher mental functions (e.g., Adams and Victor, 1985; Brodal, 1969). There are multiple interconnections between the striatum, limbic system and cerebral cortex. Gualtieri and Barnhill (1988) have recently confirmed these observations:

> Persistent TD is probably the consequence of irreversible striatal damage. But the corpus striatum is responsible for more than motor control; it is a complex organ that influences a wide range of complex human behaviors. No disease that afflicts striatal tissue is known to have only motor consequences; Parkinson's disease and Huntington's disease are only two examples. [citations deleted] (p. 150)

Underscoring the relationship between the striatum and mental function is the fact that the striatum is closely related in mammalian evolution to the development of the highest centers of the brain. The striatum increases in size parallel with the development of the cortex. The caudate and putamen of the striatum evolve from the telencephalon, the most anterior segment of embryonic development, which also gives rise to the cerebral hemispheres, including the frontal lobes and cerebral cortex. The striatum is also interconnected with the reticular activating system with its key role in the arousal and the overall emotional energy level of the individual.

Damage to the striatum and related structures, if severe enough, would be expected to produce persistent cognitive deficits and dementia, including the subcortical dementia described by Huber and Paulson (1985) [see above].

Thus, there are several related mechanisms for the development of neuroleptic-induced persistent cognitive dysfunction, tardive psychosis and tardive dementia: damage to dopamine neurons and supersensitivity of dopamine receptors in meso-limbic and cortical regions, and similar damage and dysfunction in the striatum itself, with its rich interconnections with the highest portions of the brain. It would seem inevitable that the neuroleptics would cause permanent harm to the higher mental functions, including lobotomy-like apathy or indifference.

Structural Damage to the Brain from Neuroleptic Exposure

We have briefly reviewed evidence for permanent biochemical changes (dopaminesupersensitivity) as a result of neuroleptic treatment in animals. There is corresponding evidence for permanent damage to nerve cells.

Evidence of structural brain damage, including cell degeneration and death in the basal ganglia, has been found in animals after chronic administration of neuroleptics (reviewed in Pakkenberg, Fog, and Nilakantan, 1973). Pakkenberg et al. (1973) administered long-term small doses of perphenazine (30.9 mg) to rats over a one year period and found a significant reduction in the number of cells in the basal ganglia, but not in the cortex. They related their findings to the atrophy found in neuroleptic-treated patients but claim "It is doubtful, however, whether treatment with phenothiazine derivatives also can be the cause of this, as cerebral atrophy was also found in schizophrenia before treatment with these drugs was introduced." Their conclusion is not logical: whether or not schizophrenia causes cerebral atrophy, the neuroleptics could be doing it as well. Also, as previously noted, pre-neuroleptic autopsies disclosed no consistent finding of atrophy in schizophrenics prior to the drug era. Nielsen and Lyon (1978) found cell loss in the striatum of rats after treatment for thirty-six weeks with neuroleptics. They concluded "The results further suggest that persistent irreversible anatomical changes can follow long-term neuroleptic treatment" (p. 85).

Some animal studies, usually of shorter duration, do not report damage to the basal ganglia; but nearly all of those find severe and permanent damage of a more widespread nature. Changes in the cortex of the rat were found after 1–5 weeks of trifluoperazine (Romasenko and Jacobson, 1969). Many abnormalities were found, including "homogenisation [sic] of the walls of some vessels" and an increased number of "hyperchromic and wrinkled nerve cells" (p. 26). One month after discontinuation of treatment, some of the animals no longer showed any abnormalities; but an unspecified number of others did: "More hyperchromic nerve cells were discovered in some of the experimental animals than in the control" (p. 29). There were corresponding biochemical abnormalities. The summary stated that there were "only slight changes, which, according to our morpho-histochemical study, are reversible" (p. 23). This conclusion was not warranted by the data which confirmed severe initial changes, plus some persistent pathology one month after cessation of treatment. Widespread neuropathology was found in guinea pigs after 4–13 weeks of treatment with 10 mg daily of chlorpromazine, including cell death (Mackiewicz and Gershon, 1964). "Chronic alterations of neurons were found to occur quite extensively" and included "vacuolization of the cell body, neuronophagy and concomitant glial reaction" (p. 168). The reticular formation was especially affected and the damage increased with duration of treatment. After one "comparatively low" dose of chlorpromazine, 0.5 to 5 mg per kg, Popova (1967) found structural changes in rat brains, including "swelling, chromatolysis and vacuolization of the nerve cell bodies" (p. 87) in many regions, including the sensory-motor cortex, midbrain, hypothalamus, thalamus and reticular formation. The changes in the reticular formation were related to the inhibition of its functions noted by physiologists. Coln (1975) found a reduction in the nuclear volume of cortical brain cells in rats two months after the termination of a four week treatment period with haloperidol. No attempt was made to localize the damage beyond the cerebral cortex. Reviews of animal studies can be misleading. For example, the *APA Task Force Report on TD* (APA, 1980) stated that "neuropathologic studies following acute or prolonged administration of antipsychotic drugs to animals have not convincingly and consistently demonstrated specific or localized pathological changes in the brain. . ." (p. 57). The report listed as evidence the four studies which we have reviewed in the above paragraph. Despite the APA interpretation, all four studies were convincing and consistent in one important aspect: the finding of widespread, severe, and irreversible changes in the form of neuronal damage and death.

Moreover, while the studies listed by the *Task Force* did not show consistent *localized* damage in the anticipated area, the basal ganglia, the duration of the exposure to the neuroleptics was very brief, varying from a single dose to thirteen weeks of treatment. Of great importance, animal studies with longer durations of exposure to neuroleptics − one year (Pakkenberg, Fog, and Nilakantan, 1973) and 36 weeks (Nielsen and Lyon, 1978) − showed the expected neuronal deterioration in the basal ganglia. These findings establish the capacity of the neuroleptics to produce permanent changes in basal ganglion function after chronic administration.

Not all rat studies show permanent damage. A follow-up by the Pakkenberg group (Fog, Pakkenberg, Juul, Bock, Jorgensen, and Andersen, 1976) found no irreversible changes in the rat brain with shorter duration treatments of 4 to 6 months, and concluded that the time factor was key. Similarly, Gerlach (1975) found no changes after 6 and 12 months treatment, and concluded "it may be assumed that the neuroleptics may exert an irreversible neurotoxic effect on the nigro-striatal system" (p. 53), but that the effect required aging or lengthier exposures, and that many changes might take place that were not discernable by light microscope.

In summary, most animal studies report irreversible neuronal damage, including cell death, after relatively brief exposure to neuroleptics. After longer exposure to the neuroleptics, the expected localization of damage in the basal ganglia and substantia nigra is often found. These findings in animal studies are especially striking considering the relatively short durations of treatment as well as the relatively low doses in some reports. One year is considered "long-term." Human subjects are often exposed to the neuroleptics for many years, sometimes for decades, and sometimes in very high doses. Furthermore, it is well-known that the brains of small rodents tend to be much more resistant to damage from most toxic agents than that of larger mammals.

Some human autopsy studies, reviewed earlier, have found evidence of basal ganglia deterioration and atrophy of the brain in neuroleptic-treated patients, as well as more generalized neuropathology, and are consistent with the animal reports. However, postmortem reports concerning humans have been surprisingly infrequent and somewhat inconsistent (Arai, Amano, Iseki, Yokoi, Saito, Takekawa, and Misugi, 1987; reviewed in Bracha and Kleinman, 1986; Brown et al., 1986; Rupniak Jenner, and Marsden, 1983).

Findings that the neuroleptics can permanently damage the brain structure of animals, often in the expected regions of neuroleptic impact, constitute convincing evidence that neuroleptics are the cause of the cognitive deficits and dementia found in neuroleptic-treated schizophrenic patients.

Tardive Psychosis, Tardive Dementia, and Senile Psychosis

The identification of tardive psychosis, previously discussed, bolsters more solid evidence that the neuroleptics can produce persistent cognitive dysfunction. The authors of these studies (Chouinard and Jones, 1980; Csernansky and Hollister, 1982) assign causation to the neuroleptics rather than to schizophrenia. The association of tardive psychosis with length of drug treatment and with drug withdrawal is convincing. Also, these patients frequently suffer from an organic brain syndrome, which is known to be caused by toxic drug reactions but not by schizophrenia.

Since generalized cognitive dysfunction and dementia are typically caused by an organic insult to the brain, such as toxic medication, authors of cognitive dysfunction and dementia studies usually identify the neuroleptics, rather than schizophrenia, as the probable cause (see preceding review, including DeWolfe et al., 1988; Goldberg, 1985; Grant, Adams, Carlin, Rennick, Lewis, and Schooff, 1978; Grant, Adams, Carlin, Rennick, Judd, and Schooff, 1978; Gualtieri and Barnhill, 1988; Gualtieri, et al., 1984, 1986; Ivnik, 1979; Jones, 1985; Myslobodsky, 1986; Wade et al., 1987; Wilson et al., 1983).

Psychosis in old age sometimes appears spontaneously in association with movement disorders, and the correlation between the two is probably related to deterioration of the dopamine system in the brain (Lohr and Bracha, 1988). While these disorders are produced by aging rather than by medication, the finding adds further confirmation to the fact that abnormalities of the dopamine system cause both movement disorders and mental dysfunction, and alerts us that we may reasonably expect the same untoward combination as a result of neuroleptic therapy, which also causes disturbances in dopamine neurotransmission.

Brain Imaging Studies

Studies based on the CAT, MRI and PET scans, as well as the PEG (Part I), did not prove very useful in distinguishing between schizophrenia and neuroleptics as the cause of findings of atrophy in neuroleptic-treated schizophrenics. Authors of these studies were divided in their conclusions concerning etiology, some favoring schizophrenia (Golden et al., 1980; Johnstone, Crow, Frith, Husband, and Kreel, 1976; Johnstone, Crow, Frith, Stevens, Kreel, and Husband, 1978; Shelton et al., 1988; Weinberger et al., 1979, 1980) and others favoring neuroleptics (DeMeyer, Gilmore, DeMeyer, Hendrie, Edwards, and Franco, 1984; DeMeyer, Gilmore, Hendrie, DeMeyer, and Franco, 1984; Famuyiwa et al., 1979; Sabuncu et al., 1977). Famuyiwa et al. suggested that if their findings were born out by other studies, "radical changes in drug treatment policy are indicated" (p. 504).

Sometimes claims were made that one or another study showed atrophy in unmedicated or relatively unmedicated schizophrenics; but the review disclosed that some of these studies were inadequate or misinterpreted and that the greater number of studies failed to find atrophy in schizophrenics early in their treatment. The arguments used in favor of a schizophrenic etiology by some authors of brain imaging studies will be further evaluated in the following section.

Schizophrenia as the Cause

Are there any competing reasons or evidence to bolster the alternative view that schizophrenia is the cause? Weinberger (1984) and others have argued that neuroleptics are not the cause of the brain atrophy and associated cognitive losses. The main basis for their argument is the presumed lack of correlation between lifetime intake of neuroleptics and the degree or presence of atrophy and cognitive changes. However, researchers have no direct measurement of lifetime intake of neuroleptics as a separate variable. Instead, they measure the length of psychiatric disorder, and assume that total exposure to neuroleptics increases with the duration of the psychiatric disorder.

The argument has serious flaws. First, it can be used equally well against schizophrenia as a cause. If there is no correlation between duration of psychiatric disorder (the variable actually being measured!) and the damage, then it seems unlikely that the psychiatric disorder is the cause.

Second, their premise is not wholly correct. Supporters of schizophrenia as the cause of the atrophy sometimes cite one or two studies (Schulz et al., 1983; Weinberger et al., 1982) in defending their position that untreated schizophrenics also display atrophy. We have reviewed these studies and found that they are not convincing and they are contradicted by several others (Benes et al., 1982; Iacono et al., 1988; Jernigan et al., 1982; Tanaka et al., 1981). Another study cited occasionally as demonstrating atrophy in relatively untreated patients (Nyback et al., 1982) turned out to involve patients under age forty-five, many with multiple hospitalizations and many years of treatment. Besides, the argument does not shed much light on the cause of the brain disorders, since either neuroleptic exposure or schizophrenia would presumably take time to produce its damaging effect.

Third, although a good correlation has never been made between lifetime neuroleptic ingestion and tardive dyskinesia, we know that neuroleptics cause tardive dyskinesia (APA, 1980; Fann et al., 1980; Jenner and Marsden, 1983; Jeste and Wyatt, 1982). It is therefore no surprise that it is proving difficult to make a more exact correlation between lifetime neuroleptic ingestion and atrophy or dementia.

Overall, investigators who assume that schizophrenia is the cause of brain atrophy and persistent cognitive losses do not offer convincing evidence or rational justification. On the other hand, there is a very cogent reason to believe that the atrophy found on CT scans cannot be the product of schizophrenia. Brain atrophy is far more accurately and definitively evaluated on direct postmortem pathological examination than on CT scan. The actual pathology, if it exists, can more easily be identified and accurately measured by direct observation and microscopic studies. Yet no consistent finding of brain atrophy was made in hundreds of autopsy studies performed on schizophrenics prior to the use of neuroleptics.

From the perspective of Adams and Victor (1985, p. 1150), the CT studies of the schizophrenic brain are so inferential as to be of dubious merit without confirmatory postmortem pathological studies. I believe that the mounting evidence from a combination of CT, MRI, and PET brain scans does indicate an abnormality of the brain that corresponds with many other findings we have reviewed. If the CT scans prove inconclusive, as Adams and Victor suggest, the remaining evidence would nonetheless confirm the existence of chronic cognitive dysfunction and dementia caused by neuroleptics. More pertinent, the relative insensitivity of the CT scan underscores the importance of the failure to detect similar findings on autopsy in the pre-neuroleptic era.

The search for a consistent finding as obvious as brain atrophy had been ruled out by direct postmortem pathological examination in the pre-neuroleptic days. Weinberger and Kleinman (1986) estimated that by 1950 more than 250 studies had claimed to find a gross pathological defect in schizophrenia and "the overwhelming majority of these claims were either never replicated, unreplicable, or shown to be artifacts." The task proved so frustrating that "the effort stalled in the 1950s" (p. 52).

Based on pre-neuroleptic studies, Noyes and Kolb's *Modern Clinical Psychiatry* (1958, pp. 387–389) reviewed the failure to find a consistent neuropathological problem of any kind, let alone one so gross as atrophy of the brain, and concluded that "the present trend of opinion" attributes schizophrenia to "a faulty reaction to life situations." Again drawing on pre-neuroleptic studies, in *The*

American Handbook of Psychiatry (1959), Arieti found that hopes for a neuropathology of schizophrenia "have remained unfulfilled" (p. 488). Later textbooks would not bother to mention the possibility of gross pathological changes in the brains of schizophrenics, since the question had been laid to rest by the repeated failure to find any (e.g., Nicholi's *The Harvard Guide to Modern Psychiatry*, 1978). When the *Task Force on Tardive Dyskinesia* (APA, 1980) made a brief reference to the initial CT scan findings of brain atrophy in neuroleptic-treated patients, it remarked, "this observation is quite surprising as it is not consistent with earlier neurologic evaluations of chronic schizophrenics; it requires further critical evaluation" (p. 59).

In reply to the question "do schizophrenic patients have cerebral atrophy, dilated ventricles, neurological deficits, dementia?", Lidz (1981) observed that

> . . . [F]or 100 years investigators have reported a neuropathological or physiopathological cause of schizophrenia. The trouble is that no such findings have been replicated. If the patient suffers from dementia, the diagnosis is not schizophrenia. (p. 854)

Lidz went on to link the CT scan studies to other fervent attempts by the same investigators to find a physical basis for schizophrenia. Lidz instead recommended taking into account the impact of medications and shock treatment on the brain.

The failure to obtain consistent findings of cerebral atrophy on postmortem examination prior to the drug era strongly indicates that the recent findings of atrophy on CT scans are the result, not of schizophrenia, but of some new threat to the brain of schizophrenics. The only relevant new threat is the widespread use of the neuroleptic drugs which are already known to cause one brain disease, tardive dyskinesia.

Other reasons to doubt that schizophrenics have a deteriorating brain disorder have been reviewed by Manfred Bleuler in his book *The Schizophrenic Disorders* (1978). Bleuler's analysis provides some of the basis for the following summary. First, organic disorders characterized by brain atrophy and dementia are not usually reversible. To the contrary, they are most often progressive. Yet it is well-documented by Bleuler and others that many schizophrenic patients improve over time; up to one-third or one-half show significant recovery over the years.

Second, a dementing disorder, once it has progressed, would rarely if ever clear up spontaneously. Yet clinical observations abound concerning the ability of some schizophrenics to respond to acute emergencies, such as a fire in the hospital, with temporary displays of great clarity and responsibility. As Eugen Bleuler (1924) put it, "A highly excited, especially a confused, patient, may appear entirely normal from one minute to the next, only to fall back after hours or days into the previous condition" (p. 435).

Third, Manfred Bleuler reminds us, schizophrenic patients do not show any classic signs of illness; they tend to become psychotic in the bloom of life. Over time, they do not tend to show the physical signs of deterioration usually associated with progressive neurological losses, such as premature aging, infirmity, seizures or neurological signs and symptoms. They die of the same diseases that afflict normal people. In following 208 patients for decades, Bleuler found that most of them remained in generally good health "in spite of advanced age" (p. 450).

Fourth, schizophrenic patients do not suffer from the typical signs of the earlier stages of a dementing disorder, including short-term memory problems. They are usually easy to distinguish, for example, from victims of Alzheimer's disease, multi-infarct dementia, and the dementias associated with Parkinson's disease, Huntington's chorea or multiple sclerosis. As M. Bleuler (1978) put it, "In the schizophrenic psychoses, however, the old intellectual competence, warmth, and emotional depth are discernable behind every serious state of morbidity, time and time again" (p. 453).

Fifth, schizophrenic communications suggest a very different process than the mental deterioration associated with a generalized brain disease leading to atrophy and dementia. The schizophrenic's intellectual functions do not deteriorate but rather become misdirected or psychologically and spiritually deranged. Schizophrenics often speak in unusual and complex metaphors dealing with psychological and spiritual conflicts over the meaning of love, life or God. Often they display enormous passion around the concept of their own presumed evil or exalted nature. Quite frequently only one or two specific false ideas (delusions) will appear in an otherwise normal mental life, and they will be defended with intellectual vigor and a high degree of mental acuity indicating that overall brain function itself is normal.

These points do not rule out the future discovery of a subtle biochemical cause for schizophrenia, but they do tend to rule out schizophrenia as the cause of a more gross neurological disorder leading to brain atrophy and dementia. There is almost no reason to believe that findings of brain atrophy and dementia are caused by schizophrenia, while there is considerable reason to indict neuroleptic therapy.

Other Causes of Mental Deterioration and Brain Damage

Mental deterioration in psychiatric patients, especially long-term mental hospital inmates, can be produced in a variety of ways, lending confusion to attempts to find definite causes in any particular case.

First, long-term stays in custodial mental hospitals and nursing homes can result in severe and partially irreversible losses in mental capacity on a purely psychosocial basis. Second, when psychoactive drugs suppress mental function over a long period of time, the individual may fail to develop or lose intellectual function without damage to the brain. Those who deal with the developmentally retarded have been especially concerned about permanent maturational suppression resulting from neuroleptic therapy (extensive reviews in Kuehnel and Slama, 1984; Plotkin and Rigling, 1979; also see Breggin, 1983; Hartlage, 1965).

Third, mental losses and even brain disease in chronic psychiatric patients can result from a variety of covert physical causes, as Marsden (1976), Jellinck (1976) and others have noted. These causes include malnutrition and poor medical care through self-neglect or staff-neglect, head trauma from beatings, poor sanitation, and unrecognized chronic disease. Many chronic patients are extreme abusers of cigarettes, alcohol, caffeine, and street drugs.

Due to the passage of time and inadequate or lost records, many chronic patients may be the unsuspected recipients of one or more physical treatments that might cause brain damage, such as metrazol, insulin and electric shock; psychosurgery; and various toxic agents used in psychiatry in previous decades (Breggin, 1979, 1980a, 1980b, 1980c).

Many studies that have been cited as linking schizophrenia to brain damage or dementia (e.g., Brown et al., 1986; Jeste et al., 1980; Johnstone et al., 1976, 1978; Waddington and Youssef, 1986) have drawn their subjects from among chronic patients. They cannot truly separate the effects of schizophrenia from the many other stresses in the lives of these patients.

Discussion

The term dysmentia has been used occasionally in the literature when referring to the generalized brain disorder associated with prolonged exposure to the neuroleptics. This coinage seems unnecessary, since the patients in question typically have dementia as defined in DSM-III-R. That the dementia is iatrogenic in origin should not lead us to cloud the picture with a misleading euphemism.

At present, among some authorities, there is an apparent reluctance to give consideration to the increasing evidence that the neuroleptics cause persistent cognitive deficits, dementia and brain atrophy. For example, no textbook or other source brings together the broad spectrum of evidence compiled and analyzed in this review. It took psychiatry twenty years to recognize tardive dyskinesia as an iatrogenic illness, although it afflicted a large portion of hospitalized patients (Gelman, 1984, p. 1753). Resistance to dealing adequately with tardive dyskinesia continues (Brown and Funk, 1986; Wolf and Brown, 1987). An even greater reluctance to recognize tardive dementia and brain atrophy is likely, since the damage is still more catastrophic. Furthermore, it is easier to overlook cognitive defects and dementia than to ignore dyskinesias, and easier as well to mistakenly attribute the deficits to the patient's psychiatric disorder.

A final word of caution is necessary concerning agents such as clozapine that do not cause as many acute dyskinesias as do other neuroleptics. Clozapine produces a typical neuroleptic suppression and reactive supersensitivity in A10 dopaminergic neurons that project fibers into the meso-limbic system and cerebral cortex (Chiodo and Bunney, 1983). We should not be lulled into using such drugs more freely on the unconfirmed hope of causing fewer cases of tardive dyskinesia. Because of their specificity for A10 neurons, these neuroleptics are probably an equal or greater threat in producing persistent cognitive deficits, dementia and atrophy.

Conclusion and Suggestions

There is convincing evidence to indicate that long-term treatment with neuroleptic medication frequently produces persistent cognitive deficits, dementia and atrophy of the highest centers of the brain. In addition, there is some evidence that neuroleptics also produce a reactive tardive psychosis. There is little or no reason to believe that schizophrenia causes any of these adverse effects, especially dementia and brain atrophy.

The most consistent information on prevalence has been generated by brain scans which measure brain atrophy. We can estimate a prevalence of 10–40% among neuroleptic-treated patients, increasing with duration of treatment and age.

Even if the rate turns out to be in the lower range, we are confronted with an epidemic of iatrogenic brain damage of large proportions with serious consequences. Millions of patients, some with tardive dyskinesia and some without, have developed drug-induced damage to the higher brain and mental processes. The following steps are proposed.

First, the threat of neuroleptic-induced persistent cognitive deficits, tardive dementia and brain atrophy should be recognized in the *PDR* and in drug company advertising.

Second, along with TD, persistent cognitive deficits, tardive dementia and brain atrophy should become part of the standard informed consent warning given to patients and their families before the initiation of neuroleptic treatment. The general public should also be warned about the dangers of these widely used medications.

Third, psychiatric textbooks (Nicholi, 1988; Talbot et al., 1988) and reviews should no longer relegate discussions of the issue to sections on schizophrenia and instead place them in their appropriate context among neuroleptic side effects. If textbooks and reviews consider the subject controversial, they should nonetheless present the problem as one of great importance.

Fourth, future research should focus directly on neuroleptic-induced damage to the brain and mind.

Fifth, the health professions are obliged to find and implement methods for the rehabilitation of persons suffering from iatrogenic brain damage from all sources. As a part of this, the growing movement surrounding the rehabilitation of head injury victims should be extended to encompass patients injured by neuroleptic treatment.

Sixth, the threat of damage to the highest centers of the brain constitutes one more reason for a thoroughgoing re-evaluation of the assumptions behind the use of neuroleptics. Every effort must be made to curtail their use.

Seventh, more attention should be given to non-pharmacological treatment alternatives utilizing professionals (Breggin, 1980d; Karon and Vandenbos, 1981; Mosher and Burti, 1989; Walkenstein, 1972) as well as those utilizing self-help groups (Chamberlin, 1978; Low, 1950; Zinman et al., 1987).

Finally, the patient's right to refuse treatment, well-established in general medicine, should be more thoroughly extended to psychiatry. The best safeguard against the abusive prescription of medication is a voluntary psychiatry based on informed consent.

Never before in history has the psychiatric and medical profession been confronted with an iatrogenic tragedy of such proportions as the neuroleptic-induced epidemic of tardive dyskinesia, persistent cognitive deficits, tardive dementia, and brain atrophy. It is time for the profession to take responsibility for the damage it is inflicting on millions of patients throughout the world.

References

Abrahamson, I. (1935). *Lethargic Encephalitis.* New York: privately published.

Adams, R.D., and Victor, M. (1985). *Principles of neurology.* New York: McGraw-Hill.

Alexopoulos, G.S. (1979). Lack of complaints in schizophrenics with tardive dyskinesia. *Journal of Nervous and Mental Diseases, 167,* 125–127.

American College of Neuropsychopharmacology–Food and Drug Administration Task Force. (1973). A special report: Neurological syndromes associated with antipsychotic drug use. *Archives of General Psychiatry, 28,* 463–467.

American Psychiatric Association. (1980). *Task force report: Tardive dyskinesia.* Washington, D.C.: APA.

American Psychiatric Association. (1985). *Task force on tardive dyskinesia: Letter to the membership of the Association.* Washington, D.C.: APA.

American Psychiatric Association. (1987). *DSM-III-R.* Washington, D.C.: APA.

Andreasen, N.C. (1988). Brain imaging: Applications in psychiatry. *Science, 239,* 1381–1388.

Arai, N., Amano, N., Iseki, E., Yokoi, S., Saito, A., Takekawa, Y., and Misugi, K. (1987). Tardive dyskinesia with inflated neurons of the cellular dentate nucleus. *Acta Neuropathologica (Berlin), 73,* 38–42.

Arieti, S. (1959). Schizophrenia: Other aspects; psychotherapy. In S. Arieti (Ed.), *American handbook of psychiatry, I* (pp. 455–484). New York: Basic Books.

Bartels, M., and Themelis, J. (1983). Computerized tomography in tardive dyskinesia. Evidence of structural abnormalities in the basal ganglia system. *Archive für Psychiatrie and Nervenkrankheiten, 233,* 371–379.

Benes, F., Sunderland, P., Jones, B., LeMay, M., Cohen, B.M., and Lipinski, J.F. (1982). Normal ventricles in young schizophrenics. *British Journal of Psychiatry, 141,* 90–93.

Bergen, J.A., Eyland, E.A., Campbell, J.A., Jenkings, P., Kellehear, K., Richards, A., and Beumont, J.V. (1989). The course of tardive dyskinesia in patients on long-term neuroleptics. *British Journal of Psychiatry, 154*, 523-528.

Bleuler, E. (1924). *The textbook of psychiatry.* New York: Macmillan.

Bleuler, M. (1978). *The schizophrenic disorders: Long-term patient and family studies.* New Haven: Yale University Press.

Bracha, H.S., and Kleinman, J.E. (1986). Postmortem neurochemistry in schizophrenia. *Psychiatric Clinics of North America, 9*, 133-141.

Breggin, P.R. (1979). *Electroshock: Its brain-disabling effects.* New York: Springer.

Breggin, P.R. (1980a). Disabling the brain with electroshock. In M. Dongier and E. Wittkower (Eds.), *Divergent views in psychiatry* (pp. 247-271). Hagerstown, Maryland: Harper and Row.

Breggin, P.R. (1980b). Psychosurgery as brain-disabling therapy. In M. Dongier and E. Wittkower (Eds.), *Divergent views in psychiatry* (pp. 302-326). Hagerstown, Maryland: Harper and Row.

Breggin, P.R. (1980c). Brain-disabling therapies. In E. Valenstein (Ed.), *The psychosurgery debate: Scientific, legal and ethical perspectives* (pp. 467-505). San Francisco: W.H. Freeman.

Breggin, P.R. (1980d). *The psychology of freedom: Liberty and love as a way of life.* Buffalo: Prometheus.

Breggin, P.R. (1983). *Psychiatric drugs: Hazards to the brain.* New York: Springer.

Breggin, P.R. (1989a). Addiction to neuroleptics? [letter]. *American Journal of Psychiatry, 146*, 560.

Breggin, P.R. (1989b). Dr. Breggin replies [follow-up letter on addiction to neuroleptics]. *American Journal of Psychiatry, 146*, 1240.

Breggin, P.R. (1991, in press). *Toxic psychiatry.* New York: St. Martins.

Brill, H. (1975). Postencephalitic states or conditions. In S. Arieti (Ed.), *American handbook of psychiatry* (pp. 1163-1174). New York: Basic Books.

Brodal, A. (1969). *Neurological anatomy.* New York: Oxford University Press.

Brown, P., and Funk, S.C. (1986). Tardive dyskinesia: Barriers to the professional recognition of an iatrogenic disease. *Journal of Health and Social Behavior, 27*, 116-132.

Brown, R., Colter, N., Corsellis, J., Crow, T.J., Frith, C.D., Jagoe, R., Johnstone, E.C., and Marsh, L. (1986). Postmortem evidence of structural brain changes in schizophrenia. *Archives of General Psychiatry, 43*, 36-42.

Buchsbaum, M.S., Ingvar, D.H., Kessler, R., Waters, R.N., Cappelletti, J., van Kammen, D.P., King, A.C., Johnson, J.L., Manning, R.G., Flynn, R.W., Mann, L.S., Bunney, W.E., and Sokoloff, L. (1982). Cerebral glucography with positron tomography. *Archives of General Psychiatry, 39*, 251-259.

Burke, R.E., Fahn, S., Jankovic, J., Marsden, C.D., Lang, A.E., Gollomp, S., and Ilson, J. (1982). Tardive dystonia: Late-onset and persistent dystonia caused by antipsychotic drugs. *Neurology, 32*, 1335-1346.

Chamberlin, J. (1978). *On our own: Patient-controlled alternatives to the mental health system.* New York: Hawthorn.

Chiodo, L.A., and Bunney, B.S. (1983). Typical and atypical neuroleptics: Differential effects of chronic administration on the activity of A9 and A10 midbrain dopaminergic neurons. *Journal of Neuroscience, 3*, 1607-1619.

Chouinard, G., and Jones, B. (1980). Neuroleptic-induced supersensitivity psychosis: Clinical and pharmacologic characteristics. *American Journal of Psychiatry, 137*, 16-21.

Chouinard, G., and Jones, B. (1982). Neuroleptic-induced supersensitivity psychosis, the "hump course," and tardive dyskinesia. [letter]. *Journal of Clinical Psychopharmacology, 2*, 143-144.

Chouinard, G., Jones, B., and Annable, L. (1978). Neuroleptic-induced supersensitivity psychosis. *American Journal of Psychiatry, 135*, 1409-1410.

Christensen, E., Moller, J.E., and Faurbye, A. (1970). Neuropathological investigation of 28 brains from patients with dyskinesia. *Acta Psychiatrica Scandinavica, 46*, 14-23.

Cohen, D., and Cohen, H. (1986). Biological theories, drug treatments, and schizophrenia: A critical assessment. *Journal of Mind and Behavior, 7*, 11-36.

Coln, E.J. (1975). Long-lasting changes in cerebral neurons induced by drugs. *Biological Psychiatry, 10*, 227-264.

Crane, G. (1973). Clinical psychopharmacology in its 20th year. *Science, 181*, 124-128.

Csernansky, J., and Hollister, L.E. (1982). Probable case of supersensitivity psychosis. *Hospital Formulary, 17*, 395-399.

DeMeyer, M.K., Gilmore, R., DeMeyer, W.E., Hendrie, H., Edwards, M., and Franco, J.N. (1984). Third ventricle size and ventricular/brain ratio in treatment-resistant psychiatric patients. *Journal of Operational Psychiatry, 15,* 2–8.

DeMeyer, M.K., Gilmore, R., Hendrie, H., DeMeyer, W.E., and Franco, J.N. (1984). Brain densities in treatment resistant schizophrenic and other psychiatric patients. *Journal of Operational Psychiatry, 15,* 9–16.

Deniker, P. (1970). Introduction to neuroleptic chemotherapy into psychiatry. In F. Ayd and B. Blackwell (Eds.), *Discoveries in biological psychiatry* (pp. 155–164). Philadelphia: Lippincott.

Deniker, P. (1971, October 6). Deniker recounts to symposium discovery of chlorpromazine. *Psychiatric News,* p. 6.

DeVeaugh-Geiss, J. (1979). Informed consent for neuroleptic therapy. *American Journal of Psychiatry, 136,* 959–962.

DeWolfe, A.S., Ryan, J.J., and Wolf, M.E. (1988). Cognitive sequelae of tardive dyskinesia. *Journal of Nervous and Mental Disease, 176,* 270–274.

DiMascio, A., and Shader, R.I. (1970). *Clinical handbook of psychopharmacology.* New York: Science House.

Edwards, H. (1970). The significance of brain damage in persistent oral dyskinesia. *British Journal of Psychiatry, 116,* 271–275.

Famuyiwa, O.O., Eccleston, D., Donaldson, A.A., and Garside, R.F. (1979). Tardive dyskinesia and dementia. *British Journal of Psychiatry, 135,* 500–504.

Fann, W.E., Smith, R.C., Davis, J.M., and Domino, E.F. (Eds). (1980). *Tardive dyskinesia.* New York: SP Medical and Scientific Books.

Farde, L., Wiesel, F-A., Halldin, C., and Sedvall, G. (1988). Central D2-dopamine receptor occupancy in schizophrenic patients treated with antipsychotic drugs. *Archives of General Psychiatry, 45,* 71–76.

Farkas, T., Wolf, A.P., Jaeger, J., Brodie, J.D., Christman, D.R., and Fowler, J.S. (1984). Regional brain glucose metabolism in chronic schizophrenia. *Archives of General Psychiatry, 41,* 293–300.

Fog, R., Pakkenberg, H., Juul, P., Bock, E., Jorgensen, O.S., and Andersen, J. (1976). High-dose treatment of rats with perphenazine enanthate. *Psychopharmacology, 50,* 305–307.

Forrest, F.M., Forrest, I.S., and Roizin, L. (1963). Clinical, biochemical and post mortem studies on a patient treated with chlorpromazine. *Revue Agressologie, 4,* 259–265.

Gelman, S. (1984). Mental hospital drugs, professionalism, and the constitution. *Georgetown Law Journal, 72,* 1725–1784.

Gerlach, J. (1975). Long-term effect of perphenazine on the substantia nigra in rats. *Psychopharmacologia (Berlin), 45,* 51–54.

Goetz, K.L., and van Kammen, D.P. (1986). Computerized axial tomography scans and subtypes of schizophrenia: A review of the literature. *Journal of Nervous and Mental Disease, 174,* 31–41.

Goldberg, E. (1985). Akinesia, tardive dysmentia, and frontal lobe disorder in schizophrenia. *Schizophrenia Bulletin, 11,* 255–263.

Goldberg, T.E., Weinberger, D.R., Berman, K.F., Pliskin, N.H., and Podd, M.H. (1987). Further evidence for dementia of the prefrontal type in schizophrenia. *Archives of General Psychiatry, 44,* 1008–1014.

Golden, C.J., Moses, J.A., Zelazowski, M.A., Graber, B., Zatz, L.M., Horvath, T.B., and Berger, P.A. (1980). Cerebral ventricular size and neuropsychological impairment in young chronic schizophrenics. *Archives of General Psychiatry, 37,* 619–623.

Grant, I., Adams, K.M., Carlin, A.S., Rennick, P.M., Judd, L.L., and Schooff, K. (1978). *The collaborative neuropsychological study of polydrug users.* Minneapolis: Unpublished paper delivered at the International Neuropsychological Association.

Grant, I., Adams, K.M., Carlin, A.S., Rennick, P.M., Judd, L.L., Schooff, K., and Reed, R. (1978). Organic impairment in polydrug users: Risk factors. *American Journal of Psychiatry, 135,* 178–184.

Grant, I., Adams, K.M., Carlin, A.S., Rennick, P.M., Lewis, J.L., and Schooff, K. (1978). The collaborative neuropsychological study of polydrug users. *Archives of General Psychiatry, 35,* 1063–1074.

Gross, H., and Kaltenback, E. (1968). Neuropathological findings in persistent hyperkinesia after neuroleptic long-term therapy. In A. Cerletti and F.J. Bove (Eds.), *The present status of psychotropic drugs* (pp. 474–476). Amsterdam: Excerpta Medica.

Gualtieri, C.T., and Barnhill, L.J. (1988). Tardive dyskinesia in special populations. In M.E. Wolf and A.D. Mosnaim (Eds.), *Tardive dyskinesia: Biological mechanisms and clinical aspects* (pp. 135–154). Washington, D.C.: American Psychiatric Press.

Gualtieri, C.T., Quade, D., Hicks, R.E., Mayo, J.P., and Schroeder, S.R. (1984). Tardive dyskinesia and other clinical consequences of neuroleptic treatment in children and adolescents. *American Journal of Psychiatry, 141,* 20–23.

Gualtieri, C.T., Schroeder, R., Hicks, R., and Quade, D. (1986). Tardive dyskinesia in young mentally retarded individuals. *Archives of General Psychiatry, 43,* 335–340.

Gunne, L.M., and Haggstrom, J. (1985). Experimental tardive dyskinesia. *Journal of Clinical Psychiatry, 46,* 48–50.

Gur, R.E., Resnick, S.M., Alavi, A., Gur, R.C., Caroff, S., Dann, R., Silver, F.L., Saykin, A.J., Chawluk, J.B., Kushner, M., and Reivich, M. (1987). Regional brain function in schizophrenia, I: A positron emission tomography study. *Archives of General Psychiatry, 44,* 119–125.

Gur, R.E., Resnick, S.M., Gur, R.C., Alavi, A., Caroff, S., Kushner, M., and Reivich, M. (1987). Regional brain function in schizophrenia, II: Repeated evaluation with positron emission tomography. *Archives of General Psychiatry, 44,* 126–129.

Guze, B.H., and Baxter, Jr., L.R. (1985). Neuroleptic malignant syndrome. *New England Journal of Medicine, 313,* 163–164.

Hartlage, L.C. (1965). Effects of chlorpromazine on learning. *Psychological Bulletin, 64,* 235–245.

Huber, S.J., and Paulson, G.W. (1985). The concept of subcortical dementia. *American Journal of Psychiatry, 142,* 1312–1317.

Hunt, J.I., Singh, H., and Simpson, G.M. (1988). Neuroleptic-induced supersensitivity psychosis: Retrospective study of schizophrenic inpatients. *Journal of Clinical Psychiatry, 49,* 258–261.

Hunter, R., Blackwood, W., Smith, M.C., and Cumings, J.N. (1968). Neuropathological findings in three cases of persistent dyskinesia following phenothiazine medication. *Journal of the Neurological Sciences, 7,* 263–273.

Hunter, R., Earl, C.J., and Thornicroft, S. (1964). An apparently irreversible syndrome of abnormal movements following phenothiazine medication. *Proceedings of the Royal Society of Medicine, 57,* 24–28.

Iacono, W.G., Smith, G.N., Moreau, M., Beiser, M., Fleming, J.A.E., Lin, T., and Flak, B. (1988). Ventricle and sulci size at onset of psychosis. *American Journal of Psychiatry, 145,* 820–824.

Itil, T.M., Reisberg, B., Huque, M., and Mehta, D. (1981). Clinical profiles of tardive dyskinesia. *Comprehensive Psychiatry, 22,* 282–290.

Ivnik, R.J. (1979). Pseudodementia in tardive dyskinesia. *Psychiatric Annals, 9,* 211–218.

Jancin, B. (1979, January). Could chronic neuroleptic use cause psychosis? *Clinical Psychiatry News,* p. 1.

Jellinck, E.H. (1976). Cerebral atrophy and cognitive impairment in chronic schizophrenia. *Lancet, 2,* 1202–1203.

Jellinger, K. (1977). Neuropathologic findings after neuroleptic long-term therapy. In L. Roizin, H. Shiraki, and N. Grčević (Eds.), *Neurotoxicology* (pp. 25–45). New York: Raven Press.

Jenner, P., and Marsden, C.D. (1983). Neuroleptics and tardive dyskinesia. In J.T. Coyle and S.J. Enna (Eds.), *Neuroleptics: Neurochemical, behavioral and clinical perspectives* (pp. 223–254). New York: Raven Press.

Jernigan, T.L., Zatz, L.M., Moses, J.A., and Cardellino, J.P. (1982). Computed tomography in schizophrenics and normal volunteers. I: Fluid volume. *Archives of General Psychiatry, 39,* 765–770.

Jeste, D.V., Iager, A.C., and Wyatt, R.J. (1986). The biology and experimental treatment of tardive dyskinesia and other related movement disorders. In P.A. Berger and H.K. Brodie (Eds.), *Biological psychiatry* (pp. 535–580). New York: Basic Books.

Jeste, D.V., Wagner, R.L., Weinberger, D.R., Reith, K.G.R., and Wyatt, R.J. (1980). Evaluation of CT scans in tardive dyskinesia. *American Journal of Psychiatry, 137,* 247–248.

Jeste, D.V., Wisniewski, A.A., and Wyatt, R.J. (1986). Neuroleptic-associated tardive syndromes. *Psychiatric Clinics of North America, 9,* 183–192.

Jeste, D.V., and Wyatt, R.J. (1982). *Understanding and treating tardive dyskinesia.* New York: Guilford Press.

Johnstone, E.C., Crow, T.J., Frith, C.D., Husband, J., and Kreel, L. (1976). Cerebral ventricular size and cognitive impairment in chronic schizophrenia. Lancet, 2, 924–926.

Johnstone, E.C., Crow, T.J., Frith, C.D., Stevens, M., Kreel, L., and Husband, J. (1978). The dementia of dementia praecox. Acta Psychiatrica Scandinavica, 57, 305–324.

Jones, B.D. (1985). Tardive dysmentia: Further comments. With commentary by S. Mukherjee and R.M. Bilder. Schizophrenia Bulletin, 11, 87–190.

Kalinowsky, H., and Hippius, H. (1969). Pharmacological, convulsive and other somatic treatments in psychiatry. New York: Grune and Stratton.

Karon, B., and Vandenbos, G. (1981). The psychotherapy of schizophrenia: The treatment of choice. New York: Jason Aronson.

Kelso, Jr., J.R., Cadet, J.L., Pickar, D., and Weinberger, D.R. (1988). Quantitative neuroanatomy in schizophrenia: A controlled magnetic resonance imaging study. Archives of General Psychiatry, 45, 533–541.

Koshino, Y., Hiramatsu, H., Isaki, K., and Yamaguchi, N. (1986). An electroencephalographic study of psychiatric inpatients with antipsychotic-induced tardive dyskinesia. Clinical electroencephalography, 17, 30–35.

Krishnan, K.R.R., Ellinwood, Jr., E.H., and Rayasam, K. (1988). Tardive dyskinesia: Structural changes in the brain. In M.E. Wolf and A.D. Mosnaim (Eds.), Tardive dyskinesia: Biological mechanisms and clinical aspects (pp. 165–178). Washington, D.C.: American Psychiatric Press.

Kuehnel, T.G., and Slama, K.M. (1984). Guidelines for the developmentally disabled. In K.M. Tardiff (Ed.), The psychiatric uses of seclusion and restraint (pp. 87–102). Washington, D.C.: American Psychiatric Press.

Lawson, W.B., Waldman, I.N., and Weinberger, D.R. (1988). Schizophrenic dementia: Clinical and computed axial tomography correlates. Journal of Nervous and Mental Disease, 176, 207–212.

Lehmann, H.E. (1975, Summer). Psychopharmacological treatment of schizophrenia. Schizophrenia Bulletin, pp. 25–45.

Levenson, J.L. (1985). Neuroleptic malignant syndrome. American Journal of Psychiatry, 142, 1137–1145.

Lidz, T. (1981). Psychoanalysis, schizophrenia, and the art of book reviewing [letter]. American Journal of Psychiatry, 138, 854.

Lohr, J.B., and Bracha, H.S. (1988). Association of psychosis with movement disorders in the elderly. Psychiatric Clinics of North America, 11, 61–68.

Low, A.A. (1950). Mental health through will-training. Winnetka, Illinois: Willett.

Lund, D.S. (1989, May). Tardive dyskinesia lawsuits on increase. Psychiatric Times, p. 1.

Lyon, K., Wilson, J., Golden, C.J., Graber, B., Coffman, J.A., and Bloch, S. (1981). Effects of long-term neuroleptic use on brain density. Psychiatric Research, 5, 33–37.

Mackiewicz, J., and Gershon, S. (1964). An experimental study of the neuropathological and toxicological effects of chlorpromazine and reserpine. Journal of Neuropsychiatry, 5, 159–169.

Marsden, C.D. (1976). Cerebral atrophy and cognitive impairment in chronic schizophrenia. Lancet, 2, 1079.

Matheson Commission (1939). Epidemic encephalitis. New York: Columbia University Press.

Matsubara, T., and Hagihara, B. (1968). Action mechanism of phenothiazine derivatives on mitochondrial respiration. Journal of Biochemistry, 63, 156–164.

Mosher, L.R., and Burti, L. (1989). Community mental health: Principles and practice. New York: Norton.

Mukherjee, S. (1984). Tardive dysmentia. A reappraisal. Schizophrenia Bulletin, 10, 151–152.

Mukherjee, S., and Bilder, R.M. (1985). Commentary. Schizophrenia Bulletin, 11, 189–190.

Myslobodsky, M. (1986). Anosognosia in tardive dyskinesia: "Tardive dysmentia" or "tardive dementia"? Schizophrenia Bulletin, 12, 1–6.

Myslobodsky, M.S., Tomer, R., Holden, T., Kempler, S., and Sigol, M. (1985). Cognitive impairment in patients with tardive dyskinesia. Journal of Nervous and Mental Disease, 173, 156–160.

Neuroleptics to cary FDA class warning. (1985, May 17). Psychiatric News, p. 1.

Nicholi, A.M. (Ed.). (1978). The Harvard guide to modern psychiatry. Cambridge, Massachusetts: Belknap.

Nicholi, A.M. (Ed.). (1988). The new Harvard guide to psychiatry. Cambridge, Massachusetts: Belknap.

Nielsen, E.G., and Lyon, M. (1978). Evidence for cell loss in corpus striatum after long-term treatment with a neuroleptic drug (flupenthixol) in rats. *Psychopharmachology, 59,* 85–89.

Noyes, A.P., and Kolb, L.C. (1958). *Modern clinical psychiatry* (Fifth Edition). Philadelphia: Saunders.

Nyback, H., Weisel, F.-A., Berggren, B.-M., and Hindmarsh, T. (1982). Computed tomography of the brain in patients with acute psychoses and healthy volunteers. *Acta Psychiatrica Scandinavica, 65,* 403–414.

Pakkenberg, H., Fog, R., and Nilakantan, B. (1973). The long-term effect of perphenazine enanthate on the rat brain. Some metabolic and anatomical observations. *Psychopharmacologia (Berlin), 29,* 329–336.

Paulson, G.M. (1959). Phenothiazine toxicity, extrapyramidal seizures, oculo-gyric crises. *Journal of Mental Science, 105,* 798–802.

PDR: *Physicians' Desk Reference.* (1973). Oradell, New Jersey: Medical Economics.

PDR: *Physicians' Desk Reference.* (1978). Oradell, New Jersey: Medical Economics.

Plotkin, R., and Rigling, K. (1979). Invisible manacles: Drugging mentally retarded people. *Stanford Law Review, 31,* 637–678.

Popova, E.N. (1967). On the effect of some neuropharmacological agents on the structure of neurons of various cyto-architectonic formations. *Journal für Hirnforschung, 9,* 71–89.

Roizin, L., True, C., and Knight, M. (1959). Structural effects of tranquilizers. *Research Publications of the Association for Research in Nervous and Mental Disease, 37,* 285–324.

Romasenko, V.A., and Jacobson, I.S. (1969). Morpho-histochemical study of the action of trifluoperazine on the brain of white rats. *Acta Neuropathologica (Berlin), 12,* 23–32.

Rosenbaum, A.H. (1979). Pharmacotherapy of tardive dyskinesia. *Psychiatric Annals, 9,* 205–210.

Rupniak, N.M.J., Jenner, P., and Marsden, C.D. (1983). The effect of chronic neuroleptic administration on cerebral dopamine receptor function. *Life Sciences, 32,* 2289–2311.

Sabuncu, N., Sabacin, S., Saygill, R., Kumral, K., and Ornek, T. (1977). Cortical atrophy caused by long-term therapy with antidepressive and neuroleptic drugs: A clinical and experimental study. In L. Roizin, H. Shiraki, and N. Drcevic (Eds.), *Neurotoxicology* (pp. 149–158). New York: Raven Press.

Schulz, S.C., Koller, M.M., Kishore, P.R., Hamer, R.M., Gehl, J.J., and Friedel, R.O. (1983). Ventricular enlargement in teenage patients with schizophrenic spectrum disorder. *American Journal of Psychiatry, 14,* 1591–1595.

Sellinger, O.Z., and Azcurra, J.M. (1970). The breakdown of polysomes and the stimulation of protein synthesis in cerebral mechanisms of defense against seizures. In A. Lajtha (Ed.), *Protein metabolism of the nervous system* (pp. 519–532). New York: Plenum.

Shelton, R.C., Karson, C.N., Doran, A.R., Pickar, D., Bigelow, L.B., and Weinberger, D.R. (1988). Cerebral structural pathology in schizophrenia: Evidence for selective prefrontal cortical defect. *American Journal of Psychiatry, 145,* 154–163.

Sheppard, G., Gruzelier, J., Manchanda, R., Hirsch, S.R., Wise, R., Frackowiak, R., and Jones, T. (1983). O positron emission tomography scanning of predominantly never-treated acute schizophrenic patients. *Lancet, 24,* 1448–1452.

Smith, J.M., Kuchorski, M.A., Oswald, W.T., and Waterman, M.A. (1979). A systematic investigation of tardive dyskinesia inpatients. *American Journal of Psychiatry, 136,* 918–922.

Sovner, R., DiMascio, A., Berkowitz, D., and Randolph, P. (1978). Tardive dyskinesia and informed consent. *Psychosomatics, 19,* 172–177.

Struve, F.A., and Willner, A.E. (1983). Cognitive dysfunction and tardive dyskinesia. *British Journal of Psychiatry, 143,* 597–600.

Supersensitivity psychosis thought to often follow withdrawal of neuroleptics after extended use. (1983, September 1). *Psychiatric News,* p. 39.

Talbott, J.A., Hales, R.E., and Yudofsky, S.C. (Eds.). (1988). *Textbook of psychiatry.* Washington, D.C.: American Psychiatric Press.

Tanaka, Y., Hazama, H., Kawahara, R., and Kobayashi, K. (1981). Computerized tomography of the brain in schizophrenic patients. *Acta Psychiatrica Scandinavica, 63,* 191–197.

Teller, D.N., and Denber, H.C.B. (1970). Mescaline and phenothiazines: Recent studies on subcellular localization and effects upon membranes. In A. Lajtha (Ed.), *Protein metabolism of the nervous system* (pp. 685–698). New York: Plenum.

van Sweden, B. (1984). Neuroleptic neurotoxicity: Electro-clinical aspects. *Acta Neurologica Scandinavica, 69,* 137–146.

Waddington, J.L., and Youssef, H.A. (1986). Late onset involuntary movements in chronic schizophrenia: Relationships of "tardive" dyskinesia to intellectual impairment and negative symptoms. *British Journal of Psychiatry, 149,* 616–620.

Wade, J.B., Taylor, M.A., Kasprisin, A., Rosenberg, S., and Fiducia, D. (1987). Tardive dyskinesia and cognitive impairment. *Biological Psychiatry, 22,* 393–395.

Walkenstein, E. (1972). *Beyond the couch.* New York: Crown.

Weinberger, D.R. (1984). Computed tomography (CT) findings in schizophrenia: Speculation on the meaning of it all. *Journal of Psychiatric Research, 18,* 477–490.

Weinberger, D.R., Cannon-Spoor, E., Potkin, S.G., and Wyatt, R.J. (1980). Poor premorbid adjustment and CT scan abnormalities in chronic schizophrenia. *American Journal of Psychiatry, 137,* 1410–1414.

Weinberger, D.R., DeLisi, L.E., Perman, G.P., Targum, S., and Wyatt, R.J. (1982). Computed tomography in schizophreniform disorder and other acute psychiatric disorders. *Archives of General Psychiatry, 39,* 778–783.

Weinberger, D.R., and Kleinman, J.E. (1986). Observations on the brain in schizophrenia. In A. Frances and R. Hales (Eds.), *American Psychiatric Association Annual Review* (Volume 5, pp. 42–67). Washington, D.C.: American Psychiatric Association.

Weinberger, D.R., Torrey, E.F., Neophytides, H.N., and Wyatt, R.J. (1979). Lateral ventricular enlargement in chronic schizophrenia. *Archives of General Psychiatry, 36,* 735–739.

White, F.J., and Wang, R.Y. (1983). Differential effects of classical and atypical antipsychotic drugs on A9 and A10 dopamine neurons. *Science, 221,* 1054–1056.

Wildi, E., Linder, A., and Costoulas, G. (1967). Schizophrenia and involutional cerebral senility. *Psychiatry and Neurology, 154,* 1–26.

Wilson, I.C., Garbutt, J.C., Lanier, C.F., Moylan, J., Nelson, W., and Prange, Jr., A.J. (1983). Is there a tardive dysmentia? *Schizophrenia Bulletin, 9,* 187–192.

Wojcik, J.D., Gelenberg, A.J. LaBrie, R.A., and Mieske, M. (1980). Prevalence of tardive dyskinesia in an outpatient population. *Comprehensive Psychiatry, 21,* 370–380.

Wolf, M.E., and Brown, P. (1987). Overcoming institutional and community resistance to a tardive dyskinesia management program. *Hospital and Community Psychiatry, 38,* 65–68.

Wolf, M.E., Ryan, J.J., and Mosnaim, A.D. (1982). Organicity and tardive dyskinesia. *Psychosomatics, 23,* 475–480.

Wolkin, A., Angrist, B., Wolf, A., Brodie, J.D., Wolkin, B., Jaeger, J., Cancro, R., and Rotrosen, J. (1988). Persistent cerebral metabolic abnormalities in chronic schizophrenia determined by positron emission tomography. *American Journal of Psychiatry, 142,* 564–571.

Wolkin, A., Jaeger, J., Brodie, J.D., Wolf, A., Fowler, J., Rotrosen, J., Gomez-Mont, F., and Cancro, R. (1985). Low frontal glucose utilization in chronic schizophrenia: A replication study. *American Journal of Psychiatry, 145,* 251–253.

Yassa, R., and Jones, B. (1985). Complications of tardive dyskinesia: A review. *Psychosomatics, 26,* 305–313.

Yassa, R., Nastase, C., Camille, Y., and Belzile, L. (1988). Tardive dyskinesia in a psychogeriatric population. In M.E. Wolf and A.D. Mosnaim (Eds.), *Tardive dyskinesia: Biological mechanisms and clinical aspects* (pp. 123–134). Washington, D.C.: American Psychiatric Press.

Zec, R.F., and Weinberger, D.R. (1986). Relationship between CT scan findings and neuropsychological performance in chronic schizophrenia. *Psychiatric Clinics of North America, 9,* 49–61.

Zinman, S., Howie the Harp, and Budd, S. (1987). *Reaching across: Mental health clients helping each other.* Riverside, California: California Network of Mental Health Clients.

©1990 The Institute of Mind and Behavior, Inc.
The Journal of Mind and Behavior
Summer and Autumn 1990, Volume 11, Numbers 3 and 4
Pages 465 [219] – 488 [242]
ISSN 0271-0137
ISBN 0-930195-05-1

The Political Economy of Tardive Dyskinesia: Asymmetries in Power and Responsibility

David Cohen

Université de Montréal

and

Michael M^CCubbin

York University

Tardive dyskinesia is a serious, well publicized adverse effect resulting from long-term neuroleptic drug use. However, little progress has been made during the last two decades in ensuring that these drugs are prescribed with necessary caution. Incentives and constraints operating on the major participants (patients, families, physicians, institutions, drug companies, society) in the decision-making process leading to the prescription of neuroleptics increase the likelihood that the benefits of drugs will be exaggerated and their adverse effects minimized. When combined with imbalances of power, these factors ensure that persons having little power and information to make the decision to prescribe will bear most costs of that decision. This points to the operation of an inefficient system which can be expected to yield sub-optimal results. We suggest ways to make the decision process more efficient by more closely aligning responsibility with cost. If those who hold power in the decision process are held accountable for the unwanted risks they impose upon others, both the use of neuroleptics and its inevitable iatrogenesis would probably be reduced.

Tardive dyskinesia (TD), a movement disorder induced by neuroleptic drugs and first described in 1957, has been a most controversial subject in psychiatry — extensively studied, discussed and debated since the early 1970s. Although there is no effective method to treat TD, and despite the fact that it is irreversible in many cases, the current practice of maintaining disturbing and disturbed people indefinitely on neuroleptics has only assured, as Mosher and Burti (1989) put it, the growth of a new species, the "tardive dyskinesic,

The authors wish to thank Peter R. Breggin, Phil Brown, and Robert L. Sprague for helpful suggestions on earlier drafts. Requests for reprints should be sent to David Cohen, Ph.D., Ecole de service social, Université de Montréal, C.P. 6128, succursale A, Montréal, Québec, Canada H3C 3J7.

stigmatized by the impossible-to-hide, cosmetic disfigurement of tardive dyskinesia" (p. 3). According to one estimate, up to 625,000 people per year in
the United States exhibit signs of TD (Dewan and Koss, 1989).

In response to rising concern about this public health problem, the
American Psychiatric Association (APA) in 1979 and 1985 offered guidelines
to prevent and manage TD (APA, 1985; Baldessarini, Cole, Davis, Gardos,
Preskorn, Simpson, and Tarsy, 1979). These included using neuroleptics at
minimum doses, monitoring for side effects, discussing side effects with patients and families, and reducing or withdrawing drugs if TD appears. Moreover, in a dozen well-publicized court cases between 1980 and 1988, patients
filed civil suits for damages for injury suffered as a result of TD (Slaw and
Kalachnik, 1988). Courts ruled that to prescribe drugs without monitoring
the patient, that failure to diagnose TD accurately, that failure to react appropriately to signs of TD, and that failure to inform the patient of the risks
of TD were instances of negligent practice (see summaries and commentaries
by Gualitieri, Sprague, and Cole, 1986; Mills and Eth, 1987; Mills, Norquist,
Shelton, Gelenberg, and Van Putten, 1986; Slaw and Kalachnik, 1985). In
the largest verdict, *Hedin v. United States* (1984), the plaintiff was awarded
over $2,000,000. In 1982, Pirodsky summarized the emerging consensus on the
prevention of TD: "the best way to deal with tardive dyskinesia right now
is primary prevention. This means using less medication or perhaps not using
it at all" (p. 170).

Unfortunately, a decade later, we see no indication that the incidence of
TD is about to decline. Although outpatient prescriptions of neuroleptics
in the United States have decreased about one percent a year between
1976–1985 (from 21 to 19 million) [Wysowsky and Baum, 1989], this trend is
accompanied by switches to more potent drugs (such as haloperidol) which
are prescribed in much higher chlorpromazine-equivalent doses than the
previously popular phenothiazines. Reardon, Rifkin, Schwartz, Myerson, and
Siris (1989) confirm this trend, showing that mean daily chlorpromazine-
equivalent doses of neuroleptics prescribed in institutional and community
settings have doubled between 1973 and 1982. Mosher and Burti (1989) remark
that "it is especially painful to us that, in spite of a nearly 5% annual incidence
in T.D. (i.e., in four years 20% of neuroleptic-maintained patients will have
developed it), it has become difficult to even raise the question of withdrawal
or decreased neuroleptic dosage with psychiatrists presently in the public
system" (p. 3). At the same time, nine times out of ten, TD is misdiagnosed,
even by well-trained clinicians (Dixon, Weiden, Frances, and Rapkin, 1989;
Weiden, Mann, Haas, Mattson, and Frances, 1987). In addition, "few institutions have adopted the APA guidelines, and in those that have, many professionals try to circumvent them. Even when informed consent about psychiatric treatment is seriously pursued, patients are provided little information

about side effects. When side effects are mentioned, tardive dyskinesia is frequently not among those named" (Wolf and Brown, 1988, p. 284, references omitted). These puzzling facts might be explained by dynamics in the decisions to administer neuroleptics that do not fully take into consideration the balance of costs and benefits ensuing from the use of neuroleptics.

TD is a complex problem because it results from decisions made by several parties, not just those of patients who might be physically afflicted by this disease. Furthermore, the costs and benefits of neuroleptic drug use may not be distributed in accordance with the relative power of the parties involved in the decisions to prescribe neuroleptics. For example, a voluntary mental patient not fully informed by the prescribing physician of the risks of TD, or an involuntary patient forcibly medicated, or an elderly nursing home resident who has not been told that neuroleptics were prescribed, may develop TD. Patients having little power and information available to make a decision concerning prescription often end up bearing most of the costs resulting from that decision. Disregarding the issue of moral responsibility for the production of TD, analysis of these facts from a purely economic perspective points to the operation of an inefficient system of decision-making which can be expected to yield sub-optimal results.

In this paper we discuss some of the incentives that operate on various parties (patients, families, medical and other professionals, institutions, drug companies, society) involved in the decision-making process leading to the prescription of neuroleptic drugs, and some of the constraints that limit these actors' freedom to make decisions. The structural biases in this process increase the likelihood that participants in the decision will opt in favor of using neuroleptics, will downplay their risks, and will exaggerate their benefits. These biases, when combined with imbalances of power and responsibility, result in behaviour which is inefficient in the sense that most costs are borne by participants who do not have the incentive nor the power to impose these costs.

In a number of areas linked to neuroleptic prescription and its consequences, including informed consent to treatment, civil litigation for compensation for TD, and drug information provided to prescribers, we suggest ways to make decision-making more efficient by more closely aligning responsibility with cost. If those who have the power in the decision to treat using neuroleptics are informed of and held accountable for the risks they impose, the use of neuroleptics would be reduced, with a concomitant reduction in neuroleptic-induced iatrogenesis.

Therapeutic and Iatrogenic Effects of Neuroleptics

After thirty-five years of use, the limitations of neuroleptic drugs have become acutely apparent and the subject of much debate. Some authors question whether the term "therapeutic," as applied to neuroleptic effects, has any meaning (Breggin, 1983; Cohen, 1988, 1989; Fisher and Greenberg, 1989; Lidz, 1987); some criticize psychiatry's overreliance on drugs to control "schizophrenic" patients and its systematic avoidance of psychosocial alternatives (Easton and Link, 1987; Haley, 1989; Karon, 1989; Kiesler and Sibulkin, 1987, pp. 245–248; Mosher and Burti, 1989); while others detail the visible and hidden costs of adverse effects (Dewan and Koss, 1989; Van Putten and Marder, 1987). According to Doggett and Mercurio (1989), if "schizophrenia" were less debilitating, neuroleptics "would probably be withdrawn on grounds of toxicity" (p. 121). Neurological effects alone include parkinsonism, akathisia, dystonic reactions, the potentially fatal neuroleptic malignant syndrome, supersensitivity psychosis upon drug withdrawal, tardive dementia, and tardive dyskinesia. As many as 75% to 95% of patients develop extrapyramidal symptoms during the course of treatment (Casey, 1989, p. 47).

Roughly one-fifth of patients on long-term neuroleptic treatment exhibit symptoms of TD (Gerlach and Casey, 1988), with the majority of cases rated as mild (Baldessarini et al., 1979). Among the aged and institutionalized, prevalence may be about 40% (Yassa, Nastase, Camille, and Belzile, 1988). Dewan and Koss (1989, pp. 218–219) estimate – using the figure of two million adults prescribed neuroleptics annually in the United States – that somewhere between 90,000 and 625,000 people suffer irreversible TD in a given year. Their figure does not include nursing home residents and the mentally retarded, the two most medicated groups in society (Aman and Singh, 1988; Cluxton and Hurford, 1987); hence it seems likely that more than a million Americans are suffering persistent TD today. It is difficult to estimate accurately the prevalence of TD because neuroleptics also *mask* TD: abnormal movements may emerge only during dose reduction or drug withdrawal. It is now recognized that some physicians do not reduce neuroleptic dosage because they fear that abnormal movements will emerge as a result (Bélanger, 1990).

Other physicians are reluctant to discontinue neuroleptics because of medical complications caused by TD even though they suspect or know that TD is present. Chouinard (1986) states that "a considerable number of patients, particularly those over 65 years of age, would die of complications relating to swallowing or breathing if the neuroleptic medication is withdrawn" (p. 3). Still, some authors suggest that too many discussions of TD are "alarmist" or "overreactions" (Munetz and Schultz, 1986).

Despite the known risks of neuroleptics, most psychiatrists continue to prescribe these drugs because they believe that "the unique therapeutic benefits of neuroleptics are striking and well proved . . . while the effectiveness of alternative treatments remains unproved" (Baldessarini and Cohen, 1986, p. 750). However, considerable evidence from controlled, random-assignment studies clearly shows that, *given the proper social environment*, most newly identified "schizophrenics" can be treated successfully with little or no psychotropic medication. Moreover, open studies demonstrate consistently that these types of social environments can be successfully adapted for use with veteran clients (see extensive reviews and discussions by Karon, 1989, and Mosher and Burti, 1989, pp. 109–168; see also Elizur and Minuchin, 1989).

The "striking" and "unique" benefits of neuroleptics are these drugs' unusual ability to quickly quiet down very excited persons without inducing sleep. Karon (1989) describes this short-term effect and its implications:

> Patients usually become less frightened and frightening. They also generally become less angry. They may lose some of their dramatic "positive" symptoms, like hallucinations. . . . In other cases, the hallucinations and delusions remain, but the patients are not as troubled by them. They take orders better, and comply with other people's demands better. . . . Violent patients usually become manageable, although sometimes only by dosage levels that leave the patient barely awake. The ward staff, treating physician, and family do not feel powerless. Patients are spared some of the destructive things that other people, out of fear, often used to do to schizophrenic patients, both in and out of hospitals. (p. 145)

In longer-term use, the advantages of neuroleptics are more difficult to discern. Regardless of whether patients are maintained on oral or injected neuroleptics, where compliance is ensured, two-year relapse rates in random assignment double-blind studies run about 70–80% for placebo-treated patients and 40–50% for neuroleptic-maintained patients. Combined with a 5% annual incidence of tardive dyskinesia in the latter group, the risk/benefit ratio does *not* seem to favor long-term maintenance (Mosher and Burti, 1989, p. 44). Easton and Link (1987) state that they "have been making long-term observations of patients who do and do not relapse – with high doses, low doses or no doses, and clinically, there has not appeared to be any particular relationship between neuroleptic intake and relapse diminution" (p. 49). Long-term outcome in "schizophrenia" is no better today than it was before the introduction of neuroleptics, when two-thirds of "schizophrenics" recovered without drugs (see Haley, 1989; Mosher and Burti, 1989, p. 3).

We therefore find plausible Karon's (1989) conclusion at the end of his own detailed review of psychosocial treatments for "schizophrenics," that "unfortunately, political and economic factors and a concentration on short-term cost-effectiveness, rather than the scientific findings, currently seem to dictate the type of treatment" (p. 146). One may question the logic and practice of maintaining "schizophrenics" on indefinite maintenance treatment with neuroleptics and exposing them to the known toxicities of these chemicals. Nevertheless, inadequacies in the structure of the mental health system continue to suppress honest appraisals and implementations of alternatives to drug treatments. Drugs are easy to administer – initiating and maintaining supportive, well-staffed social environments is difficult and expensive.

The use of neuroleptic drugs generates difficult dilemmas which patients, physicians, families and other parties face continually. Allocating responsibility for TD and compensating its victims are problems that these participants — and the rest of society — will have to address soon (Appelbaum, Schaffner, and Meisel, 1985).

The Ideal Prescribing Situation

One ethical assumption underlies our analysis: that a person does not have the right to interfere in another person's decisions if these decisions do not affect the first person tangibly.[1] Given this principle, we would not consider the production of drug-induced diseases problematic on a social level if the conditions implicit in Adam Smith's welfare-maximizing free market (Smith, 1924, p. 400) were to exist. These conditions are as follows: individuals are "rational," in that they will attempt to maximize their welfare; all persons have equal access to all available information on the drugs; all persons have an equal ability to understand this information and its implications; no externalities arise from a person's decision to use or not use a neuroleptic, that is to say, this decision has a tangible impact — positive or negative — only on that person[2]; and finally, all citizens have equal access to the drug at a free market price. If all these conditions were met, this would result in a situation where no intermediaries need be involved in the decision to use neuroleptics. Hence, in this situation, responsibility for the consequences of drug use lies with the individual who alone possesses power to decide to take the drug. On a societal level, this abstract situation could not be improved upon by policy intervention.

In reality, of course, these conditions do not hold fully. The decision to use neuroleptics is made in different contexts with varying degrees of adherence to the above "ideal" conditions. We examine some typical contexts in which neuroleptics are used, assess the extent to which participants in the decision to prescribe neuroleptics impose externalities on others, and suggest how these variations from the "ideal" result in sub-optimal consequences. The ensuing

---

[1]We do not attempt the difficult task of defining explicitly what qualifies objectively as a "tangible" interest other than to note that it inevitably involves some further ethical assumptions about what interests are invalid. For example, do persons who are offended because their neighbor sits on his or her porch in pajamas have a *valid* interest in that particular behavior, even if such behavior might affect their property values? (We think not.)

[2]Meade (cited in Cornes and Sandler, 1986, p. 29) has offered the following definition of externality which fits this context well: "an event which confers an appreciable benefit (inflicts an appreciable damage) on the decision or decisions which led directly or indirectly to the event in question." The existence of an externality implies transaction costs and/or imperfect information resulting in a sub-optimal allocation of resources relative to what could be achieved with a change in institutional/government policies (see Dahlman, 1988).

policy recommendations are designed to render the decision-making process more efficient, that is, more likely to yield benefits exceeding costs. We avoid directly addressing the moral issues inherent in the decision-making process leading to use or avoidance of neuroleptics as moral issues per se, concentrating instead on an efficiency criterion.[3] We do not ignore the difference between a moral problem and a technical problem, but we believe it may be very difficult indeed to arrive at a consensus about moral responsibility for TD. We also find that most technical discussions of socio-legal implications of TD fail to address technical issues that might illuminate some of the moral dilemmas (but see Appelbaum et al., 1985; Breggin, 1983; Brown and Funk, 1986; Crane, 1982; Wolf and Brown, 1988).

We use a "political economy" approach in explaining the circumstances under which neuroleptics are prescribed; economic in the sense that actions and transactions by individuals are assumed comprehensible given identified interests (security, money, power, status, etc.), political in recognizing that individuals and groups act to influence the setting of rules which alter the incentive and constraint structure within which the decisions of concern are made. The two terms are put together in recognition that the *same* people act in the political and economic spheres, and that there exists a dynamic relationship between the two spheres. The foregoing is essentially how Buchanan (1972) described the "theory of public choice," a new field whose practitioners frequently term their approach as "political economy," using a broader and more traditional sense of the term than that used by Marxist authors who adopt a class structure analysis.

Power, Information and Incentives in the Prescription of Neuroleptic Drugs

Neuroleptic drugs are prescribed to members of two broad and overlapping categories which can be loosely characterized as "psychiatric patients" and "the institutionalized dependent." The first category contains persons diagnosed with acute or chronic psychotic disorders, for whom neuroleptics are officially indicated (included in this category are those diagnosed with manic-depression; between 1976-1985, there was a nine-fold increase in the number of neuroleptic prescriptions for this subgroup of patients [Wysowsky and Baum, 1989]). The second category contains more or less helpless and

---

[3]"Efficiency" becomes a less clear-cut concept when combined with considerations of power allocations (see Turk, 1983). Economics typically considers power as a given, and the efficiency criterion that of Pareto-optimality, a situation where no one could improve without someone else becoming worse off. Policy recommendations that result in redistributions of initial power could result in a violation of the Pareto-optimality criterion. Our notion of efficiency is modified Pareto-optimality which allows for redistribution of power endowments in accordance with our above-stated ethical assumption regarding non-interference by a person without a tangible interest.

institutionalized persons, with or without psychiatric diagnoses, such as the elderly in nursing homes, the mentally disadvantaged in community residential facilities and the indigent ex-patients in board and care homes. Today, after nearly three decades of psychiatric transinstitutionalization, most persons prescribed neuroleptics fall within the second category.

In this section we describe — using as examples psychiatric patients and nursing home residents — the situations in which neuroleptic drugs are prescribed, with attention to attributes of power/constraints, information, and incentives with respect to the major participants in the medication process (e.g., patients, doctors, institutions and their staff, families, drug companies, society/government). Our arguments would also apply to other groups receiving neuroleptics, but with some modifications. For example, although the level of neuroleptic use among residents of facilities for the mentally disadvantaged is very high (Buck and Sprague, 1989), this level appears to have dropped significantly during the last decade (see analyses by Aman and Singh, 1988; Beyer, 1988; Schroeder, 1988).[4]

Neuroleptics for Psychiatric Patients

Patients. Over 90% of hospitalized persons with a diagnosis of schizophrenia are prescribed neuroleptic drugs (Ban, Guy, and Wilson, 1984). For what reasons are they given drugs? Diamond (1985) mentions that drugs relieve some of patients' pain and suffering, protect patients from unbearable stresses, help patients to sleep or to work, and help patients to shut out unpleasant thoughts. A few first-person accounts of the benefits provided by neuroleptic drugs have been published. For example, Bockes (1985), a graduate student diagnosed as schizophrenic, first resisted taking drugs, but later accepted medication after several hospitalizations. Periodically she experiences hallucinations, but knows when these are coming and uses neuroleptics "before things get out of hand" (p. 489). In sum, neuroleptic drugs, like other drugs, are sought after by certain people who have learned to derive distinct benefits from their use.

Other patients take neuroleptics not because they appreciate their psychophysical benefits but because drugs come with a role these individuals must assume to buttress a claim of disability (perhaps one of the few career options they have). Still other patients do not particularly wish to take neuroleptics,

---

[4]This may be the result of several interacting factors, such as the fact that one of the first tardive dyskinesia lawsuits involved a mentally disadvantaged resident of a residential facility; the entrenched advocacy movement on behalf of the institutionalized mentally disadvantaged; the focus on objective behavioral criteria to justify medication; the increasing application of medication-reducing and medication-monitoring programs in these facilities; and — compared to nursing homes — a greater involvement of trained professionals in the care offered to the mentally disadvantaged.

but feel they must because of implicit or explicit threats. These patients may be threatened with new or prolonged incarceration, with loss of financial benefits (some welfare agencies will dispense funds only upon proof that neuroleptics have been injected), with eviction from one's lodgings, with removal of family affection, with the belief that they will forever remain "mentally ill." There is also an undetermined number of veteran patients who cannot be weaned off neuroleptics either "because their dopamine receptors are starved or because of a real addiction-like withdrawal syndrome which includes what *looks like* the beginning of an exacerbation of psychosis" (Mosher and Burti, 1989, p. 47; see also Breggin, 1989). Finally, some psychiatric patients refuse to take neuroleptic drugs. Professionals often assert that these patients are "delusional" or "deny their illness," though when the patients themselves are given a forum to express their reasons, they usually cite the unpleasantness of adverse effects (Burstow and Weitz, 1988; Van Putten, 1974).[5] It is difficult to estimate how many persons on neuroleptics do not wish to take them. We do know that in 1980, 26% of inpatient psychiatric admissions in the United States were classified as involuntary (cited in Roth, 1989). This statistic is, of course, misleading, since many other less formal but equally effective degrees of coercion of patients co-exist in the mental health system as a whole.

Families. Families of patients have numerous incentives to encourage the use of neuroleptic drugs. Families may support drug use because they seek to support a claim of disability and thus formally enlist the help of the state in supporting their relative/patient. Many patients are "failures," in that they lack basic work and educational skills. In another vein, family members have strong and obvious interests in suppressing the outward signs of psychosis in one of their own, especially if this member lives with them, is dependent on them, and disturbs them with angry, withdrawn, or unpredictable behaviour. The stigma, embarrassment, stresses and sorrows of being related to someone who acts incomprehensibly or erratically are extremely difficult to bear (Lefley, 1989).

Families also come to believe what they are told about their relatives, that they suffer from a brain disease which responds to treatment with neuroleptic drugs (see Johnson, 1989; Rose, 1988). Drug treatment is therefore seen as an enlightened, loving response to psychological distress. In the past, psycho-social formulations of the "causes" of "schizophrenia" implicitly or explicitly blamed families for producing behaviour then labelled "schizo-

---

[5]It is astonishing to note the paucity of published professional discussions envisaging TD from the patient's point of view. Dearing's (1982) short piece is an exception. Accounts from patients themselves appear in Skov (1985) and Steinman (1979), the latter a magazine article on neuroleptics. Finally, TD patients presented their stories in the CBS Evening News programs of November 21–23, 1983.

phrenic." It is well-accepted today that the main reason families of persons with mental illness hold as a central tenet that "schizophrenia" is a brain disease is that this view places no blame on the family (Buie, 1989; Johnson, 1989). Perhaps the most vocal, well-organized and influential lobby group in mental health is the National Alliance for the Mentally Ill (NAMI), an organization of nearly 80,000 relatives of psychiatric patients, which has successfully oriented publicly-funded research toward defining "schizophrenia" as a disease of the brain (see McLean, 1990). For the fiscal year 1990, NAMI is actively lobbying for "at least a $500 million budget for NIMH, with a special emphasis on brain research" (Buie, 1989, p. 26).

Society. The definition and management of misbehaviour and unhappiness as mental health problems constitute an important characteristic of our society. This is reflected in, among other things, monopoly licensing of medical practitioners to diagnose and treat various conditions classified by these practitioners as illnesses. From a societal perspective, drug treatment appears much less costly than any other alternative, cheaper perhaps than even funding *research* into alternatives. Some policy advantages of using drugs are the simplicity of the policy itself and the ease with which it can be communicated to decision makers and the public, the existence of a large network of prescribers, and the ease of training these prescribers (see Kiesler and Sibulkin, 1987, p. 246).

Brown and Cooksey (1989) and Morreim (1990) have discussed two major trends in the new economics of psychiatry and mental health in the United States: the growth of corporate entrepeneurial activities which aim to raise revenues by expanding one's products, services, and clienteles; and reciprocal pressures to contain costs. "The economic pressure to fill beds translates into a commensurate pressure on the profession to expand the concept of psychiatric illness, and with it the criteria for hospitalization and other extensive (revenue-producing) care. . . . Conversely, [with] cost-containment . . . psychiatrists may be pressured to emphasize only those forms of care that are easiest to document and cheapest to deliver" (Morreim, 1990, p. 98).

To the extent that government and third parties pay the cost of health care, they are justified in influencing the decision whether or not to treat with drugs. However, governments are often short-sighted, failing to consider in their policy decisions some of the longer-term costs of neuroleptic treatment should TD develop in substantial numbers of patients. Clearly, neuroleptic treatment in the short run saves the costs of institutionalization, professional services, and policing deviance, but in the longer run such costs may still have to be paid. Severe TD implies severe disability, mental and physical (Engle, Whall, Dimond, and Bobel, 1985; Gardos, Cole, Salomon, and Schneilbock, 1987), including possibly tardive psychosis and tardive dementia. This, in turn, implies institutionalization or extensive home care support. Discussions on the short- and long-term costs of neuroleptic use are rare (but see Dewan and Koss, 1989), and these costs remain unexplored despite the numbers of TD cases.

The paucity of discussions on long-term costs may reflect the belief that drugs are justified because of the medical nature of the problems drugs are said to treat. This belief — roughly translated as "the medical model" — constitutes one of the ideological underpinnings of our modern age and necessarily shapes possible responses to TD. For example, Munetz and Schultz (1986), who claim to adopt a balanced, rational approach to TD, state that the proposition "schizophrenia is a serious brain disease," "need[s] to be accepted before TD can be responded to objectively" (p. 168). Similarly, Rose (1988, p. 1) believes that only "a change in the way schizophrenia is perceived in America will help to make antipsychotic medicine more acceptable." This is an unusual assertion, since prescribers, families, institutions, drug companies, and society widely praise, endorse, use, advertise and accept neuroleptics. If anyone needs to accept neuroleptics more than at present, patients themselves appear to be the prime candidates.

Not unexpectedly, patients are the least represented parties in public policy debates and lobbying. This is partly a result of the "free rider" problem, which increases as group size increases (i.e., people are individually likely to invest fewer resources in lobbying the more dispersed are the benefits arising from such lobbying). Therefore, by virtue of numbers alone, we cannot expect patient advocacy groups to enjoy an advantage over competing groups with smaller membership (Katz, Nitzan, and Rosenberg, 1990). The drug industry has less of a free rider problem than patient groups since the relatively few firms benefit directly from investing to influence public perceptions and government policies. Psychiatric associations, for their part, have defeated the free rider problem among their members by enforcing membership (with legal sanction); the group as a whole has the power to levy members for contributions for lobbying purposes. While families have a free rider problem similar to that of patients, family associations have been very successful in inducing families to join their lobby groups and to make a membership contribution. Some of their success, relative to that of patient groups, can be attributed to patients' limited socio-political skills, education, and access to financial resources.

Groups representing patients' interests are very small, loosely organized and receive, at best, haphazard funding. On Our Own, an association of current and ex-psychiatric patients in Toronto, constitutes the only such group in Canada to consistently offer guidelines for the use of biological treatments in psychiatry. However, their magazine, *Phoenix Rising*, is regularly threatened with dissolution due to underfunding. The privation of patient groups weakens their ability to participate in public policy debates and leaves a greater role to the other parties involved. Two former On Our Own activists put it this way: "Those who have experienced [neuroleptics] rarely have the resources to combat the propaganda churned out by the medical establishment and its allies – they can't launch an advertising campaign to counter the deceptive schizophrenia posters found on the Toronto Transit Commission vehicles" (Burstow and Weitz, 1990, p. 8). Mental patients, as with other relatively helpless and unempowered people, thus often must rely on *others* to protect their public interests. It is natural to think that families are best-suited for this role, but there is no reason to assume that the interests of patients and the interests of families coincide. On the contrary, common sense suggests that patient and family concerns may conflict – and personal observation confirms that they usually do. This simple fact is rarely acknowledged, which helps explain why so few concerned persons press to ensure that points of view unique to patients are reflected in public debates.

Physicians. The most powerful incentive for psychiatrists to prescribe neuroleptics derives from their professional identity as physicians. For most practicing psychiatrists, "functional" psychoses are soon-to-be-discovered brain diseases or the symptoms of such diseases. Though practitioners recognize the importance of social, psychological and environmental factors on the causes, courses and outcomes of many conditions they treat, their practice relies almost exclusively on psychotropic drugs. According to Mosher and Burti (1989), "the drug treatment of schizophrenia seems to be subject to the greatest intensity of dogmatism. . . . [W]ithdrawing neuroleptics from persons with this label is extraordinarily difficult. . . . The party line that schizophrenia is a chronic illness treatable only with medication has the field firmly in its grasp" (p. 40).

Brown and Funk (1986) have also pointed out the importance of physician-patient differences in the perception of medication efficacy: "Physicians usually perceive medication in terms of symptom reduction and/or illness cure, whereas patients typically are more concerned about its effects on daily living routines. . . ." These authors believe physician concern "with narrow medical issues rather than broader sociomedical ones . . . demonstrates some important shortcomings of [medical] training," notably, an "emphasis on individual pathology without regard for social components of the experience of illness" (pp. 126–127).

In a similar vein, Szasz (1977) pointed out that psychiatrists do not give money to their poor patients or friendship to the lonely. Today, the only visible sign of their power to heal is the drug and the regimen with which the drug is prescribed (Montagne, 1988). It is not difficult to see why, as Munetz (1985) suggested, it is psychologically painful for a clinician to recognize that medication he or she has prescribed may cause severe or irreversible harm. Yet, even if such recognition occurs, what is an ordinary, well-intentioned physician schooled in the medical model to do? Well-organized psychosocial healing contexts are so rare or inaccessible as not even to rate as a viable alternative (Elizur and Minuchin, 1989).[6] At the present time, aside from hospitalization and neuroleptic drugs, the only real option in the treatment of a "schizophrenic" patient is to do nothing. Yet, to do nothing or to re-move neuroleptics, even in a research project, may leave the physician ex-posed to charges of unethical practice (Engstrom, 1988). Even expressing views concerning the danger of neuroleptics may lead to serious repercussions. "When a psychiatrist (Dr. Peter Breggin) acknowledged on a television inter-view . . . that patients' concerns about [TD] were justified, that this was a serious problem, and that patients should seek out professionals who are in-terested in helping the patients understand themselves, and not professionals who are interested in only medicating, an attempt was made to silence him" (Karon, 1989, p. 107). NAMI, assisted by the American Psychiatric Associa-tion, filed charges with the medical licensing board of Maryland to revoke Dr. Breggin's medical license (the charges were eventually dismissed).

Thus, every general bias that we are able to identify in the practitioner increases the likelihood of prescribing drugs. Moreover, if − in the doctor's mind − information given to the patient about drug risks leads to the patient's refusal to take the drug, then the doctor also has an incentive *not* to inform. Benson (1984) reported that one-third of psychiatrists disclosed risks for signifi-cant adverse effects and TD to patients on neuroleptics, and one-tenth thought it better not to discuss this with patients. One recent trend, however, repre-sents a potential incentive to prevent TD: the threat of malpractice litiga-tion. Recent, well-publicized cases have set precedents and − in theory at least − have constrained psychiatric practice. Yet, as we have seen, established guidelines such as APA's "have been honored more in the breach than the keeping" (Gualtieri et al., 1986, p. 206).

Generally, doctors are assumed to act "in the best interests" of their pa-tients. In our view, this should mean acting *as the patient would act* if fully competent and possessing the knowledge possessed by the doctor. The doc-tor, however, brings in more than his or her knowledge in reaching the deci-sion. The doctor also brings in his or her own values, which may or may not correspond with the patient's, including values attached to the medical model − a model which constitutes more than a theory but which may be

---

[6]It is beyond the scope of this paper to analyze why "community mental health," which was seen as a viable alternative by many physicians in the 1960s and early 1970s, has greatly declined and why choice of treatment is now posed as a simple dichotomy of drug/no drug. Suffice it to say that this change may be due to the strong rightward trend of American politics during this period, a trend characterized in the field of mental health by the application of narrow perspectives to larger social problems and by the downplaying of real and potential fears about the effects of psychotechnology expressed by target populations and other critics (see analyses by Brown, 1985; Mosher and Burti, 1989).

in fact a self-serving attitude/paradigm for the profession [see Engel, 1977]). *Drug companies.* Drug companies profit from drug sales and cannot be expected to have incentives other than aiming for increased consumption of their products. The symbiotic relationship between drug companies, medical associations and regulatory bodies has been extensively discussed (Silverman and Lee, 1974). Drug companies are directly involved in the decision to prescribe drugs via the information they provide to doctors and the funds they contribute to professional psychiatric associations. This information includes advertisements in psychiatric journals, package inserts, and other forms of labeling and promotion. In the standard by which most investigators judge the quality of prescription practices, the *Physicians' Desk Reference*, listings themselves — which must be approved by the Food and Drug Administration (FDA) — are forms of labeling *and* promotion, or a form of paid advertising distributed freely to physicians (Silverman, 1976). A recent example of drug promotion is an unprecendented ten-page advertisement by Sandoz Pharmaceuticals Corporation for the neuroleptic clozapine (Clozaril) — used for a decade in Europe and recently introduced into the United States — in the January 1990 issue of the *American Journal of Psychiatry* and other journals. The ad, which resembles a newspaper insert, comes complete with the Statue of Liberty announcing "A beacon of hope for thousands of problem schizophrenic patients and their psychiatrists" (clozapine is thought to be superior than typical neuroleptics for nonresponders and almost free of extrapyramidal symptoms). The amount of money multinational drug companies can spend on advertising creates an imbalance in the sort of information physicians are exposed to. Simply, information provided by independent observers and anti-drug advocates does not get nearly as much publicity (see also McDonnell, 1986; Mintz, 1985).

Neuroleptics for Elderly Nursing Home Residents

The staple use of neuroleptics in nursing homes is well-documented (Bishop, 1989; Cluxton and Hurford, 1987). In a recent study of all 33,351 Illinois long-term adult nursing home residents who are Medicaid recipients, Buck (1988) found that 45% received neuroleptic drugs. Most neuroleptics had mean lengths of administration of six months or more, "implying that once individuals are placed on such medications, they continue to receive them" (p. 417). If we estimate a conservative 20% prevalence rate of neuroleptic use in nursing homes, approximately 400,000 institutionalized elderly in the United States are receiving these drugs.

Most experts agree that neuroleptics are administered to nursing home residents because the drugs effectively control disruptive and agitated behaviour (Fauteux, 1988). On a daily basis, one-fifth of elderly nursing home residents may exhibit "problem behaviours," such as disorientation, aggression, wandering, noisiness (Rockwood, Stolee, and Robertson, 1989). One study found that neuroleptics were prescribed more frequently to "physically incapacitated people together with wandering and aggressive ones" (Nygaard, Bakke, and Breivik, 1990, p. 170). To what extent is this practice justified? It is well to remember that few persons are officially committed to nursing homes and treatment is thus ostensibly on a "voluntary" basis for most residents. Thus, in only a few situations might there exist some legal controls that would apply to compensate for the general helplessness of the resident.

Residents. Many residents of nursing homes — perhaps even the typical resident — have less than full mental capacity, and many incompetent patients receive neuroleptic drugs without recognition of their incompetency by a court of law (Hoffman, 1989). It is reasonable to assume that most of these persons do not have any incentives to take neuroleptics. We cannot imagine that neuroleptics make them feel better physically. Generally, we do not see the possibility that neuroleptics present any benefits for these individuals. However, neuroleptics have a cost: the onset of TD — of which increasing age is the single most widely accepted risk factor (Gerlach and Casey, 1988). The available evidence clearly supports the conclusion that nursing home residents are usually not informed of the risks of drugs and that the rationale offered for prescribing the drugs — if one is offered — is simplistic or misleading. The investigators in one study — which attempted to determine how prescribers obtained informed consent from their nursing home patients — summarized part of their findings as follows: "The results indicate that physicians in nursing homes do not inform their patients of the risks of neuroleptics, do not seek consent, and do not consider competency to be even an issue" (Gurian, Baker, Jacobson, Lagerbom, and Watts, 1990, p. 37).

Institutions. By 1980, 81% of nursing homes in the United States were privately owned (Hawes and Phillips, 1986). These facilities operate in a highly competitive market, increasingly dominated by large proprietary chains. Possibly the strongest incentive for these institutions to remain competitive is to keep their costs as low as is legally possible (see Grimaldi, 1985, pp. 80–81). Service competition is restricted to the few elite homes which charge more than the competitive minimum to clients or families who are relatively wealthy. However, over 50% of nursing home expenditures in the United States are financed by direct or indirect government funding (Eckholm, 1990). For these institutions most revenues are legally fixed and profit lies in cutting costs.

Third-party payers can be expected to be less concerned about service than the client but more concerned about price. Therefore, it may be the rare institution that will maintain staff and standards beyond the minimum legal requirements. There is a very high patient-staff ratio, and minimum standards in fact operate as *average* standards of care (Waxman, Klein, and Carner,

1985). A recent study estimates that there are only 1.5 licensed nursing staff per 100 patients in United States nursing homes, compared to one registered nurse for 4.5 patients in acute care ("Hospitalization," 1989).

According to Waxman et al. (1985), "psychotropic drugs are used less for the treatment of ailing patients than for the treatment of an ailing institution – the long-term care industry" (p. 886). Pay is low, physical conditions are often poor, work is demanding, frequently degrading. Nursing home staff are consequently less qualified than those in other health care settings. Physicians are usually not present. More than 90% of the patient care in nursing homes is actually delivered by nurses' aides, who, in terms of education and wages, fall at the bottom of the nursing home hierarchy; job turnover among aides averages nearly 40% annually in the United States (pp. 886–887). Under these conditions, "it is not difficult to understand how psychotropic drugs, particularly [neuroleptics], are quite effective in reducing the burden on the staff. Patients who are drowsy, asleep, or slowed down are simply less of a management problem" (p. 887). According to other studies, overdrugging of residents is especially common on weekends, when homes are apt to be short-staffed (Bishop, 1989; see also Lempinen, 1987).

How do staff responsibilities correlate with staff knowledge of psychotropic drugs? Avorn, Dreyer, Connelly, and Soumerai (1989), in a survey of 55 rest homes in Massachusetts, assessed staff competence and found a low level of comprehension of the purpose and side effects of commonly used psychotropics. The neuroleptic chlorpromazine (Thorazine, Largactil) was identified as a minor tranquilizer by 47% and as an antidepressant by 12%, while 19% did not know its purpose. In response to a straightforward clinical vignette, nearly half the respondents failed to recognize the primary manifestation of TD, attributing the symptoms to a stroke (15 percent), mental illness (11 percent), a heart condition (6 percent), or blood pressure problems (3 percent), or gave no response (12 percent). Among the residents with movement disorders noted on examination by surveyors, only 17% had any mention of TD in their records.

Engle et al. (1985) showed that among residents in foster care homes on neuroleptics, as the number of TD symptoms increase, there is a corresponding decrease in the ability to perform activities. This suggests that medicating nursing home residents in order to reduce the time it takes to care for them is an option that may not be fully balanced by information concerning the increased disability of these residents, and thus the increased efforts to minister to them.

Physicians may be paid by the resident, institution, a government agency, families, or insurance companies, but they are hired by the institution. It is unlikely that residents of nursing homes have much say concerning who their doctor will be. Much of the information the physician receives about the residents will come by necessity from the staff. The power of nurses and other staff is considerable: Avorn et al. (1989) found nearly half of prescriptions for neuroleptics to be written "as needed," thereby placing the decision to administer in the hands of the nurses. Ray, Blazer, Schaffner, and Federspiel (1987) — reporting on the failure of an educational visit aiming to reduce neuroleptic prescriptions by nursing home physicians — concluded that "in the nursing home, nursing staff may have a key part in therapeutic decisions. Alternate methods of behavior management can require increased commitment of time by nurses and physicians or resources by the facility, a commitment which may be difficult to make in the present-day nursing home environment" (p. 1449).

As noted, many people who enter nursing homes have limited capacity, a condition magnified further by residing in an institution. It is easy for physicians in such a situation to treat the consent process lightly, and that appears to be the reality in most nursing homes. Their own biases, as noted earlier, in addition to the institutional pressures, would militate against disclosing risks such as TD or explaining why a neuroleptic is needed. The fear of malpractice would be much lower than in more supervised settings, and when TD symptoms emerge, these might be attributed by staff to the resident's generally disabled condition.

Institutional pressures, delegation of health care responsibilities to facility staff, and an insufficient recognition of the risk of TD lead us to the conclusion that the effect of physicians' neuroleptic prescription practices in nursing homes reflects more the interests of institutions than of residents. In the short term at least, the decision to use neuroleptics in a nursing home imposes a cost to the resident and a benefit to the institution. The latter is often funded by third parties, supposedly acting on behalf of the resident, to provide shelter, care, and supervision. Such funding does not justify the *modification* of the resident through the administration of neuroleptics. Unfortunately, an institution that does not encourage the indiscriminate use of neuroleptics may believe itself to be at a competitive disadvantage to an institution that does, since the latter practice may cut costs and may be more attractive to potential payers. However, if neuroleptic use were drastically curtailed and all institutions changed their practices, costs would be increased equitably for all. Hence, regulating the administration of neuroleptics might not face institutional opposition — as long as regulations are enforced and institutions are compensated for increased care costs.

Policy Recommendations

Our brief examination of the contexts within which neuroleptic drugs are prescribed reveals systematic pressures, constraints, and biases leading participants to opt for neuroleptics without sufficient attention to the costs imposed by their use. In our view, this situation calls for countervailing pressures and policy interventions.

The Medical Model

There is a pressing need for public debate about the legitimacy of the medical model (i.e., that the phenomena termed "mental illnesses" are actual diseases requiring eradication or management by mental health professionals [Engel, 1977]). In our view, society can best represent its interests if it becomes more aware of the controversy surrounding issues of definition of misbehaviour, and if it attempts to critically rethink the claims of biological psychiatry (see Fisher and Greenberg, 1989). To that end, we suggest, as a first step, that patients and patient advocate groups receive far greater assistance to represent and present their points of view to the general public. Such assistance would help to counterbalance the advantages enjoyed by groups with competing perspectives, particularly by professional associations, who have reduced their free-rider problem due to government regulation sanctioning professional monopolies (see, for example, Kilbane and Beck, 1990).

Standard of Care

The incentives facing institutions and doctors are such that, by itself, *information on TD is not sufficient to produce major changes in neuroleptic prescription practices.* Unquestionably, adherence to the American Psychiatric Association's 1979 guidelines would reduce the incidence and prevalence of TD and other adverse effects. Fewer persons would be treated with neuroleptics, and fewer persons on neuroleptics would receive high doses. Constant monitoring for TD through periodic dose reduction or drug withdrawal would uncover early signs and lead to proper management and prevention of the condition. The results of litigation thus far have established little in the way of judicially created standards for the administration of neuroleptics. We believe the American Psychiatric Association guidelines should immediately form the basis for such standard. In our view, not adhering to these guidelines without valid reason constitutes grounds for malpractice action. Specific regulations should be considered regarding certain aspects of neuroleptic use: for example, if "as needed" prescriptions are not banned altogether, time restrictions must be imposed on them. The APA should yearly re-issue its guidelines with a warning that contravenors could be liable to disciplinary action (e.g., license suspension or revocation, fine, re-education, removal of prescription privileges) if a complaint is substantiated. All persons — particularly nursing home staff and aides – who have a role in prescribing and administering the drugs should have a role in monitoring for TD.

Informed Consent

Informed consent remains at the heart of ethical medical practice. In our view, consent, not the presence of illness, constitutes the only morally justifiable basis for medical treatment. If a patient appears incompetent, it is incumbent upon the health professional not to treat and to obtain a court order to do so.

For a condition as severe as TD, a signed consent form should be a minimum requirement. A consent form may in some instances serve to cover up the failure to obtain true informed consent, but a consent form need not simply explain risks and benefits of neuroleptics. A consent form should specify the physician's duties as given in the APA guidelines, and it should be signed by the prescriber. The consent form should also indicate that the prescriber's professional actions are suitably monitored, and be signed by the administrator (see, for example, Kalachnik and Slaw's [1986, p. 5] discussion of written informed consent policy variables). Failure to abide by the conditions of consent forms would constitute, in the absence of mitigating circumstances, sufficient grounds for courts to find malpractice.

Civil Litigation

Civil litigation is a means of reducing externalities so that those who impose unwanted costs on others are made to compensate the affected persons. In this context it means that physicians and institutions who improperly impose or maintain neuroleptic treatments, for example, without the patient's full informed consent, should compensate the patient who develops TD as a result. However, since litigation is available to a very few, court decisions have a limited impact. On the other hand, court decisions inform patients and families of the risks of TD and warn physicians and administrators of the risks *they* may face if the patient develops TD.

Some observers of the judicial process, while supporting the concept of malpractice litigation, decry "excessive" awards to plaintiffs. In any individual case such awards may be excessive, but overall they amount to a minute fraction of what "justifiably" would be awarded if all aggrieved TD sufferers were to litigate. Malpractice awards are paid for by professionals' insurance companies and are reflected in the fees for insurance. To the extent that these fees approach the cost of TD borne by patients who were not properly treated or informed, doctors and administrators can be expected to moderate their use of neuroleptics. Since the vast majority of potentially successful litigants will never go to court, individual awards should more than compensate successful litigants for all identifiable costs, including loss of earnings, loss of enjoyment of life, loss of companionship borne by the victim and by family members. In cases of negligence, a punitive award should also be levied. If anything, such litigation should be encouraged, including using existing government funding mechanisms, such as provision of legal aid and/or justice department funding to monitor relevant court cases and help provide precedents to aspiring litigants.

Drug Information

Professional medical and psychiatric associations should recognize the flagrant conflict of interest in accepting paid advertisements for drugs in their official journals as well as in the practice of financial support of their professional and scientific activities. While any individual practitioner might with good conscience deny the impact of such drug company subsidies in their own practice, these subsidies, combined with the high rate of psychotropic drug prescription by physicians, create a clear impression of at least systematic or unconscious bias.

Physicans are subject to extremely large quantities of information (in the form of advertisements, samples, brochures, and other promotional material) from drug companies operating with a purely financial incentive. Should not physicians also receive information from the naysayers? By means of voluntary compliance or regulation, drug company information should be made more balanced by inclusion of references to controversies regarding therapeutic and adverse effects of neuroleptics.

Conclusion

Although we believe that our recommendations, if implemented, will help reduce the problems we have outlined in this paper, we realize that decision-makers are likely to consider them only in a social and economic environment which reflects a commitment to scientific and professional responsibility, and to individual autonomy (see Mosher and Burti, 1989). Thus, as long as psychosocial alternatives to drug treatment of "schizophrenics" do not exist widely, drug treatment is inevitable. As long as non-medical health professionals continue to defer to physicians when medication decisions are contemplated and avoid learning more about the documented values and limitations of drug treatment, prescription abuses will persist. As long as mental health interventions continue to be dominated by mental hospitalization, the preservation of personal power of patients will be eroded and will lead to further dependency and iatrogenic injury.

References

Aman, M.G., and Singh, N.N. (1988). Patterns of drug use: Methodological considerations, measurement techniques, and future trends. In M.G. Aman and N.N. Singh (Eds.), *Psychopharmacology of the developmental disabilities* (pp. 1–28). New York: Springer-Verlag.

American Psychiatric Association. (1985). APA statement on tardive dyskinesia. *Hospital and Community Psychiatry, 36,* 902.

Appelbaum, A., Schaffner, K., and Meisel, A. (1985). Responsibility and compensation for tardive dyskinesia. *American Journal of Psychiatry, 142,* 806–810.

Avorn, J., Dreyer, P., Connelly, K., and Soumerai, S.B. (1989). Use of psychoactive medication and the quality of care in rest homes: Findings and policy implications of a statewide survey. *The New England Journal of Medicine, 320,* 227–232.

Baldessarini, R.J., and Cohen, B.M. (1986). Regulation of psychiatric practice [Editorial]. *American Journal of Psychiatry, 143,* 750–751.

Baldessarini, R.J., Cole, J.D., Davis, J.M., Gardos, G., Preskorn, S.H., Simpson, G.M., and Tarsy, D. (1979). *Tardive dyskinesia: Report the of the American Psychiatric Association task force on late neurological effects of antipsychotic drugs.* Washington, D.C.: American Psychiatric Association.

Ban, T.A., Guy, W., and Wilson, W.H. (1984). Pharmacotherapy of chronic hospitalized schizophrenics: Diagnosis and treatment. *Psychiatric Journal of the University of Ottawa, 9,* 191–195.

Bélanger, M. (1990). Les neuroleptiques à long terme: Les pierres d'achoppement [Long-term neuroleptic treatment: The stumbling blocks]. *L'actualité médicale,* 1, 74–76.

Benson, P.R. (1984). Informed consent: Drug information is closed to patients prescribed antipsychotic medication. *Journal of Nervous and Mental Disease, 172,* 642–653.

Beyer, H.A. (1988). Litigation and use of psychoactive drugs in developmental disabilities. In M.G. Aman and N.N. Singh (Eds.), *Psychopharmacology of the developmental disabilities* (pp. 29–57). New York: Springer-Verlag.

Bishop, K. (1989, March 13). Studies find drugs still overused to control nursing home elderly. *New York Times,* pp. A-1; A-12.

Bockes, Z. (1985). First person account: "Freedom" means knowing you have a choice. *Schizophrenia Bulletin, 11,* 487–489.

Breggin, P.R. (1983). *Psychiatric drugs: Hazards to the brain.* New York: Springer.

Breggin, P.R. (1989). Addiction to neuroleptics [letter]. *American Journal of Psychiatry, 146,* 560.

Brown, P. (1985). *The transfer of care: Psychiatric deinstitutionalization and its aftermath.* London: Routledge & Kegan Paul.

Brown, P., and Cooksey, E. (1989). Mental health monopoly: Corporate trends in mental health services. *Social Science and Medicine, 28,* 1129–1138.

Brown, P., and Funk, S.C. (1986). Tardive dyskinesia: Professional barriers to the recognition of an iatrogenic disease. *Journal of Health and Social Behavior, 27,* 116–132.

Buchanan, J.M. (1972). Toward analysis of closed behavioral systems. In J.M. Buchanan and R.D. Tollison (Eds.), *Theory of public choice: Political applications in economics* (pp. 11–23). Ann Arbor, Michigan: University of Michigan Press.

Buck, J.A. (1988). Psychotropic drug practice in nursing homes. *Journal of the American Geriatrics Society, 36,* 409–418.

Buck, J.A., and Sprague, R.L. (1989). Psychotropic medication of mentally retarded residents in community long-term care facilities. *American Journal of Mental Retardation, 93,* 618–623.

Buie, J. (1989, July). Families of mentally ill have advocate in Flynn. *The APA Monitor,* p. 26.

Burstow, B., and Weitz, D. (1988). (Eds.). *Shrink resistant.* Vancouver, British Columbia: New Star Books.

Burstow, B., and Weitz, D. (1990, January 8). The tragic myth of schizophrenia. *The Toronto Globe and Mail,* p. A8.

Casey, D.E. (1989). Clozapine: Neuroleptic-induced EPS and tardive dyskinesia. *Psychopharmacology, 99* (Supplement), 47–53.

Chouinard, G. (1986). Advances in the management of acute mania and bipolar manic-depressive illness. In The Medicine Publishing Foundation (Ed.), *New concepts in mania and panic disorder:*

Focus on clonazepam: Proceedings of a symposium held in Vancouver, Canada, September, 1986 (pp. 3–14). Oxford: Medicine Publishing.

Cluxton, R.J., and Hurford, B. (1987). Medicating the elderly. In C. Chambers, J. Lindquist, O. White, and M. Harters (Eds.), *The elderly: Victims and deviants* (pp. 72–109). Athens, Ohio: Ohio University Press.

Cohen, D. (1988). Social work and psychotropic drug treatments. *Social Service Review, 63,* 576–599.

Cohen, D. (1989). Author's reply: Good intentions are not enough. *Social Service Review, 64,* 660–664.

Cornes, R., and Sandler, R. (1986). *The theory of externalities, public goods and club goods.* Cambridge: Cambridge University Press.

Crane, G.E. (1982). Medical and legal responsibilities of physicians prescribing neuroleptics. In J. DeVeaugh-Geiss (Ed.), *Tardive dyskinesia and related involuntary movement disorders: The long-term effects of anti-psychotic drugs* (pp. 189–191). Boston: John Wright PSG.

Dahlman, C.J. (1988). The problem of externality. In T. Cowen (Ed.), *The theory of market failure: A critical examination* (pp. 209–234). Fairfax, Virginia: George Mason University Press.

Davidson, M., Keefe, R., Mohs, R., Siever, L., Bergman, R.L., Losonczy, M.F., Horvath, T., and Davis, K.L. (1988). Dr. Davidson and colleagues reply [letter]. *American Journal of Psychiatry, 145,* 388.

Dearing, B. (1982). Patient perspectives on iatrogenic disease. In J. DeVeaugh-Geiss (Ed.), *Tardive dyskinesia and related involuntary movement disorders: The long-term effects of anti-psychotic drugs* (pp. 195–198). Boston: John Wright PSG.

Dewan, M.J., and Koss, M. (1989). The clinical impact of the side effects of psychotropic drugs. In S. Fisher and R. Greenberg (Eds.), *The limits of biological treatments for psychological distress: Comparisons with psychotherapy and placebo* (pp. 189–234). Hillsdale, New Jersey: Lawrence Erlbaum Associates.

Diamond, R.L. (1985). Drugs and the quality of life: The patient's point of view. *Journal of Clinical Psychiatry, 46,* 49–35.

Dixon, L., Weiden, P.J., Frances, A., and Rapkin, B. (1989). Management of neuroleptic-induced movement disorders: Effects of physician training. *American Journal of Psychiatry, 146,* 104–106.

Doggett, N.S., and Mercurio, G.G. (1989). Calcium blockers in tardive dyskinesia [letter]. *American Journal of Psychiatry, 146,* 121–122.

Easton, K., and Link, I. (1987). Do neuroleptics prevent relapse? Clinical observations in a psychosocial rehabilitation program. *Psychiatric Quarterly, 53,* 42–50.

Eckholm, E. (1990, March 27). Haunting issue for U.S.: Caring for the elderly ill. *New York Times,* pp. A1; A18.

Elizur, J., and Minuchin, S. (1989). *Institutionalizing madness: Families, therapy, and society.* New York: Basic Books.

Engel, G.L. (1977). The need for a new medical model: A challenge for biomedicine. *Science, 196,* 129–136.

Engle, V.F., Whall, A., Dimond, C., and Bobel, L. (1985). Tardive dyskinesia: Are your older clients at risk? *Journal of Gerontological Nursing, 11,* 25–27.

Engstrom, F.W. (1988). Ethical issues in drug studies [letter]. *American Journal of Psychiatry, 145,* 387–388.

Fauteux, A. (1988, December 6). Tranquilizers used just to keep elderly patients quiet, experts say. *The Montreal Gazette,* p. A-4.

Fisher, S., and Greenberg, R.P. (1989). A second opinion: Rethinking the claims of biological psychiatry. In S. Fisher and R.P. Greenberg (Eds.), *The limits of biological treatments for psychological distress: Comparisons with psychotherapy and placebo* (pp. 309–336). Hillsdale, New Jersey: Lawrence Erlbaum Associates.

Gardos, G., Cole, J.O., Salomon, M., and Schneilbock, S. (1987). Clinical forms of severe tardive dyskinesia. *American Journal of Psychiatry, 144,* 895–902.

Gerlach, J., and Casey, D.E. (1988). Tardive dyskinesia. *Acta Psychiatrica Scandinavica, 77,* 369–378.

Grimaldi, P.L. (1985). *Setting rates for hospital and nursing home care.* Jamaica, New York: Spectrum.

Gualtieri, C.T., and Sprague, R.L. (1984). Preventing tardive dyskinesia and preventing tardive dyskinesia litigation. *Psychopharmacology Bulletin, 24,* 346–348.

Gualtieri, C.T., Sprague, R.L., and Cole, J.O. (1986). Tardive dyskinesia litigation and the dilemmas of neuroleptic treatment. *The Journal of Psychiatry and Law*, Spring/Summer, 187–216.

Gurian, B.S., Baker, E., Jacobson, S., Lagerbom, B., and Watts, P. (1990). Informed consent for neuroleptics with elderly patients in two settings. *Journal of the American Geriatrics Society*, 38, 37–44.

Haley, J. (1989). The effect of long-term outcome studies on the therapy of schizophrenia. *Journal of Marital and Family Therapy*, 15, 127–132.

Hawes, C., and Phillips, C.D. (1986). The changing structure of the nursing home industry and the impact of ownership on quality, cost, and access. In B.H. Gray (Ed.), *For-profit enterprise in health care* (pp. 492–541). Washington, D.C.: National Academy Press.

Hedin v. United States. United States District Court, Minnesota, Fifth Division, No. 5-83-3 (1984).

Hoffman, B. (1989). Future trends in the legal rights of patients in nursing homes. *Canadian Medical Association Journal*, 141, 21–25.

Hospitalization of nursing home patients costs millions. (1989, November 29). *UC Clip Sheet*, 65, 1.

Johnson, D.L. (1989). Schizophrenia as a brain disease: Implications for psychologists and families. *American Psychologist*, 44, 553–555.

Kalachnik, J.E., and Slaw, K.M. (1986). Tardive dyskinesia: Update for the mental health administrator. *Journal of Mental Health Administration*, 13, 1–8.

Karon, B.P. (1989). Psychotherapy versus medication for schizophrenia: Empirical comparisons. In S. Fisher and R.P. Greenberg (Eds.), *The limits of biological treatments for psychological distress: Comparisons with psychotherapy and placebo* (pp. 105–150). Hillsdale, New Jersey: Lawrence Erlbaum Associates.

Katz, E., Nitzan, S., and Rosenberg, J. (1990). Rent-seeking for pure public goods. *Public Choice*, 65, 49–60.

Kiesler, C., and Sibulkin, A. (1987). *Mental hospitalization: Myths and facts about a national crisis*. Beverly Hills: Sage.

Kilbane, S.C., and Beck, J.H. (1990). Professional associations and the free rider problem: The case of optometry. *Public Choice*, 65, 181–187.

Lefley, H.P. (1989). Family burden and family stigma in major mental illness. *American Psychologist*, 44, 556–560.

Lempinen, E.W. (1987, June 16). San Mateo nursing home fined for deaths, injuries. *San Francisco Chronicle*, p. 4.

Lidz, T. (1987). Editorial book review: The effective treatment of schizophrenic patients. *Journal of Nervous and Mental Disease*, 175, 447–449.

McDonnell, K. (1986). (Ed.). *Adverse effects: Women and the pharmaceutical industry*. Toronto: Women's Educational Press.

McLean, A. (1990). Contradictions in the social production of clinical knowledge: The case of schizophrenia. *Social Science and Medicine*, 30, 969–985.

Mills, M.J., and Eth, S. (1987). Legal liability with psychotropic drug use: Extrapyramidal syndromes and tardive dyskinesia. *Journal of Clinical Psychiatry*, 48 (Supplement), 28–33.

Mills, M.J., Norquist, G.S., Shelton, R.C., Gelenberg, A.J., and Van Putten, T. (1986). Consent and liability with neuroleptics: The problem of tardive dyskinesia. *International Journal of Law and Psychiatry*, 8, 243–252.

Mintz, M. (1985). *At any cost: Corporate greed, women, and the Dalkon Shield*. New York: Pantheon.

Montagne, M. (1988). The metaphorical nature of drugs and drug-taking. *Social Science and Medicine*, 26, 417–424.

Morreim, E.H. (1990). The new economics of medicine: Special challenges for psychiatry. *Journal of Medicine and Philosophy*, 15, 97–119.

Mosher, L., and Burti, L. (1989). *Community mental health: Principles and practice*. New York: Norton.

Munetz, M.R. (1985). Overcoming resistance to talking to patients about tardive dyskinesia. *Schizophrenia Bulletin*, 12, 168–172.

Munetz, M.R., and Schultz, S.C. (1986). Minimization and overreaction to tardive dyskinesia. *Schizophrenia Bulletin*, 12, 168–172.

Nygaard, H.A., Bakke, K.J., and Breivik, K. (1990). Mental and physical capacity and consumption of neuroleptic drugs in residents of homes for aged people. *Acta Psychiatrica Scandinavica*, 80, 170–173.

Pirodsky, D.M. (1982). Prediction and prevention of tardive dyskinesia: Panel discussion. In J. DeVeaugh-Geiss (Ed.), *Tardive dyskinesia and related involuntary movement disorders: The long-term effects of anti-psychotic drugs* (pp. 170-171). Boston: John Wright PSG.

Ray, W.A., Blazer, D.G., Schaffner, W.S., and Federspiel, C.F. (1987). Reducing antipsychotic drug prescribing for nursing home patients: A controlled trial of the effect of an educational visit. *American Journal of Public Health, 77*, 1448-1450.

Reardon, G.T., Rifkin, A., Schwartz, A., Myerson, A., and Siris, S.G. (1989). Changing patterns of neuroleptic dosage over a decade. *American Journal of Psychiatry, 146*, 726-729.

Rockwood, K., Stolee, P., and Robertson, D. (1989). The prevalence of problem behaviour in elderly residents of long term care institutions. *Canadian Journal of Public Health, 80*, 302-303.

Rose, R. (1988). Schizophrenia, civil liberties, and the law. *Schizophrenia Bulletin, 14*, 1-6.

Roth, L.H. (1989). Four studies of mental health commitment [Editorial]. *American Journal of Psychiatry, 146*, 135-137.

Schroeder, S.R. (1988). Neuroleptic medications for persons with developmental disabilities. In M.G. Aman and N.N. Singh (Eds.), *Psychopharmacology of the developmental disabilities* (pp. 82-100). New York: Springer-Verlag.

Silverman, M. (1976). *The drugging of the Americas: How multinational drug companies say one thing about their products to physicians in the United States, and another thing to physicians in Latin America.* Berkeley: University of California Press.

Silverman, M., and Lee, P.R. (1974). *Pills, profits, and politics.* Berkeley: University of California Press.

Skov, J. (1985). Recovering from psychiatry. *Phoenix Rising, 5*, 5-8.

Slaw, K.M., and Kalachnik, J.E. (1985). Tardive dyskinesia: Facts the mental health administrator may not know. *Journal of Mental Health Administration, 12*, 22-27.

Slaw, K.M., and Kalachnik, J.E. (1988). *Litigation involving tardive dyskinesia.* Unpublished manuscript.

Smith, A. (1924). *An inquiry into the nature and causes of the wealth of nations* [Chapter II, Book IV]. New York: J.M. Dent & Sons.

Steinman, M. (1979, March 18). The catch-22 of antipsychotic drugs. *New York Times Magazine*, pp. 114-118.

Szasz, T.S. (1977). *The theology of medicine: The political-philosophical foundations of medical ethics.* New York: Harper-Colophon.

Turk, J. (1983). Power, efficiency and institutions: Some implications of the debate for the scope of economics. In A. Francis, J. Turk, and P. Willman (Eds.), *Power, efficiency and institutions* (pp. 189-204). London, England: Heinemann Books.

Van Putten, T. (1974). Why do schizophrenic patients refuse to take their drugs? *Archives of General Psychiatry, 31*, 67-72.

Van Putten, T., and Marder, S.R. (1987). Behavioral toxicity of antipsychotic drugs. *Journal of Clinical Psychiatry, 48* (Supplement), 13-19.

Waxman, H.M., Klein, M., and Carner, E.A. (1985). Drug misuse in nursing homes: An institutional addiction? *Hospital and Community Psychiatry, 36*, 886-887.

Weiden, P.J., Mann, J.J., Haas, G., Mattson, M., and Frances, A. (1987). Clinical nonrecognition of neuroleptic-induced movement disorders: A cautionary study. *American Journal of Psychiatry, 144*, 1148-1153.

Wolf, M.E., and Brown, P. (1988). Overcoming institutional and community resistance to a tardive dyskinesia management program. In M.E. Wolf and A.D. Mosnaim (Eds.), *Tardive dyskinesia: Biological mechanisms and clinical aspects* (pp. 281-290). Washington, D.C.: American Psychiatric Press.

Wysowsky, D.K., and Baum, C. (1989). Antipsychotic drug use in the United States, 1976-1985. *Archives of General Psychiatry, 46*, 929-932.

Yassa, R., Nastase, C., Camille, Y., and Belzile, Y. (1988). Tardive dyskinesia in a psychogeriatric population. In M.E. Wolf and A.D. Mosnaim (Eds.), *Tardive dyskinesia: Biological mechanisms and clinical aspects* (pp. 123-133). Washington, D.C.: American Psychiatric Press.

©1990 The Institute of Mind and Behavior, Inc.
The Journal of Mind and Behavior
Summer and Autumn 1990, Volume 11, Numbers 3 and 4
Pages 489 [243] – 512 [266]
ISSN 0271-0137
ISBN 0-930195-05-1

Electroshock: Death, Brain Damage, Memory Loss, and Brainwashing

Leonard Roy Frank

San Francisco, California

Since its introduction in 1938, electroshock, or electroconvulsive therapy (ECT), has been one of psychiatry's most controversial procedures. Approximately 100,000 people in the United States undergo ECT yearly, and recent media reports indicate a resurgence of its use. Proponents claim that changes in the technology of ECT administration have greatly reduced the fears and risks formerly associated with the procedure. I charge, however, that ECT as routinely used today is at least as harmful overall as it was before these changes were instituted. I recount my own experience with combined insulin coma-electroshock during the early 1960s and the story of the first electroshock "treatment." I report on who is now being electroshocked, at what cost, where, and for what reasons. I discuss ECT technique modifications and describe how ECT is currently administered. I examine assertions and evidence concerning ECT's effectiveness and ECT-related deaths, brain damage, and memory loss. Finally, I describe "depatterning treatment," a brainwashing technique developed in Canada during the 1950s, drawing a parallel between electroshock and brainwashing.

In October 1962, at the age of 30, I had a run-in with psychiatry and got the worst of it. According to my hospital records (Frank, 1976), the "medical examiners," in recommending that I be committed, wrote the following: "Reportedly has been showing progressive personality changes over past 2 or so years. Grew withdrawn and asocial, couldn't or wouldn't work, & spent most of his time reading or doing nothing. Grew a beard, ate only vegetarian food and lived life of a beatnik – to a certain extent" (p. 63). I was labeled "paranoid schizophrenic, severe and chronic," denied my freedom for nine months and assaulted with a variety of drugs and 50 insulin-coma and 35 electroshock "treatments."

Each shock treatment was for me a Hiroshima. The shocking destroyed large parts of my memory, including the two-year period preceding the last

Requests for reprints should be sent to Leonard Roy Frank, 2300 Webster Street, San Francisco, California 94115.

shock. Not a day passes that images from that period of confinement do not float into consciousness. Nor does the night provide escape, for my dreams bear them as well. I am back there again in the "treatment room"; coming out of that last insulin coma (the only one I remember); strapped down, a tube in my nose, a hypodermic needle in my arm; sweating, starving, suffocating, struggling to move; a group of strangers around the bed grabbing at me; thinking — where am I, what the hell is happening to me?

Well into the shock series, which took place at Twin Pines Hospital in Belmont, California, a few miles south of San Francisco, the treating psychiatrist wrote to my father:

> In evaluating Leonard's progress to date, I think it is important to point out there is some slight improvement but he still has all his delusional beliefs regarding his beard, dietary regime and religious observances that he had prior to treatment. We hope that in continuing the treatments we will be able to modify some of these beliefs so that he can make a reasonable adjustment to life. (p. 77)

During the comatose phase of one of my treatments, my beard was removed — as "a therapeutic device to provoke anxiety and make some change in his body image," the consulting psychiatrist had written in his report recommending this procedure. He continued, "Consultation should be obtained from the TP attorney as to the civil rights issue — but I doubt that these are crucial. The therapeutic effort is worth it — inasmuch that he can always grow another" (p. 76). Earlier, several psychiatrists had tried unsuccessfully to persuade me to shave off my beard. "Leonard seems to attach a great deal of religious significance to the beard," the treating psychiatrist had noted at the time. He had even brought in a local rabbi to change my thinking (p. 75), but to no avail. I have no recollection of any of this: it is all from my medical records.

> Genuine religious conversions are also seen after the new modified lobotomy operations. For the mind is freed from its old strait-jacket and new religious beliefs and attitudes can now more easily take the place of the old. (Sargant, 1957, p. 71)

> At the "Mental Health Center" [in Albuquerque] where I work, there is a sign on the wall near the inpatient wards that reads: "PATIENTS' RIGHTS: Patients have the right to religious freedom unless clinically contraindicated." (Jones, 1988, p. 2).

One day, about a week after my last treatment, I was sitting in the "day room," which was adjacent to the shock-treatment wing of the hospital building. It was just before lunch and near the end of the treatment session (which lasts about five hours) for those being insulin-shocked. The thick metal door separating the two areas had been left slightly ajar. Suddenly, from behind the door, I heard the scream of a young man whom I had recently come to know and who was then starting an insulin course. It was a scream like nothing I had ever heard before, an all-out scream. Hurriedly, one of the nurses closed the door. The screams, now less audible, continued a while longer. I do not remember my own screams; his, I remember.

> [The insulin-coma patient] is prevented from seeing all at once the actions and treatment of those patients further along in their therapy. . . . As much as possible, he is saved the trauma of sudden introduction to the sight of patients in different stages of coma — a sight which is not very pleasant to an unaccustomed eye. (Gralnick, 1944, p. 184)

During the years since my institutionalization, I have often asked myself how psychiatrists, or anyone else for that matter, could justify shocking a human being. Soon after I began researching my book *The History of Shock Treatment* (1978) I discovered Gordon's (1948) review of the literature in which he compiled 50 theories purporting to explain the "healing" mechanism of the various forms of shock therapy then in use, including insulin, Metrazol, and electroshock. Here are some excerpts:

> Because prefontal lobotomy improves the mentally ill by destruction, the improvement obtained by all the shock therapies must also involve some destructive processes. . . .
> They help by way of a circulatory shake up. . . .
> It decreases cerebral function. . . .
> The treatments bring the patient and physician in closer contact. . . .
> Helpless and dependent, the patient sees in the physician a mother. . . .
> Threat of death mobilizes all the vital instincts and forces a reestablishment of contacts with reality. . . .
> The treatment is considered by patients as punishment for sins and gives feelings of relief. . . .
> Victory over death and joy of rebirth produce the results. . . .
> The resulting amnesia is healing. . . .
> Erotization is the therapeutic factor. . . .
> The personality is brought down to a lower level and adjustment is obtained more easily in a primitive vegetative existence than in a highly developed personality. Imbecility replaces insanity. (pp. 399–401)

One of the more interesting explanations I found was proposed by Manfred Sakel, the Austrian psychiatrist who in 1933 introduced insulin coma as a treatment for schizophrenia. According to Sakel (cited in Ray, 1942, p. 250),

> with chronic schizophrenics, as with confirmed criminals, we can't hope for reform. Here the faulty pattern of functioning is irrevocably entrenched. Hence we must use more drastic measures to silence the dysfunctioning cells and so liberate the activity of the normal cells. This time we must *kill* the too vocal dysfunctioning cells. But can we do this without killing normal cells also? Can we *select* the cells we wish to destroy? I think we can. (italics in original)

Electroshock may be considered one of the most controversial treatments in psychiatry. As I document below, the last decade has witnessed a resurgence of ECT's popularity, accompanied by assertions from proponents concerning its effectiveness and safety — assertions which deny or obscure basic facts about the historical origins of ECT, the economic reasons behind its current popularity, as well as its potential for destroying the memories and lives of those subjected to it.

The First Electroshock

Electroshock was introduced in Rome in 1938. Psychiatrist Ugo Cerletti (1956) administered the first electroshock to an Italian man identified as S.E., a 39-year-old engineer sent to him for observation by the Police Commissioner of Rome. An accompanying note stated that S.E. had been arrested at the railroad station "while wandering about without a ticket on trains ready for departure" and did not appear "to be in full possession of his mental faculties" (p. 93). S.E. was diagnosed as "schizophrenic" based on "his passive behavior, incoherence, low affective reserves, hallucinations, deliriant ideas of being influenced, neologisms" (p. 93). Having found a suitable subject, Cerletti readied the experiment. Surrounded by several colleagues, he applied the first shock which — because the voltage had been set too low — failed to induce a convulsion. As the doctors discussed what to do next, S.E., "who evidently had been following the conversation, said clearly and solemnly, without his usual gibberish: 'Not another one! It's deadly!' " (p. 93). In spite of this plea, Cerletti ordered a second and larger jolt, which caused S.E. to have a seizure.

This example of psychiatric experimentation had a theatrical quality to it which Cerletti excluded from his account. For this, one has to turn to Lothar B. Kalinowsky, the dean of American electroshock. Born in 1899, Kalinowsky left Germany in 1933 for Italy, where he eventually became associated with Cerletti, who, according to another electroshock colleague (Accornero, 1988, p. 42), was then referred to as "Maestro." Kalinowsky missed the first electroshock experiment but was present for the second. In a recent interview (Abrams, 1988b), Kalinowsky commented on these early events in the history of electroshock:

> Cerletti had been worried that something might go wrong with the first treatment, and it was given in secret. . . . When the first treatment went well, we were allowed to attend the second treatment. We were called together for the treatment with a trumpet! (p. 30)

Asked for his impression of ECT on seeing it for the first time, Kalinowsky replied,

> According to my wife — because I don't remember it exactly — she claims that when I came home I was very pale and said "I saw something terrible today — I never want to see that again!" (p. 30)

Kalinowsky, however, overcame his initial distaste for electroshock and during 1939–1940 went on to help introduce the procedure in France, England, the Netherlands, and the United States. Cerletti's first impression of electroshock was similar to Kalinowsky's:

> When I saw the patient's reaction, I thought to myself: This ought to be abolished! Ever since I have looked forward to the time when another treatment would replace electroshock. (cited in Ayd, 1963, p. A7)

Electroshock Facts and Figures

Since 1938 between 10 and 15 million people worldwide have undergone electroshock. While no precise figure is available, it is estimated that about 100,000 people in the United States are electroshocked annually (Fink, cited in Rymer, 1989, p. 68). Moreover, the numbers appear to be increasing. Recent media accounts report a resurgence of ECT interest and use. One reason for this is the well-publicized enthusiasm of such proponents as Max Fink, editor-in-chief of *Convulsive Therapy*, the leading journal in the field. Fink was recently cited as saying that "[ECT should be given to] all patients whose condition is severe enough to require hospitalization" (Edelson, 1988, p. 3).

A survey of the American Psychiatric Association (APA) membership focusing on ECT (APA, 1978) showed that 22% fell into the "User" category. Users were defined as psychiatrists who had "personally treated patients with ECT," or "recommended to residents under their supervision that ECT be used on patients," during the last six months (p. 5). If valid today, this figure indicates that approximately 7,700 APA members are electroshock Users.

A survey of all 184 member hospitals of the National Association of Private Psychiatric Hospitals (Levy and Albrecht, 1985) elicited the following information on electroshock practices from the 153 respondents (83%) who answered a 19-item questionnaire sent to them in 1982. Fifty-eight percent of the respondents used electroshock (3% did not use electroshock because they considered it to be "inappropriate treatment for any illness"). The hospitals using ECT found it appropriate for a variety of diagnoses: 100% for "major depressive disorder," 58% for "schizophrenia," and 13% for "obsessive-compulsive disorder." Twenty-six percent of the ECT-using hospitals reported no contraindications in the use of the procedure. Darnton (1989) reported that the number of private free-standing psychiatric hospitals grew from 184 in 1980 to 450 in 1988. In addition, nearly 2,000 general hospitals offer inpatient psychiatric services (p. 67). While the use of ECT in state hospitals has fallen off sharply over the last 20 years, the psychiatric wards of general hospitals have increased their reliance on ECT in the treatment of their adult inpatients (Thompson, 1986).

In cases of depression, an ECT series ranges from six to 12 seizures — in those of schizophrenia, from 15 to 35 seizures – given three times a week, and usually entails four weeks of hospitalization. In 72% of the cases, according to the APA (1978, p. 8) survey cited above, electroshock costs are paid for by insurance companies. This fact led one psychiatrist to comment, "Finding that the patient has insurance seemed like the most common indication for giving electroshock" (Viscott, 1972, p. 356). The overall cost for a series of electroshock in a private hospital ranges from $10,000 to $25,000. With room rates averaging $500 to $600 a day, and bed occupancy generally falling, some hospitals have obtained considerable financial advantage from their use of ECT. A regular ECT User can expect yearly earnings of at least $200,000, about twice the median income of other psychiatrists. _Electroshock is a $2–3 billion-a-year industry._

More than two-thirds of electroshock subjects are women, and a growing number are elderly. In California, one of the states that requires Users to report quarterly the number and age categories of electroshock subjects, "the percentage 65 and over" being electroshocked increased gradually from 29% to 43% between 1977 and 1983 (Warren, 1986, p. 51). More recently, Drop and Welch (1989) reported that 60% of the ECT subjects in a recent two-year period at the Massachusetts General Hospital in Boston were over 60 years and 10% were in their eighties (p. 88). There are published reports of persons over 100 years old (Alexopoulos, Young, and Abrams, 1989) and as young as 34½ months (Bender, 1955) who have been electroshocked. In the latter case, the child had been referred in 1947 to the children's ward of New York's Bellevue Hospital "because of distressing anxiety that frequently reached a state of panic . . . . The child was mute and autistic." The morning after admission he received the first of a series of 20 electroshocks and was discharged one month later. "The discharge note indicated a 'moderate improvement,' since he was eating and sleeping better, was more freindly with the other children, and he was toilet trained" (pp. 418–419).

Children continue to be electroshocked. Black, Wilcox, and Stewart (1985) reported on "the successful use of ECT in a prepubertal boy with severe depression." Sandy, 11 years old, received 12 unilateral ECTs at the University of Iowa Hospitals and Clinics in Iowa City. He "improved remarkably" and "was discharged in good condition. Follow-up over the next 8 years revealed five more hospitalizations for depression" (p. 98).

Some of the better known people who have undergone shock treatment include: Antonin Artaud, Thomas Eagleton, Claude Eatherly, Frances Farmer, Zelda Fitzgerald, James Forrestal, Janet Frame, Ernest Hemingway, Vladimir Horowitz, Bob Kaufman, Seymour Krim, Vivien Leigh, Oscar Levant, Robert Lowell, Vaslav Nijinsky, Jimmy Pearsall, Robert Pirsig, Sylvia Plath, David Reville, Paul Robeson, Gene Tierney, and Frank Wisner.

In the early 1970s electroshock survivors – together with other former psychiatric inmates/"patients" — began forming organizations aimed at regulating or abolishing electroshock and other psychiatric practices which they believed were harmful. In 1975 one group, the Network Against Psychiatric Assault (San Francisco/Berkeley), was instrumental in the passage of legislation that regulated the use of electroshock in California. Since then more than 30 states have passed similar legislation.

In 1982 the Coalition to Stop Electroshock led a successful referendum campaign to outlaw ECT in Berkeley, California. Although the courts overturned the ban six weeks after it went into effect, this was the first time in American history that the use of any established medical procedure had been prohibited by popular vote.

The Committee for Truth in Psychiatry (CTIP), all of whose members are electroshock survivors, was formed in 1984. Thus far, it has successfully opposed the APA's efforts to have the Food and Drug Administration (FDA) reclassify ECT devices from the dangerous, high-risk category (Class III) of medical devices to the low-risk category (Class II). The 1979 law governing medical devices requires the FDA to investigate Class III devices preliminary to reclassifying or banning them. However, CTIP's call for the FDA to fulfill its full investigative mandate has thus far gone unheeded.

Method of Administration

Typically, modified ECT (see below) is administered in the following manner. The subject is not allowed to eat or drink anything for at least six hours before treatment. Tranquilizers or sedatives may be used during this period to lessen the subject's fears and sometimes his or her physical resistance to treatment. About 30 minutes before the convulsion, Atropine — a conventional preanesthetic medication — is administered to maintain heart activity and dry secretions in the mouth and air passages, thus reducing the risk of suffocation or other complications that could develop from swallowing one's own saliva. Bladder and bowels should be emptied; dentures, hairpins, and sharp-edged jewelry are removed.

The subject is then brought to the "treatment room" and put on a bed, gurney, or thickly padded table. Electrolyte jelly, applied to the areas where the electrodes are to be placed, increases conductivity and prevents burns. A short-acting barbiturate, commonly Brevital (methohexital), renders the subject unconscious in a few moments. The muscle relaxant Anectine (succinylcoline) is then administered to reduce the risk of bone dislocations and fractures during the convulsion. It virtually paralyzes the entire body, including the respiratory system. Consequently, while this agent is in effect, the subject's breathing must be maintained artificially. After a rubber gag is inserted into the subject's mouth, the electrodes are put in place. Electrode placement is a matter of controversy among Users (see below). During the procedure blood pressure, heart rate and other functions are monitored.

The User now presses a button on the shock device releasing between 100 and 150 volts of electricity into the subject's brain for anywhere from one-half second to two seconds. This produces a *grand mal* convulsion lasting between 30 and 60 seconds. The immediate possible complications include apnea, cyanosis, and heart problems such as arrhythmias and cardiac arrest.

The convulsion is followed by a period of coma, from which the subject awakens with a number of the following effects: confusion, disorientation, amnesia, apathy, dizziness, headache, nausea, muscle ache, physical weakness, and delirium. Most of these gross effects usually subside after a few hours, but amnesia, apathy ("emotional blunting"), learning difficulties, and loss of creativity, drive and energy may last for weeks and months. In many instances they are in some measure permanent. The intensity, number, and spacing of the individual electroshocks in a series greatly influence the severity and persistence of these effects.

Claims of Electroshock Effectiveness

Virtually all the psychiatrists who evaluate, write about and do research on electroshock are themselves Users. This partially explains why claims regarding ECT's effectiveness abound in the professional literature — while the risks associated with the procedure are consistently understated or overlooked. User estimates of ECT's effectiveness in the treatment of the affective disorders (i.e., depression, mania, and manic-depression) usually range from 75% to 90%. Two important questions, however, need to be addressed: What is meant by effectiveness and how long does it last?

Breggin (1979, p. 135; 1981, pp. 252–253) has proposed a "brain-disabling hypothesis" to explain the workings of electroshock. The hypothesis suggests that ECT "effectiveness" stems from the brain damage ECT causes. As happens in cases of serious head injury, ECT produces amnesia, denial, euphoria, apathy, wide and unpredictable mood swings, helplessness and submissiveness. Each one of these effects may appear to offset the problems which justified the use of ECT in the first place. Amnesia victims, having forgotten their problems, tend to complain less. Denial serves a similar purpose: because of their embarrassment, ECT subjects tend to discount or deny unresolved personal problems as well as ECT-caused intellectual deficits. With euphoria, the subject's depression seems to lift. With apathy, the subject's "agitation" (if that had been perceived as part of the original problem) seems to diminish. Dependency and submissiveness tend to make what may have been a resistive, hostile subject more cooperative and friendly. In hailing the wonders of electroshock, psychiatrists often simply redefine the symptoms of psychiatrogenic brain damage as signs of improvement and/or recovery.

Electroshock advocates themselves unwittingly provide support for the brain-disabling hypothesis. Fink, Kahn, and Green (1958) offered a good example when describing a set of criteria for rating improvement in ECT subjects: "When a depressed patient, who had been withdrawn, crying, and had expressed suicidal thoughts, no longer is seclusive, and is jovial, friendly and euphoric, denies his problems and sees his previous thoughts of suicide as 'silly,' a rating of 'much improved' is made" (p. 117). Two additional illustrations are given below; see Cleckley (cited in Thigpen, 1976) and Hoch (1948).

On the question of duration of benefit from ECT, Weiner (1984) − in one of the most important review articles on ECT published during the last decade − was unable to cite a single study purporting to show long-term, or even medium-term, benefits from ECT. Opton (1985) drew this conclusion from the Weiner review: "In this comprehensive review of the literature, after fifty years of research on ECT, no methodologically sound study was found that reported beneficial effects of ECT lasting as long as four weeks" (p. 2). Pinel (1984), in his peer commentary on the Weiner article, accepted Weiner's conclusion that "the risks of ECT-related brain damage are slight" and then added, "it is difficult to justify any risks at all until ECT has been shown unambiguously to produce significant long-term therapeutic benefits" (p. 31).

The following excerpt from an article in *Clinical Psychiatry News* reveals the short-range outlook of many ECT Users:

> The relapse rate after successful treatment for affective disorders is very high, from 20% to 50% within 6 months after a *successful* course of ECT, according to Dr. Richard Abrams [a well-known ECT proponent]. "I think it is reasonable and appropriate to always initiate maintenance in the form of a tricyclic [an antidepressant drug] or lithium," he said. For patients who relapse despite adequate drug therapy, maintenance ECT [periodic single electroshocks, spaced several weeks or months apart] has been used successfully. (Klug, 1984, p. 16) [italics added]

The underlying assumption of this approach is that affective disorders are for the most part chronic and irreversible. There is a popular saying among psychiatrists, "Once a schizophrenic, always a schizophrenic." While not a maxim, "Once a depressive, always a depressive," is nevertheless a core belief among many ECT Users. It "explains" so much for them. From this perspective, there are hardly any ECT failures, only patients with recurring depressive episodes who require ongoing psychiatric treatment, intensive and maintenance by turns.

Proponents also claim, but cannot demonstrate, that ECT is effective in cases of depression where there is a risk of suicide. They often cite a study by Avery and Winokur (1976) to support their position. But this study makes no such claim, as we can see from the authors' own conclusion: "In the present study, treatment [ECT and antidepressants] was not shown to affect the suicide rate" (p. 1033). Nevertheless, Allen (1978), in the very first paragraph of his article on ECT observed, "Avery and Winokur showed that suicide mortality in patients afflicted with psychotic depression was lower in patients treated with ECT than in those who were not" (p. 47).

Death from Electroshock

Proponents claim that electroshock-caused death is rare. Alexopoulos et al. (1989) cited studies published in 1979 and 1985 indicating that the death rate from ECT was between 1 and 3 per 10,000 persons treated (0.01%– 0.03%) – considerably lower than estimates for the early years of ECT and, according to the authors, "probably related to the introduction of anesthesia and muscular relaxants" (p. 80). On the other hand, Kalinowsky (1967), who reported a death rate of up to 1 per 1,000 for the period before the premedicative drugs were being routinely used, had "the definite impression that the anesthesia techniques increased the number of fatalities" (p. 1282). Crowe (1984a, p. 164) cited a study conducted during 1972–1973 in Denmark which reported a rate of 2.9 deaths per 10,000 cases (0.029%).

Can any of these figures be relied upon? In researching my book on shock treatment (Frank, 1978, p. 153–156), I found reports of 384 electroshock-related deaths published between 1941 and 1977 in English-language sources, among which were a number of reports and studies with much higher death rates than those cited above. For example: three deaths in 150 cases – 2% (Lowinger and Huddleson, 1945); four deaths in 276 cases – 1.4% (Granlick, 1946); five deaths in 356 cases – 1.4% (Martin, 1949); two deaths in 18 cases – 11.1% (Weil, 1950); three deaths in 700 cases – 0.4% (Gaitz, Pokorny, and Mills, 1956); three deaths in 90 cases – 3.3% (Kurland, Hanlon, Esquibel, Krantz, and Sheets, 1959); three deaths in 1,000 cases – 0.3% (McCartney, 1961); two deaths in 183 cases – 1.1% (Freeman and Kendell, 1980).

In the broadest and most informative study on ECT-related deaths, Impastato (1957) reported 254 deaths: 214 from published accounts and 40 previously unpublished. Most of the fatalities had received unmodified ECT. He estimated an overall death rate of 1 per 1,000 (0.1%) and 1 per 200 (0.5%) in persons over 60 years of age. Impastato was able to determine the cause of death in 235 cases. There were 100 "cardiovascular deaths" (43%), 66 "cerebral deaths" (28%), 43 "respiratory deaths" (18%), and 26 deaths from other causes (11%) (p. 34).

Impastato's estimate of an ECT death rate among elderly persons five times higher than the overall death rate – coupled with his finding that cardiovascular failure was responsible for 43% of the deaths – should be very troubling in light of the growing tendency toward shocking the elderly. To justify this practice, Users usually point to the serious risks of cardiac complications and death involved in treating the elderly depressed – particularly those with heart disease – with antidepressant drugs. In current standard psychiatric practice, these drugs constitute basically the only alternative to electroshock.

Whether ECT or antidepressants offer less risk of fatality for these persons remains an open question, but Users assume ECT is less risky. In addition to the Impastato findings, other evidence suggests that Users are underestimating the dangers of using ECT on the elderly. Freeman and Kendell (1980) found that of 183 persons subjected to ECT in 1976 at the Royal Edinburgh Hospital in Scotland, two women aged 69 and 76 had died 24 and 48 hours respectively after each had received her 13th electroshock. Autopsies revealed myocardial infarction in both cases (p. 10). A more recent study (Gerring and Shields, 1982) also calls attention to the risks of ECT for elderly persons with heart problems. Of 42 persons undergoing modified ECT during a one-year period (1975–1976) at the Payne Whitney Clinic in New York City, 17 (40%) had presented with heart disease. Twelve of the 17 (70%) developed heart complications. Eleven of the 12 were over age 60. Nine of the 12 developed arrythmias. "Four of the complications in this series were life-threatening. . . . Patient E.S. sustained a cardiopulmonary arrest 45 minutes after her fifth treatment" and died (pp. 140–141).

The Impastato findings have embarrassed the electroshock camp. As a result, this essential research has been largely neglected in the literature on electroshock since then. Thus, in three key review books authored or co-authored by Kalinowsky (Kalinowsky, 1959; Kalinowsky and Hippius, 1969; Kalinowsky and Hoch, 1961), the Impastato study was nowhere mentioned, although Impastato's other works were frequently cited. Kalinowsky is not alone in this regard. Crowe's (1984a) ECT-review article – because it was published in the influential *New England Journal of Medicine* – must be considered among the most important of the 1980s. Citing a paper by Maclay (1953), Crowe wrote that "the largest reported series of deaths included 62 from the years 1947–1952" (p. 164), but Crowe neither referred to the Impastato study in his ECT mortality section nor cited it among his 80 references.

Weiner's (1984) extensive ECT review article, cited above, was accompanied by comments from 22 professionals (almost all of whom were favorably disposed to ECT) and more than 350 references. Weiner discussed, briefly and dissimissively, autopsy reports of ECT-related brain damage. The Impastato study, however, was nowhere cited. A study published in 1957 and reporting 66 "cerebral deaths" in 235 ECT-related deaths was certainly relevant to Weiner's review (titled, "Does Electroconvulsive Therapy Cause Brain Damage?"), despite the fact that respiratory assistance and muscle relaxants were not routinely used until the 1960s. The relevance of the Impastato study to Weiner's review was further borne out by his inclusion of two other less incriminating and much smaller studies from the same time period (p. 7).

These clinical studies and review works, along with the following considerations, suggest that the psychiatric profession is overlooking, downplaying and underreporting ECT deaths:

1. Users are reluctant to report such deaths because they reflect unfavorably upon their own professional competence, and may invite lawsuits and public criticsm of the psychiatric profession.

2. Users, because of personal commitment, professional pride, and financial interest, are sometimes unwilling to recognize deaths almost surely related to ECT.

3. Psychiatric journals — in order to maintain the status of the profession and avoid discord within its ranks — may not be printing some of the ECT death reports submitted to them. Published reports fell off sharply soon after publication of the Impastato (1957) study. For the 1960–1977 period, I was able to find reports of only 24 ECT deaths, compared with 360 for the 1941–1959 period (Frank, 1978, pp. 153–156). In addition, there have been very few death-survey articles published since 1960. In general, according to Grimm (1978), "there has been a dramatic drop in the number of published accounts of any problems with the practice of ECT, especially deaths. There is an erie silence in a literature that hitherto was substantial and extremely useful in questions of morbidity and mortality" (p. 30).

4. Post-mortem reports are often inconclusive. It is difficult to establish a causal relationship between ECT and a subsequent death. What one coroner regards as causal, another might see as only contributory or irrelevant.

5. ECT review articles—almost always undertaken by ECT proponents—underestimate ECT death rates by citing as corroborative evidence the studies and estimates most favorable to their position.

6. Family members — due to grief, guilt, or other reasons — sometimes do not allow autopsies to determine cause of death following ECT or other psychiatric treatments.

Brain Damage from Electroshock

One does not need a medical degree to recognize the destructive potential of passing 100 to 150 volts of electricity through the human brain. The same amount of current used to produce a seizure in ECT, if applied to the chest, would be fatal (Task Force, 1977, p. 1).

Fifteen years before the Impastato study (1957) which reported 66 "cerebral deaths," and four years after the introduction of ECT, Alpers and Hughes (1942) commented on their findings in an autopsy performed on a woman who had died following electroshock:

> The foregoing case is the first reported instance, so far as we now, of hemorrhages in the brain attributable to electrical convulsion treatment. . . . [T]he importance of the

case lies in that it offers a clear demonstration of the fact that electrical convulsion treatment is followed at times by structural damage of the brain. (p. 177)

Hoch (1948), a well-known ECT proponent, likening electroshock to lobotomy, claimed that the brain damage each produced was beneficial:

This brings us for a moment to a discussion of the brain damage produced by electroshock. . . . Is a certain amount of brain damage not necessary in this type of treatment? Frontal lobotomy indicates that improvement takes place by a definite damage of certain parts of the brain. (pp. 48–439)

Psychiatrist and neurophysiologist Pribram commented in a 1974 interview:

I'd much rather have a small lobotomy than a series of electroconvulsive shocks. . . . I just know what the brain looks like after a series of shocks — and it's not very pleasant to look at. (p. 9)

The American Psychiatric Association's (1978) ECT survey, cited earlier, reported that 41% of the psychiatrist-respondents agreed with the statement, "It is likely that ECT produces slight or subtle brain damage." Only 26% disagreed. In their review of the literature, Templer and Veleber (1982) concluded "that ECT caused and can cause permanent brain pathology" (p. 65). Sament (1983), a neurologist, published his views on ECT's brain-damaging effects in a letter to the editor of a professional journal:

I have seen many patients after ECT, and I have no doubt that ECT produces effects identical to those of a head injury. After multiple sessions of ECT, a patient has symptoms identical to those of a retired, punch-drunk boxer. After one session of ECT the symptoms are the same as those of a concussion (including retrograde and anterograde amnesia). After a few sessions of ECT the symptoms are those of a moderate cerebral contusion, and further enthusiastic use of ECT may result in the patient functioning at a subhuman level. (p. 11)

Sackeim (1986) also describes in a straightforward manner the effects of ECT:

The ECT-induced seizure, like spontaneous generalized seizures in epileptics and most acute brain injury and head trauma, results in a variable period of disorientation. Patients may not know their names, their ages, etc. When the disorientation is prolonged, it is generally referred to as an organic brain syndrome. (p. 482)

Heath (1984), in his commentary on the Weiner (1984) review, quoted with disapproval a prominent psychoanalyst who often stated publicly that "ECT fried the brain." In the next paragraph, however, Heath himself wrote that "Electroconvulsive therapy has a shotgun effect on the brain" (p. 28). Also, in their commentary on the Weiner review, ECT proponents Small and Small (1984) suggested this explanation for the increasing use of ECT:

"ECT may . . . have gained in popularity because of the increasing recognition of long-lasting and sometimes irreversible impairments in brain function induced by neuroleptic drugs. (In this instance the evidence of brain damage is not subtle, but is grossly obvious even to the casual observer!)" (p. 34). We have here both an acknowledgement that ECT causes "subtle" brain damage and a rationale for continuing its use based on evidence that brain damage from one of its chief competing treatments, the neuroleptics, is "grossly obvious."

Despite evidence of ECT-caused brain damage, most fully documented by Breggin (1979), proponents continue to claim that ECT does not cause brain damage. Here are some recent examples:

> The good news is that no evidence of brain damage [from ECT] has been found. (Crowe, 1984b, p. 13A)

> There is no scientific evidence of irreversible brain damage. ("Electroconvulsive therapy," 1987, p. 3)

> The possibility of brain damage is absolutely refuted by brain scans, by neuropsychological studies, by autopsies, by animal studies, and by analysis of cerebrospinal fluid and blood chemicals. (Peterson, cited in Rymer, 1989, p. 71)

> I can't prove there's no brain damage [from ECT]. I can't prove there are no other sentient beings in the universe either. But scientists have been trying for thirty years to find both, and so far they haven't come up with a thing. (Fink, cited in Rymer, 1989, p. 71)

In a recent 216-page document, *The Practice of ECT: Recommendations for Treatment, Training and Privileging,* the Task Force on ECT (APA, 1989) dismissed the critical issue of electroshock-caused brain damage with two sentences. The first, "Cerebral complications are notably rare" (p. 63), is false. The second, which concluded the Task Force's recommendations for information to be provided in the formal consent document for ECT — "In light of the available evidence, 'brain damage' need not be included as a potential risk" (p. 77) — is falsely premised. From this latter statement we see that the report's authors not only denied the possibility of ECT-caused brain damage, but found the very notion of such damage so *unthinkable* that they placed the term in quotation marks.

Memory Loss from Electroshock

The most serious and common effect of electroshock as reported by survivors is memory loss. The loss stretching backward in time from the treatment period is called retrograde amnesia and may cover many months or years. The memory loss from the treatment period forward in time is called anterograde amnesia and usually covers several months, often including the treatment period itself. The amnesia may be global or patchy; some memories return, others are permanently lost. These losses affect one's entire personality and are often experienced as a diminution of self. They not only impair one's ability to function in everyday affairs but also in higher realms of spiritual and creative activity.

Herskovitz (cited in Philadelphia Psychiatric Society, 1943) reported finding memory defects among 174 people treated with ECT at the Norristown State Hospital, Pennsylvania, "to be rather general and often prominent. Therefore, patients whose occupation requires intellectual ability are selected for treatment with caution" (p. 798). In 1972, at the age of 48 Marilyn Rice (cited as Natalie Parker, a pseudonym, in Roueché, 1974) underwent a series of eight ECTs at the Psychiatric Institute of Washington. Soon afterwards, ECT-caused disability forced her into early retirement from her job as an economist. She described her return to work following electroshock:

> I came home from the office after that first day back feeling panicky. I didn't know where to turn. I was terrified. All my beloved knowledge, everything I had learned in my field during twenty years or more was gone. I'd lost the body of knowledge that constituted my professional skill. . . . I'd lost my experience, my knowing. But it was worse than that. I felt I'd lost myself. (pp. 95–96)

Andre (1988) described her memory losses following a series of 15 ECTs at New York Hospital in New York City in 1984 when she was 24 years old:

> My behavior was greatly changed; in a brain-damaged stupor, I smiled, cooperated, agreed that I had been a very sick girl and thanked the doctor for curing me. I was released from the hospital like a child just born. I knew where I lived, but I didn't recognize the person I lived with. I didn't know where I had gotten the unfamiliar clothes in the closet. I didn't know if I had any money or where it was. I didn't know the people calling me on the phone. . . . Very, very gradually – because you can't know what you don't remember – I realized that three years of my life were missing. Four years after shock, they are still missing. (p. 2)

Between February 1977 and October 1978 Freeman and Kendell (1980) interviewed 166 patients who had ECT during either 1971 or 1976 in Edinburgh. Of this group, 64% reported "memory impairment" (25% "thought symptom severe," 39% "thought symptom mild") [p. 13]. Twenty-eight percent agreed with the statement that "ECT causes permanent changes to memory" (p. 14). Squire (1982, 1983) reported findings of his three-year follow-up study of 35 people who had received an average of 11 bilateral ECTs (see next section). Of the 31 people available for interview, 18 (58%) answered "no" to the question, "Do you think your memory now is as good as it is for most people your age?" All but one of the 18 attributed their memory difficulties to ECT (1982, p. 1221).

Abrams (1988a) summarized his chapter on memory functioning after ECT as follows: "A remarkable amount has been learned in the past decade about the effects of ECT on memory, and the day is now past when the physician administering bilateral ECT can blithely assure his patient that 'the memory-loss will only be temporary' " (p. 153). Abrams favors unilateral ECT, claiming that it causes little or no "memory disturbance" and that "whatever dysmnesia does occur will be transient and probably undetectable 6 months later" (p. 154).

Over the years, ECT Users have tried to discount the significance of amnesia reports from electroshock survivors. Kalinowsky and Hoch (1952) gave an early explanation: "All patients who remain unimproved after ECT are inclined to complain bitterly of their memory difficulties" (p. 139). Implicit in this remark is the suggestion to Users that an ECT series should continue until the subject's memory "complaints" cease. In the same vein, the APA's 1978 report on ECT lent its weight to the notion that ECT "might lead many individuals . . . to have persistent illusion of memory impairment" (p. 68).

More recently, Users have been arguing that the culprit responsible for memory problems is more likely to be the depression, not the electroshock (Crowe, 1984a). They assert that memory loss is a component of depression. Where the ECT subject is elderly, Users are likely to regard reports of memory loss as a normal sign of the aging process and, in the more severe cases, as symptomatic of senility. It is interesting to note that the Janis (1950) study — which concluded that ECT caused persistent amnesia (p. 372) — included very few depressed persons (only 3 of 30 subjects). More significantly on this point, the control group of 19 "depressed patients" who had not undergone ECT in the Squire (1983) study, cited above, "reported no memory problems at all at follow-up" (p. 6).

Electroshock Modifications

In recent years, to allay growing public fears concerning the use of electroshock, proponents have launched a media campaign, claiming among other things that with the introduction of certain modifications in the administration of ECT the problems once associated with the procedure have been solved, or at least substantially reduced. These techniques center around the use of anesthetics and muscle relaxants, changes in electrode placement, and the use of brief-pulse electrical stimulation. However, investigation and common sense indicate that while these modifications may offer some advantages — for example, muscle relaxants prevent the subject's thrashing about, thereby greatly reducing the risk of bone and spinal fractures and making the procedure less frightening to watch — the basic facts underlying the administration of electroshock have not changed at all. The nature of the human brain and that of electricity are no different today than they were more than 50 years ago when ECT was introduced. Whatever may be the ameliorating factors of the newer delivery techniques, when a convulsogenic dose of electricity is applied to the brain, there is going to be a certain amount of brain damage, some of which will be permanent. There is even evidence that the drug modifications make ECT more destructive than ever, for, as central nervous system depressants, anesthetics and muscle relaxants raise the subject's convulsive threshold, which in turn makes it necessary to apply a larger dose of electricity to set off the convulsion. And, the more current applied, the more amnesia and brain damage. As Reed (1988) noted, "The amnesia directly relating to ECT depends on the amount of current used to trigger the generalized convulsion" (p. 29).

Other problems are associated with the use of premedications in ECT. In his study of 254 ECT deaths, Impastato (1957) reported that 13 of 66 persons from the "cerebral death" group had received muscle relaxants and that these "appear to play a major role in the death of some of these patients" (p. 42). There were also five other patients who died immediately after receiving muscle relaxants but before being given the electric shock. These figures are from a period when muscle relaxants were not widely used. More recently, Ulett (1972) concurred with Impastato on the danger of muscle relaxants in ECT: "The objection to the use of muscle relaxants is that, although decreasing the rate of fracture complication, they unquestionably increase the chance of fatal accident" (p. 284). Given the paucity of ECT-death studies in recent years, it is difficult to gauge the extent of this problem in current practice.

Another modification, unilateral ECT, has received much attention since its introduction in the late 1950s but has not replaced — and is not likely to replace — bilateral ECT as the standard technique. According to the APA survey on ECT (1978, p. 6), 75% of the Users reported using bilateral electrode placement exclusively. In bilateral ECT the electrodes are placed on the subject's temples so that the current passes through the brain's frontal lobe area. In unilateral ECT one electrode is placed on a temple and the other just above the back of the neck on the same (usually the nondominant) side of the head. Unilateral placement, proponents claim, results in less memory loss. But proponents of bilateral ECT assert that unilateral ECT is less effective and therefore requires more treatments (Gregory, Shawcross, and Gill, 1985). Cleckley (cited in Thigpen, 1976) offered this explanation for the ineffectiveness of unilateral ECT: "My thought about unilateral stimulation is that it fails to cure. I think this failure to cure is in direct proportion to the avoidance of memory loss" (p. 40). During his interview with Abrams (1988b), Kalinowsky made this comment about unilateral ECT: "My experience is completely negative and if patients improve at all, it's probably due to the repeated anesthesia induction with methohexital" (p. 38). Given the need for "somewhat more current to produce a seizure" in each treatment session (Fink, 1978, p. 79) and for more treatment sessions per series, unilateral ECT may be more brain damaging in some cases than bilateral ECT.

The problems associated with brief-pulse stimulation, another innovation in ECT administration, are similar to those associated with unilateral ECT. While brief-pulse stimulation may cause less amnesia than the routinely used sine-wave stimulation, the newer technique "may be insufficient to induce an adequate generalized seizure" (Reed, 1988, p. 29). What Ulett (1972) wrote about unidirectional current stimulation (a supposed advance in ECT technology introduced by Liberson [1948]) may also apply to brief-pulse stimulation, and to unilateral ECT as well: "[I]t is often necessary to give a greater number of these milder treatments to achieve the desired therapeutic result" (p. 287).

Electroshock and Brainwashing

The term "brainwashing" came into the language during the early 1950s. It originally identified the technique of intensive indoctrination developed by the Chinese for use on political dissidents following the Communist take-over on the mainland and on American prisoners of war during the Korean War. The method involves the systematic application of sleep and food deprivation, prolonged interrogation, brow-beating, and physical punishment to force captives to renounce their beliefs. Once "brainwashed," they are reprogrammed to accept the beliefs of their captors.

While electroshock is not overtly used against political dissidents, it is used against cultural dissidents, social misfits and the unhappy, whom psychiatrists diagnose as "mentally ill" in order to justify ECT as a medical intervention. Indeed, electroshock is a classic example of brainwashing in the most meaningful sense of the term. Brainwashing means washing the brain of its contents. Electroshock destroys memories and ideas by destroying the brain cells in which memories and ideas are stored. A more accurate name for what is now called electroconvulsive therapy (ECT) would be electroconvulsive brainwashing (ECB).

> Sometimes the confusion [following intensive ECT] passes rapidly and patients act as if they had awakened from dreaming; their minds seem like clean slates upon which we can write. (Kennedy and Anchel, 1948, p. 381)

> This recent memory loss [from standard ECT] could be compared to erasing a tape recording. (Arnot, 1975, p. 500)

> I do not know of any formal use of [shock treatment] in brain washing [sic] but it seems possible it could be so used. One can conjure up an image of large groups of dissidents in a police state being kept in a contented state of apathy by shock treatment. (Peck, 1974, p. 35)

Given this potential for social control, electroshock was almost destined to gain the attention of certain government agencies charged with "national security" responsibilities. On August 2, 1977 *The New York Times* carried a front-page story about the Central Intelligence Agency's [CIA] MKULTRA "mind control" project which had been set up secretly in the early 1950s. During the late 1950s, CIA funding for one of the programs went to psychiatrist D. Ewen Cameron, a former president of the American Psychiatric Association, who directed the Allan Memorial Institute in Montreal. The program centered around what Cameron named "depatterning treatment" and "psychic driving." Between 1956 and 1962 he published detailed descriptions of these methods in leading psychiatric journals (Cameron, 1956, 1957, 1960; Cameron, Lohrenz, and Handcock, 1962; Cameron and Pande, 1958).

In the lead section of the first article on depatterning Cameron and Pande (1958) wrote: "We are presenting a method of treatment [for "chronic paranoid schizophrenia"] which we have found to be more successful than any hitherto reported" (p. 92). The procedure combined drug-induced continuous sleep, intensive ECT, and large doses of the neuroleptic Thorazine. Cameron used the Page-Russell method of ECT administration (Page and Russell, 1948) in twice-daily sessions. Each session consisted of six 150-volt electroshocks of one-second duration, spaced so closely together that "the clonic phase [of the convulsion] does not become established until the end of the sixth electrical impulse" (Cameron et al., 1962, p. 68). The intention was to continue the sessions until the subject reached "the third stage" of depatterning, which happened after between 30 and 40 sessions (between 180 and 240 electroshocks). The shocks were then continued on a progressively reduced scale till the subject was discharged from the hospital, and once a month thereafter during a two-year follow-up period (pp. 68–69).

Cameron (1960) described the subject's condition in the third stage of depatterning: "He lives in the immediate present. All schizophrenic symptoms have disappeared. There is complete amnesia for all events of his life" (p. 27). Years later, Macdonald (1988) — who underwent depatterning in 1963 at the age of 23 — confirmed Cameron's observation:

> I have no memory of existing prior to October 1963, and the recollections I do have of events of the following years until 1966 are fuzzy and few. . . . My parents were introduced to me. . . I did not know them. [My five] children came back from wherever they had been living. I had no idea who they were. (pp. 206–209)

A "period of reorganization" followed the third stage (Cameron et al., 1962). Marks (1980) described the "psychic driving" technique which Cameron used during this period. "Once Cameron had produced the blank mind, he could then program in new patterns of behavior," or so he claimed. It was this aspect of depatterning that the CIA was most interested in. Psychic driving entailed bombarding the subjects with tape recorded, emotionally loaded messages repeated 16 hours a day. For this purpose, Cameron installed speakers under

508 [262] FRANK

pillows in "sleep rooms" where his subjects were kept. Several weeks of negative messages were followed by two to five weeks of positive ones. Cameron established the effect of the negative tapes by "running wires to [the subjects'] legs and shocking them at the end of the message" (pp. 136–137). Cameron's brainwashing methods — about which the psychiatric profession had detailed information at the time — became a scandal only after public disclosure of the CIA's financial involvement.

While electroshock cannot, of course, be used to reshape reality, it — like brainwashing — can and has been used to reshape the subject's perception of reality. Warren (1988) reported on interviews with ten married women 26–40 years old, from the San Francisco Bay Area who had undergone ECT between 1957 and 1961. The salient feature of ECT for these women was memory loss: "Troubling life-events and relationships commonly forgotten by these women included the existence of their husbands and children, their own names, and their psychiatrists" (p. 292). Some of the husbands, Warren reported, "used their wives' memory loss to establish their own definitions of past situations in the marital relationship." Other relatives found they "could freely re-define past situations without challenge" (p. 294). Warren comments: "When the recollections of one [marital] partner are to some degree erased, the dynamic reconstruction of reality shifts a little, or a lot" (p. 297).

Those who define reality usually control it. What had shifted here was power — away from the electroshock survivor. Without referring to brainwashing as such, Warren shows that electroshock and brainwashing serve similar ends. Electroconvulsive brainwashing is psychiatry's cleansing ritual; its method for controlling painful, unhappy memories and false or unpopular beliefs by destroying them.

Conclusion

Mystification and conditioning have undoubtedly played an important role in shaping the public's tolerant attitude toward electroshock. But it is not only the uninformed and misinformed public that has stood by silently during the electroshock era. There has hardly been a voice of protest from the informed elite — even when one of its own has been victimized.

While undergoing a series of involuntary electroshocks at the famed Mayo Clinic in 1961, Ernest Hemingway told visitor A.E. Hotchner, "Well, what is the sense of ruining my head and erasing my memory, which is my capital, and putting me out of business? It was a brilliant cure but we lost the patient. It's a bum turn, Hotch, terrible. . ." (cited in Hotchner, 1967, p. 308). A few days after his release from the Mayo Clinic following a second course of ECT, Hemingway killed himself with a shotgun. With all that has been written about him since his death, no recognized figure from the world of literature, academia, law, religion or science has spoken out against those responsible for this tragedy. As might have been expected, the psychiatric profession has also been silent. Not only did the psychiatrist who electroshocked Hemingway escape the censure of his colleagues, but a few years later they elected him president of the American Psychiatric Association.

Since ancient times physicians have been trying to cure epilepsy. One might therefore think that they would object to the use of artificially-induced seizures as a method of treatment. But no such objection has been forthcoming. On the contrary, the medical profession's passive acquiescence to the use of electroshock has recently turned to active support:

> The AMA [American Medical Association] has endorsed the use of electroconvulsive therapy (ECT) "as an effective treatment modality in selected patients, as outlined by the American Psychiatric Association. . . ." [The AMA] recognized ECT as "a safe procedure in proper hands." (ECT, Animal rights, 1989, p. 9)

ECT User Robert Peck titled his book *The Miracle of Shock Treatment* (1974). Antonin Artaud (cited in Sontag, 1976), the French actor and playwright, who was electroshocked in the early 1940s, wrote afterwards: "Anyone who has gone through the electric shock . . . never again rises out of its darkness and his life has been lowered a notch" (p. 530). In which perspective — or at what point between these two perspectives — is the truth to be found? This is no trivia question. For some, it will be the gravest question they will ever have to answer.

References

Abrams, R. (1988a). *Electroconvulsive therapy.* Oxford: Oxford University Press.

Abrams, R. (1988b). Interview with Lothar Kalinowsky, M.D. *Convulsive Therapy, 4,* 25–39.

Accornero, F. (1988). An eyewitness account of the discovery of electroshock. *Convulsive Therapy, 4,* 41–49.

Alexopoulos, G.S., Young, R.C., and Abrams, R.C. (1989). ECT in the high-risk geriatric patient. *Convulsive Therapy, 5,* 75–87.

Allen, M.R. (1978). Electroconvulsive therapy: An old question, new answers. *Psychiatric Annals, 8,* 47–65.

Alpers, B.J., and Hughes, J. (1942). The brain changes in electrically induced convulsions in the human. *Journal of Neuropathology and Experimental Neurology, 1,* 173–180.

American Psychiatric Association. (1978). *Electroconvulsive therapy.* Task Force Report 14. Washington, D.C.: American Psychiatric Association.

American Psychiatric Association. (1989, December 18). *The practice of ECT: Recommendations for treatment, training and privileging.* Task Force on ECT. Washington, D.C.: American Psychiatric Association.

Andre, L. (1988, May 13). ECT: The politics of experience. Testimony given before the Quality of Care Conference, Albany, New York.

Arnot, R.E. (1975). Observations on the effects of electric convulsive treatment in man — psychological. *Diseases of the Nervous System, 36,* 449–502.

Avery, D., and Winokur, G. (1976). Mortality in depressed patients treated with electroconvulsive therapy and antidepressants. *Archives of General Psychiatry, 33,* 1029–1037.

Ayd, F.J., Jr. (1963). Guest editorial: Ugo Cerletti, M.D. 1877–1963. *Psychosomatics, 4,* A6–A7.
Bender. L. (1955). The development of a schizophrenic child treated with electric convulsions at three years of age. In G. Caplan (Ed.), *Emotional problems of early childhood* (pp. 407–425). New York: Basic Books.
Black, D.W., Wilcox, J.A., and Stewart, M. (1985). The use of ECT in children: Case report. *Journal of Clinical Psychiatry, 46,* 98–99.
Breggin, P.R. (1979). *Electroshock: Its brain-disabling effects.* New York: Springer.
Breggin, P.R. (1981). Disabling the brain with electroshock. In M. Dongier and E.D. Wittkower (Eds.), *Divergent views in psychiatry* (pp. 247–271). Hagerstown, Maryland: Harper & Row.
Cameron, D.E. (1956). Psychic driving. *American Journal of Psychiatry, 112,* 502–509.
Cameron, D.E. (1957). Psychic driving: Dynamic implant. *Psychiatric Quarterly, 31,* 703–712.
Cameron, D.E. (1960). Production of differential amnesia as a factor in the treatment of schizophrenia. *Comprehensive Psychiatry, 1,* 26–34.
Cameron, D.E., Lohrenz, J.G., and Handcock, K.A. (1962). The depatterning treatment of schizophrenia. *Comprehensive Psychiatry, 3,* 65–76.
Cameron, D.E., and Pande, S.K. (1958). Treatment of the chronic paranoid schizophrenic patient. *Canadian Medical Association Journal, 78,* 92–96.
Cerletti, U. (1956). Electroshock therapy. In A.M. Sackler, M.D. Sackler, R.R. Sackler, and F. Marti-Ibanez (Eds.), *The great physiodynamic therapies in psychiatry: An historical reappraisal* (pp. 91–120). New York: Hoeber-Harper.
Crowe, R.R. (1984a). Electroconvulsive therapy: A current perspective. *New England Journal of Medicine, 311,* 163–167.
Crowe, R.R. (1984b, April 7). Shock-therapy controversy needs look at the research. *Des Moines Register,* p. 13A.
Darnton, N. (1989, July 31). Committed youth. *Newsweek,* pp. 66–72.
Drop, L.J., and Welch, C.A. (1989). Anesthesia for electroconvulsive therapy in patients with major cardiovascular risk factors. *Convulsive Therapy, 5,* 88–101.
ECT, animal rights among topics discussed at AMA's Dallas meeting. (1989, January 20). *Psychiatric News,* p. 9; 23.
Edelson, E. (1988, December 28). ECT elicits controversy – and results. *Houston Chronicle,* p. 3.
Ehrenberg, R., and Gullingsgrud, M.J.O. (1955). Electroconvulsive therapy in elderly patients. *American Journal of Psychiatry, 111,* 743–747.
Electroconvulsive therapy. (1987, December). *Harvard Medical School Mental Health Letter, 4,* 1–4.
Fink, M. (1978). Electroshock therapy: Myths and realities. *Hospital Practice, 13,* 77–82.
Fink, M., Kahn, R.L., and Green, M. (1958). Experimental studies of electroshock process. *Diseases of the Nervous System, 19,* 113–118.
Frank, L.R. (1976). The Frank papers. In J. Friedberg, *Shock treatment is not good for your brain* (pp. 62–81). San Francisco: Glide Publications.
Frank, L.R. (1978). *The history of shock treatment.* San Francisco: Frank.
Freeman, C.P.L., and Kendell, R.E. (1980). ECT: I. Patients' experiences and attitudes. *British Journal of Psychiatry, 137,* 8–16.
Gaitz, C.M., Pokorny, A.D., and Mills, M. (1956). Death following electroconvulsive therapy. *Archives of Neurology and Psychiatry, 75,* 493–499.
Gerring, J.P., and Shields, H.M. (1982). The identification and management of patients with a high risk for cardiac arrythmias during modified ECT. *Journal of Clinical Psychiatry, 43,* 140–143.
Gordon, H.L. (1948). Fifty shock therapy theories. *Military Surgeon, 103,* 397–401.
Gralnick, A. (1944). Psychotherapeutic and interpersonal aspects of insulin treatment. *Psychiatric Quarterly, 18,* 177–196.
Gralnick, A. (1946). A three-year survey of electroshock therapy: Report on 276 cases; comparative value of insulin-coma therapy. *American Journal of Psychiatry, 102,* 583–593.
Gregory, S., Shawcross, C.R., and Gill, D. (1985). The Nottingham ECT study: A double-blind comparison of bilateral, unilateral and simulated ECT in depressive illness. *British Journal of Psychiatry, 146,* 520–524.
Grimm, R.J. (1978, January). Convulsions as therapy: The outer shadows. *Psychiatric Opinion, 15,* 30–31; 45–47.

Heath, R.G. (1984). An overdue comprehensive look at a maligned treatment: Electroconvulsive therapy. *Behavioral and Brain Sciences, 7*, 27-28.

Hoch, P.H. (1948). Discussion and concluding remarks. *Journal of Personality, 17*, 48-51.

Horrock, N.M. (1977, August 2). Private institutions used in C.I.A. effort to control behavior. *New York Times*, pp. 1; 16.

Hotchner, A.E. (1967). *Papa Hemingway*. New York: Bantam.

Impastato, D. (1957). Prevention of fatalities in electroshock therapy. *Diseases of the Nervous System, 18* [supplement], 34-75.

Janis, I.J. (1950). Psychologic effects of electric convulsive treatments (1. Post-treatment amnesias). *Journal of Nervous and Mental Disease, 3*, 359-381.

Jones, T. (1988, June). Letter. *Dendron* [Eugene, Oregon], p. 2.

Kalinowsky, L.B. (1959). Convulsive shock treatment. In S. Arieti (Ed.), *American handbook of psychiatry* (Volume II, pp. 1499-1520). New York: Basic.

Kalinowsky, L.B. (1967). The convulsive therapies. In A.M. Freedman and H.I. Kaplan (Eds.), *Comprehensive textbook of psychiatry* (pp. 1279-1285). Baltimore: Williams & Wilkins.

Kalinowsky, L.B., and Hippius, H. (1969). *Pharmacological, convulsive and other somatic treatments in psychiatry*. New York: Grune and Stratton.

Kalinowsky, L.B., and Hoch, P. (1952). *Shock treatments, psychosurgery and other somatic treatments in psychiatry*. New York: Grune and Stratton.

Kalinowsky, L.B., and Hoch, P. (1961). *Somatic treatments in psychiatry*. New York: Grune and Stratton.

Kennedy, C.J.C., and Anchel, D. (1948). Regressive electric shock in schizophrenics refractory to other shock therapies. *Psychiatric Quarterly, 22*, 317-320.

Klug, J. (1984, June). Benefits of ECT outweigh risks in most patients. *Clinical Psychiatry News*, p. 16.

Kurland, A.A., Hanlon, T.E., Esquibel, A.J., Krantz, J.C., and Sheets, C.S. (1959). A comparative study of hexafluorodiethyl ether (Indoklon) and electroconvulsive therapy. *Journal of Nervous and Mental Diseases, 129*, 95-98.

Levy, S.D., and Albrecht, E. (1985). Electroconvulsive therapy: A survey of use in the private psychiatric hospital. *Journal of Clinical Psychiatry, 46*, 125-127.

Liberson, W.T. (1948). Brief stimuli therapy: Physiological and clinical observations. *American Journal of Psychiatry, 105*, 28-39.

Lowinger, L., and Huddleson, J.H. (1945). Results of electric shock therapy in the first 150 cases at the Veterans Facility, Northport, New York. *Miltary Surgeon, 97*, 271-277.

Macdonald, L. (1988). Breakthrough. In B. Burstow and D. Weitz (Eds.), *Shrink resistant: The struggle against psychiatry in Canada* (pp. 206-210). Vancouver, British Columbia: New Star Books.

Maclay, W.S. (1953). Death due to treatment. *Proceedings of the Royal Society of Medicine, 46*, 13-20.

Marks, J. (1980). *The search for the "Manchurian Candidate": The CIA and mind control*. New York: McGraw-Hill.

Martin, P.A. (1949). Convulsive therapies: Review of 511 cases at Pontiac State Hospital. *Journal of Nervous and Mental Disease, 109*, 142-157.

McCartney, J.L. (1961). Private psychiatric practice since the end of World War II. *Diseases of the Nervous System, 22*, 547-554.

Opton, E.M., Jr. (1985, June 4). Letter to the members of the panel. National Institute of Health Consensus Development Conference on Electroconvulsive Therapy.

Page, L.G.M., and Russell, R.J. (1948, April 17). Intensified electrical convulsion therapy in the treatment of mental disorders. *Lancet*, pp. 597-598.

Peck, R.E. (1974). *The miracle of shock treatment*. Jericho, New York: Exposition Press.

Philadelphia Psychiatric Society. (1943). Symposium: Complications of and contraindications to electric shock therapy. *Archives of Neurology and Psychiatry, 49*, 786-791.

Pinel, J.P.J. (1984). After forty-five years ECT is still controversial. *Behavioral and Brain Sciences, 7*, 30-31.

Pribram, K. (1974, September-October). From lobotomy to physics to Freud: An interview with Karl Pribram. *The APA Monitor*, p. 9.

Ray, M.B. (1942). *Doctors of the mind: The story of psychiatry*. Indianapolis and New York: Bobbs-Merrill.

Reed, K. (1988). Electroconvulsive therapy: A clinical discussion. *Psychiatric Medicine*, 6, 23–33.

Roueché, B. (1974, September 9). As empty as Eve. *The New Yorker*, pp. 84–100.

Rymer, R. (1989, March-April). Electroshock. *Hippocrates*, pp. 65–72.

Sackeim, H.A. (1986). Acute cognitive side effects of ECT. *Psychopharmacology Bulletin*, 22, 482–484.

Sament, S. (1983, March). Letter. *Clinical Psychiatry News*, p. 11.

Sargant, W. (1957). *Battle for the mind: A physiology of conversion and brainwashing*. Baltimore: Penguin.

Small, J.G., and Small, I.F. (1984). Current issues in ECT practice and research. *Behavioral and Brain Sciences*, 7, 33–34.

Sontag, S. (Ed.). (1976). *Antonin Artaud: Selected writings*. Berkeley, California: University of California Press.

Squire, L.R. (1982). Memory and electroconvulsive therapy [Letter]. *American Journal of Psychiatry*, 139, 1221.

Squire, L.R. (1983). Electroconvulsive therapy and complaints of memory dysfunction: A prospective three-year follow-up study. *British Journal of Psychiatry*, 142, 1–8.

Task Force of the Colorado Psychiatric Society. (1977, October). *Report and recommendations of a Task Force of the Colorado Psychiatric Society*.

Templer, D.I., and Veleber, D.M. (1982). Can ECT permanently harm the brain? *Clinical Neuropsychology*, 4, 62–66.

Thigpen, C.H. (1976). Letter. *Convulsive Therapy Bulletin*, 1, 40.

Thompson, J.W. (1986). Utilization of ECT in U.S. psychiatric facilities, 1975 to 1980. *Psychopharmacology Bulletin*, 22, 463–465.

Ulett, G.A. (1972). *A synopsis of contemporary psychiatry*. St. Louis: C.V. Mosby.

Viscott, D. (1972). *The making of a psychiatrist*. Greenwich, Connecticut: Faucett.

Warren, C.A.B. (1986). Electroconvulsive therapy: "New" treatment of the 1980s. *Research in Law, Deviance and Social Control*, 8, 41–55.

Warren, C.A.B. (1988). Electroconvulsive therapy, the self, and family relations. *Research in the Sociology of Health Care*, 7, 283–300.

Weil, P.L. (1950). "Regressive" electroplexy in schizophrenics. *Journal of Mental Science*, 56, 514–520.

Weiner, R.D. (1984). Does electroconvulsive therapy cause brain damage? *Behavioral and Brain Sciences*, 7, 1–22 [peer commentary section, pp. 22–54].

©1990 The Institute of Mind and Behavior, Inc.
The Journal of Mind and Behavior
Summer and Autumn 1990, Volume 11, Numbers 3 and 4
Pages 513 [267] – 530 [284]
ISSN 0271-0137
ISBN 0-930195-05-1

Behavior in a Vacuum:
Social-Psychological Theories of Addiction That Deny the Social and Psychological Meanings of Behavior

Stanton Peele

Mathematica Policy Research

Social psychologists have been in the forefront of the development of modern theories of cigarette smoking and obesity. These theories are reductionist: they account for behavior in purely physiological terms and regard cognitive, value, personality, and social class factors as secondary or irrelevant. Yet, from their beginnings, these theories have failed to account for major aspects of the behaviors under investigation, aspects apparently related to personal intention and social background. While it may seem surprising that work by social psychologists denies social and psychological reality, the theories discussed here actually reflect broader trends in social psychology, trends with rather large implications for our ideas about individual and social efforts at change.

Since the late 1960s, three theoretical models associated with Stanley Schachter and his students have dominated the study of eating and smoking behavior. Schachter's (1968) internal-external model, which proposed that obese persons relied primarily on external cues to regulate their eating, built upon Schachter's earlier laboratory research designed to provide succinct, mathematical explanations of human behavior. The internal-external model was superceded by Nisbett's (1972) set-point model of eating behavior, which postulated that a biological mechanism defends the innate body weight of each individual. The set-point model of obesity was complemented in the area of smoking behavior by Schachter's (1977, 1978) research showing that smokers in the laboratory strove to maintain habitual levels of cellular nicotine, a finding Schachter generalized into his nicotine-regulation model of addictive smoking. The nicotine-regulation model has become prominent along with the recognition that smoking and overeating have major similarities with alcoholism, narcotic addiction, and other appetitive-addictive conditions (Peele, 1985).

Requests for reprints should be sent to Stanton Peele, Mathematica Policy Research, Inc., P.O. Box 2393, Princeton, New Jersey 08543-2393.

Yet, all of the models developed by the Schachter group in the area of appetitive-addictive behaviors have demonstrated severe limitations in predicting the behavior of human beings in natural settings. Schachter (1982) himself later found that over 60 percent of respondents in a survey of two community groups who had ever smoked or been overweight, but who had attempted to modify their behavior, were no longer obese or smokers. Ironically, both the set-point and nicotine-regulation models had been devised primarily to explain why overeating and smoking seem so resistant to efforts at change. The models' failures in this instance reflect the inherent inadequacies of explanations of addiction that refuse to incorporate social-psychological facts as fundamental determinants of behavior (Peele, 1981). These failures are especially noteworthy in the case of the Schachter group's work since this work grew out of core areas of social psychological research, and might thus be thought unlikely to fall prey to a reductionist oversight. Instead, the work of Schachter and his students in the areas of smoking and obesity reveals that strong reductionist assumptions characterize social psychology: namely, the dominant theme in contemporary social psychology is that human beings are fundamentally unaware of and unable to influence the sources of their behavior (Nisbett and Ross, 1980). For example, according to Schachter (1980), purely biological models are "already capable of revolutionizing our understanding of the nature of a presumably psychological or social phenomena" (p. 132; the two main examples Schachter offered for this observation were smoking and alcoholism).

The research on which these ideas are based is laboratory bound. I argue in this paper that models of addiction have failed precisely because they have ignored social-psychological dimensions of behavior, as revealed most clearly by naturalistic studies (Peele, 1985). I propose further that the internal-external, set-point, and nicotine-regulation models mirror broader trends in social psychology, trends which downplay the ability of individuals to modify their own behavior according to their intentions, conscious awareness of their environments, and social settings. Psychological theories are influential in shaping our images of humanity. The models discussed in this paper have vast implications for our understanding of the sources of behavior, for how we attack social problems as a society, for how we attempt to remedy individual behavioral problems (such as smoking or eating too much), and for our conception of what being human means and our belief about the goals to which individuals and societies can aspire.

Social Psychological Models of Smoking and Eating Behavior

Schachter and his students presented results from several experiments in the 1960s showing that normal-weight people ate when hungry but obese people were unable to determine when they were full and relied instead on external cues to tell them when to eat (Nisbett, 1968; Schachter, Goldman, and Gordon, 1968; Schachter and Gross, 1968). Schachter (1971b) then explored similarities between the behavior of obese humans and ventromedial-lesioned rats, leading Schachter and Rodin (1974) to an expanded external-ity model of obesity that proposed that overweight humans (and rats) were hyperemotional and hyper-responsive to immediate stimuli of all kinds, and not just food. Eventually, Rodin (1980, 1981) rejected the internal-external model, primarily because there were internally and externally responsive eaters at all weight levels. While recognizing that a range of factors influence eating behavior, Rodin sought mainly to identify neurological mechanisms that might account for "arousal-related overeating without relying on psychodynamic factors" (1981, p. 368).

The set-point model was developed by another Schachter student, Richard Nisbett, who had been exploring parallels betwen human and animal obesity and physiological mechanisms in overweight. Nisbett (1972) proposed that the hypothalamus is set to defend a given body weight established for each individual by heredity and/or feeding during childhood. The set-point hypo-thesis has been extremely influential both in obesity research (cf. Stunkard, 1980) and in popular conceptions about overweight (cf. Bennett and Gurin, 1982). Polivy and Herman (1983) eventually suggested that people may get their weight below its set-point-determined level through conscious restraint of eating but that this is an inherently unstable and ultimately futile resolu-tion of overweight.

Although Schachter endorsed both the set-point and restrained-eating models (cf. Bennett and Gurin, 1982, p. 44), he disengaged from eating experimenta-tion in the 1970s to turn his attention to research on smoking behavior in which he initially replicated earlier designs from his work on obesity. For ex-ample, he found smokers were less willing to tolerate shocks than non-smokers, the same difference his team found between obese and normal-weight subjects. Smokers were also more distractible when nicotine-depleted, another difference that held between obese and normal-weight subjects. Obese subjects ate more when fearful and tense (Schachter et al., 1968), similar to findings that smokers smoke more under such conditions (Gilbert, 1979). Yet, whereas Schachter conceived the externality of the obese as a seemingly inbred constitutional factor, he viewed continued cigarette smoking as an acquired dependence on nicotine. What was constant in both lines of research was the idea that behavior was almost entirely biologically or pharmacologically determined, and that smoking and overeating were not responses to psychological forces.

The Regulation of Calorie and Nicotine Intake

The set-point and nicotine-regulation models explain human behavior in terms of the need to keep food (or calorie) and nicotine intake at a constant level. Evidence supporting these models includes the short-term regulation of cellular nicotine in experimental studies of smokers and the tendency, over periods of months and years, for humans to return to a constant weight level. Arrayed against this evidence are findings, which I present and discuss below, that nicotine regulation, even in the laboratory, is variable and influenced by nonpharmacological factors; that weight levels and eating do respond to environmental factors; that over the long term, weight and smoking do vary considerably and that, in particular, people have a strong tendency to cease smoking and to eliminate overweight. The set-point and nicotine-regulation models also do not consider such nonpharmacological and nonbiological relationships as that between social class and obesity and the high correlation between smoking and other substance abuse and health-risk behaviors.

Schachter (1977) found that heavy smokers presented with cigarettes containing less-than-accustomed amounts of nicotine smoked more cigarettes, confirming earlier findings that smokers regulate their intake of nicotine to keep their plasma nicotine levels constant. However, other research has shown nonpharmacological considerations are essential to understanding smoking behavior and nicotine intake. For example, nicotine administered directly (through injection or orally) does not have nearly the impact that inhaled nicotine does for habitual smokers, who continue to smoke even when they have achieved their accustomed level of cellular nicotine via capsule (Jarvick, Glick, and Nakamura, 1970). This may be why this type of research has found smokers' regulation of nicotine levels to be inexact and only approximate (McMorrow and Foxx, 1983; Schachter, 1977). As Leventhal and Cleary (1980) noted, Schachter himself found that a 77% reduction in nicotine content produced only a 17%–25% increase in cigarette consumption.

Leventhal and Cleary also suggested that Schachter's model assumes "a direct and automatic step from changes in plasma nicotine level to craving and smoking" (p. 390) without considering any other intentional or situational factors that might intervene. As an example of such a factor, Schachter (1978) himself remarked that Orthodox Jews regularly gave up smoking "without a qualm" on the sabbath. This observation might seem to introduce the entire realm of competing values and motivations in smoking behavior, including those which eventually cause many smokers to quit. Schachter did not pursue this discovery, however, since, for him, smokers' pharmacological addiction means they will undergo intense discomfort from any diminution of their nicotine intake and will ceaselessly strive to regain habitual nicotine levels, or else suffer intense discomfort from the failure to do so. For Schachter, in this work on nicotine regulation, it would seem that no one could ever comfortably forgo habitual smoking. In the following passage, he graphically described what might be the result of efforts to quit smoking:

> Whan a large portion of an addicted population is attempting to quite smoking . . . , a very large number of people in that population will be in withdrawal. Given what we

know of withdrawal, this means large numbers of people simultaneously in a state of irritability, irascibility, short temper, and so on. One could with reason anticipate high rates of divorce, assault, and general mayhem in such a population. (1980, pp. 156–157)

Actually, there is little evidence that avoidance of withdrawal is a major motivation for the continuation of smoking, since smokers frequently quit only to relapse long after they have endured peak periods of withdrawal distress (Bernstein, 1969). When nonsmokers (along with other former addicts) do relapse, they rarely do so because of sensations of physical discomfort. Instead, relapse most often results from emotional tensions and environmental pressures and former addicts' subjective reactions to these (Marlatt and Gordon, 1980). It is for this reason that blue-collar workers are better able to quit smoking when they are middle-aged, when they report experiencing less tension in their jobs (Caplan, Cobb, and French, 1975). In the naturalistic study in which he later was to discover that nearly two-thirds of those who had ever tried to quit smoking had succeeded, Schachter (1982) himself found no difference in remission rates for heavy and light smokers, although in earlier work he had claimed that those heavily addicted should be least able to overcome their need for their regular nicotine levels.

The surprisingly high percentage of formerly overweight respondents Schachter discovered had undergone an average weight loss of 35 pounds, which they had maintained for an average of 11 years. This finding is, of course, strong evidence against the set-point theory, which likens efforts to reduce weight levels to undergoing voluntary starvation. Indeed, Polivy and Herman (1983) described weight loss to be almost a physical impossibility, since "for the foreseeable future, we must resign ourselves to the fact that we have no reliable way to change the natural weight that an individual is blessed or cursed with" (p. 52). These authors actually discussed Schachter's findings of "relatively common" remission in obesity, but attributed this result to the fact that most respondents in the Schachter research were not at their set-point when they had been obese. In this case, the question is why their weight rose above set-point in the first place. And is it really true that those with "nonset-point" overweight find it easier to lose weight than those whose obesity is "natural"? Polivy and Herman presented no data to this point; in the Schachter study, remission from obesity was equally likely for those who had been 30% and more overweight and those only 15% overweight.

Rodin (1980, 1981), while sympathetic to biological interpretations of obesity in general, rejected the set-point theory on the grounds that those who lost weight were *not* more responsive to food cues than others (Rodin, Slochower, and Fleming, 1977). The original internal-external model research showed overweight people to be more responsive to external cues in eating, and Rodin and Slochower (1976) found that externally responsive subjects put on more weight than others in a food-rich environment. However, those hyper-

responsive subjects who had been of normal weight before entering this environment also displayed a tendency to lose this added weight when they
returned home. The sensitivity to external cues of many who became
overweight and their resulting fluctuation in weight level contrasts with the
idea that people adhere to a strict weight range based on internal biological
mechanisms.

Both immediate social influences and background social attitudes have been
shown to have a strong impact on an individual's weight. Garn, Cole, and
Bailey (1979) coined the phrase "cohabitational effect" to describe the strong
family-line resemblances in weight levels they found in family members
whether or not — or no matter to what extent — they were related biologically.
Community and epidemiological studies have also repeatedly demonstrated
that social class and ethnicity are major factors in obesity (Garn, Bailey, and
Higgins, 1980; Goldblatt, Moore, and Stunkard, 1965). Such social differences in weight are often enormous: Strunkard, d'Aquili, Fox, and Filion
(1972) found girls from lower-SES homes were nine times as likely to be
obese by age six as girls from upper-class homes. Social class differences appear in other health behaviors in addition to smoking and overeating. The
tendency toward excessive consumption also bridges specific substances for
the same individuals. For example, smoking and consumption of caffeine and
alcohol are correlated, especially at the highest levels of consumption (Istvan
and Matarazzo, 1984). Appetitive behavior is more than pharmacologically
bound, since drinking, smoking, and drug-taking are also related to risk-taking
behavior other than substance use, such as buckling automobile safety belts
(Mechanic, 1979).

Since Polivy and Herman (1983) suggest childhood obesity as the mark of
true set-point obesity, such findings have important implications for our views
on the maintenance of overweight. The relationship between social
background and overweight disputes set-point notions, however, by finding
social differences — almost by definition — not to be permanent. Stunkard
and his co-workers found those from ethnic groups with heightened tendencies toward overweight approximated ordinary weight levels the more they
assimilated and adopted middle-class American values. Garn, LaVelle, and
Pilkington (1984) observed that family-line resemblances disappeared the longer
family members lived apart, approaching a statistical limit of zero correlation. Indeed, large-scale, long-term epidemiological studies emphasize the im-
permanence of weight as an individual characteristic. Garn, Pilkington, and
LaVelle (1984), measuring 2575 individuals over two decades, found a strong
regression to the mean effect — those who were most lean initially showed
the greatest weight gain and those most obese typically showed the greatest
weight loss.

Longitudinal and survey studies reveal substantial tendencies for people to overcome obesity: Garn, Bailey, and Cole (1980) found that over half of initially obese men (although only 20% of obese women) were no longer overweight when measured a decade later. Combined with evidence of large-scale remission in smoking (Pierce, Fiore, Novotny, Hatziandrev, and Davis, 1989), such data suggest a substantial human tendency toward the elimination of excessive and self-destructive patterns of behavior. Clinical observations, on the other hand, have found that most therapy patients do not achieve long-term weight loss or cessation of smoking (Leventhal and Cleary, 1980; Wing and Jeffery, 1979). This difference may have to do with the nature of therapy-seeking populations. In the Schachter study, those who never attended therapy for overweight had a higher remission rate than those who had, leading Schachter (1982) to suggest that therapy may be counterproductive to overcoming these appetitive-addictive conditions.

Interviews with former heroin addicts and alcoholics who have quit addictions without the aid of therapy often reveal that addicts resolve to change their lifestyles and develop personal strategies to do so (Biernacki, 1986; Tuchfeld, 1981). Few data are available on the subjective experience of smokers and the obese who have attained remission on their own. Schachter (1982) did not report the methods his respondents used to change their behavior. However, in a brief side-bar to a report on the Schachter study in *Psychology Today* (Gerin, 1982), an editor reviewed the original interviews for such methods. The prototypical response for ex-smokers was "I decided to stop." And, although the formerly obese gave a wider range of explanations for their success, most of their descriptions amounted simply to eating less high-calory food and less food overall.

These descriptions do not prove that respondents found it easy to change their behavior. But they do suggest that people can often bring their behavior into line with strongly-held values, even when this means defying impulses to maintain high caloric or nicotine intake levels. This would seem to be the case with the Orthodox Jewish smokers observed to regularly abstain from smoking on the sabbath. Something similar may have been operating in the Rodin and Slochower (1976) study, where hyper-responsive girls of normal weight at first gained poundage in a camp where food was abundant, but managed to lose much of the weight even before leaving the camp. As Rodin (1981) noted, "these data suggest that other factors may be more important than external responsiveness in influencing the final levels of body weight attained" (p. 364). These girls seem eventually to have learned how to control their eating patterns at camp because they wanted to be a certain weight. Rodin would be unlikely to summarize the data in exactly this way, however, since she finds the idea of conscious restraint of eating to be "only a descriptive term and not a mechanism" in eating and overweight. However, intentional and social factors often appear to be essential for understanding appetitive-addictive behaviors and their modification, even if the set-point and nicotine-regulation models refuse to acknowledge such factors.

Recent Research in Relation to Larger Trends in Social Psychology

Reductionist models of overeating and smoking predate the research of selected social psychologists, of course. What is noteworthy is how social psychology has failed to bring social and psychological factors into focus when examining these behaviors. Social psychologists have been prominent opponents of purely biological or pharmacological explanations of addiction and alcoholism (cf. Chein, Gerard, Lee, and Rosenfeld, 1964; McClelland, Davis, Kalin, and Wanner, 1972). In the case of alcoholism, the division between social-psychological and disease views has created an almost war-like state (Peele, 1984a). This tension has not been present in the social-psychological study of smoking and obesity. That social psychologists conducting research in these areas accept mainstream reductive assumptions about eating and smoking behavior suggests that the set-point and nicotine-regulation models may offer basic insights into the direction of social psychology as a whole.

Veterans of the heady period at the turn of the half-century when Kurt Lewin and Henry Murray were the dominant figures in social psychology often regret developments in the field since that era (Cartwright, 1978; Katz, 1978; Kelley, 1980; Pepitone, 1981; Sarason, 1981), including the failures to consider the larger social unit and conscious intention in behavior, and the over-reliance on experimental research designed to permit convenient statistical analysis. In the area of obesity and smoking, experimental and field research often give entirely different views of behavior. Findings of social causality, of the relationships among health behaviors, and of natural remission are unlikely in the laboratory. For example, physician Albert Stunkard's (1976) shift in emphasis from social class to physiological sources of obesity coincided with his shift from epidemiological to experimental research. The contemporary field research of physical anthropologist Stanley Garn exists in total isolation from the laboratory investigations that shape current views of obesity (cf. Stunkard, 1980).

On the basis of their externality experiments, Schachter and Rodin (1974) declared: "almost any fat person can lose weight; few can keep it off" (p. 1). Rodin (1981, p. 361) repeated this sentiment. (Although Rodin's subsequent research was not limited to the laboratory, it was extremely limited in time frame.) Schachter's (1982) study of obesity over the life span, on the other hand, found long-term weight loss to be a common occurence. This same dichotomy in results occurs with the divergent research perspectives on drug use. Under laboratory conditions, addicts may appear to be totally wed to their drug of choice. However, studies of the natural history of drug addiction and alcoholism have found both that substance use varies substantially from time to time and that most alcoholics and addicts quit their habits for good (Cahalan, 1970; Maddux and Desmond, 1981; Nurco, Cisin, and Balter, 1981; Vaillant, 1983). Such anomalies led one biologically oriented researcher to announce perplexedly:

> The foundation is set for the progression of the alcohol dependence syndrome by virtue of its biologically intensifying itself. One would think that, once caught up in the process, the individual could not be extricated. However, and for reasons poorly understood, the reality is otherwise. Many, perhaps most, do free themselves. The withdrawal process, and the associated desire and drive to drink, collide with the totality of the individual and the whole of life. (Gross, 1977, p. 121)

Sometimes, anomalous views of human behavior collide within the same study and the investigator is forced to choose one version of "reality." In their study of the effects of manipulating the clock time apparent to obese and normal-weight subjects, Schachter and Gross (1968) predicted the obese would eat more when they believed it was later, while normal-weight subjects would eat the same amount no matter what time they thought it was. In fact, normal-weight subjects ate less when they thought it was later, apparently because – "aware they would eat dinner very shortly" – they were "unwilling to spoil their dinner" by filling up on the crackers the experimenters offered them (Schachter, 1968, p. 754). One might decide this was a significant aspect of the eating behavior of those who are not fat, the kind of eating restraint that may be passed along through social background or that overweight people must learn in order to loose weight. Yet Schachter (1971a, p. 96) dismissed this finding as the "spoil dinner artifact," maintaining that only the eating of the obese is cognitively influenced (albeit in a faulty way).

Nisbett (1968) examined how prefeeding subjects in an experiment would affect their reactions to better- and worse-tasting food. He found that both obese subjects and subjects who were formerly obese over-reacted to the prefeeding by eating *more* food later. Nisbett felt that "the theoretical and practical consequences of these data on the formerly overweight are considerable." Since the obese responded "to food and eating in ways which are enduring," even after they had lost weight, Nisbett concluded that "the long-range prognosis is very poor" for the obese (p. 116). This is, of course, the idea underlying set-point theory. On the other hand, it could seem a strange deduction – on the basis of finding that subjects overate under conditions of experimental forced feeding – to decide that the obese are doomed to overeat forever. After all, the formerly obese subjects had demonstrated by their actual weight loss that they were able to regulate their behavior in a desired direction over a considerable period of time outside the laboratory. The notion that laboratory behavior is somehow "truer" than other expressions of human nature traces back to developments in social psychology in the 1950s, and particularly to the formulation of the research ideal of experiments in which extraneous influences are controlled in order to observe the impact on behavior of carefully calibrated variables (Festinger, 1953). This approach marked a distinct departure from the Lewinian research model combining laboratory and field observations of global variations in behavior. Stanley Schachter was to play a seminal role in these research developments, through his early work on group influences on attitudes (Festinger, Schachter, and Back, 1950; Schachter, 1951), his studies (Schachter, 1959) on affiliation (which found that people sought the company of others under conditions of arousal and uncertainty), his classic work on the labeling of arousal states as emotions based on convenient if misleading social cues (Schachter, 1964), and his view of obesity as a reliance on external cues to determine when one is hungry and should eat.

The Schachter experiments were typical, if extreme, examples of the belief that keeping subjects off balance produces more valid results. For example, in Schachter and Singer's (1962) evocation of drug reactions, subjects who were misled about the effects of a drug injection picked up the mood of a paid experimental stooge with whom they were closeted. Such studies were not ones in which subjects had the opportunity to develop reasoned responses to familiar dilemmas or, certainly, to manipulate their environments as to be able to control their outcomes. As a result, behavior in these experiments appeared highly malleable, where people seemed in the throes of forces they were little aware of and even less able to control. This fundamental disbelief in people's ability to enact courses of action based on conscious goals and the processing of available information carried over to Schachter's (1968) and Nisbett's (1968) work in obesity and later research.

Nisbett and Wilson (1977), for example, examined data from several key social-psychology experiments and noted that subjects were rarely able to identify the experimental manipulations that prompted their behavior. Nisbett and Wilson (1977) and Nisbett and Ross (1980) created a basic model of human functioning out of this view that cognition is inescapably after-the-fact, suggestible, inaccurate, and impotent. Yet this conclusion stems from experiments designed specifically to be as noncommonsensical and as indecipherable by subjects as possible. Rather than detecting anything fundamental about human conduct, these psychologists may simply have been reifying into general laws findings that appear mainly under the very specialized laboratory conditions in which they were observed. Nevertheless, the current academic climate seems especially receptive to this point of view. Christensen-Szalanski and Beach (1984) found in their literature survey that studies showing poor judgmental performance were cited six times as often as comparable research indicating that people make accurate judgments; examples of poor judgment recalled by a group of researchers came invariably from laboratory studies, usually with college students as subjects, while most of the recalled studies of good judgments were conducted in natural settings.

Funder (1987) has argued that social-psychological studies of judgmental processes are not designed to assess actual accuracy of judgment, and that errors measured using artifical stimuli in the laboratory may not comprise faulty judgmental processes in broader social contexts. (Funder points by way of analogy to perception studies that find perceptual errors of the parlor-game variety translate into sound judgmental rules under ordinary observational conditions.) The most oft-cited judgmental error in the contemporary literature is the so-called fundamental attribution error (Ross, 1977), according to which observers consistently over-rate the importance of personality traits relative to situational determinants of behavior. This error has been uncovered regularly in laboratory studies where people judge others they do not know, or who indeed do not exist but are fabricated by experimenters to express a "canned" opinion.

It would seem quite natural in these circumstances that people's reliance on personality attributions should prove misguided. When people have the chance to form relationships and to observe each other over time, however, a sensitivity to the personality characteristics of others could be quite useful (Peele, 1983, 1984b). Funder and Dobroth (1987) reported that correlations between peer and parental assessments of subjects and such subject behavior as delay of gratification regularly achieve the same order of predictive power as do potent situational factors in typical social-psychology experiments. They noted further that industrial psychologists have repeatedly validated relationships between personnel assessments and job performance. Mischel (1984), who has been associated with the view that personality is impermanent and maybe nonexistent, declared on the basis of his research review that people often make quite sound attributions based on complex personality-situation assessments.

Social-Psychological Sources of Behavior and Our Image of Humanity

The fundamental attribution error and other portrayals of human beings as myopic and misdirected may reflect philosophical and moral assumptions as much as empirical results. Prominent and popular thought in social psychology has found people to be unaware of — and thus unable to control — the causes of their actions. This image of the wellsprings of behavior is similar to that which many theorists have proposed to account for obesity and smoking, as well as alcohol and drug addiction. In the latter two cases, the individual is thought to act only in order to maintain alcohol or heroin intoxication. All other motivations are seen to have lost any meaning for the person, now in an animal-like state (cf. Peele, 1985). From a contrasting perspective, other theorists conceive of addiction as an effort by the individual to modify psychological states and to adjust to specific environmental conditions (Alexander and Hadaway, 1982).

These opposing notions present different images of the human being and can affect how people conceive of themselves and their possibilities for regulating their behavior. Oddly, those most likely to describe themselves as being unable to control their drug or alcohol use and to believe that only medical or biological interventions can "save" them may be those who are most likely to become addicted in the first place (Peele, 1985). The same may hold for obesity and smoking. For example, research with smokers has found that those who believe they have the most internal control over their smoking, regardless of the actual level of their addiction, are better able to quit smoking (Shiffman, 1985). What then is the result of speculation such as the following by Polivy and Herman (1983): "As research progresses, we will eventually be able to imagine . . . biological interventions – even including genetic manipulations" – in order to " 'change the setting' for natural weight" (p. 52). The emphasis on smoking as a process of chemical dependence (Krasnegor, 1979) leads to analogous proposals that smoking is best quit through nicotine weaning or replacement techniques. Recently, however, Hughes, Gust, Keenan, Fenwick, and Healy (1989) performed a systematic comparative trial between Nicarette (a nicotine gum) and a placebo, and found negligible differences in abstinence rates for smoking between the treatment and control groups at the end of a year.

The idea that addiction is an external form of enslavement that can strike anyone and that medical "operations" are the only possible ways to remove or combat an addiction bespeak a frightening world view, one that sees it as hopeless for people to try to control their own lives or habits. It is doubly distressing to find that these ideas are being presented as if they were the results of scientific investigations when, in fact, the bulk of the evidence runs in a contrary direction – that is, that personal outlook and social setting are the crucial elements in creating and maintaining or fighting addiction. The practical implications of this difference in scientific or public health perspectives are endless. For example, when President George Bush announced (in September of 1989) a multi-billion dollar program to combat overseas drug production and commerce, he found the money for his drug war in such domestic programs as housing and juvenile justice, which are meant to support inner-city residents in their efforts to overcome poverty and the pressure toward criminal life styles. If self-efficacy, and the outlook and environments that make this possible, are crucial to establishing resistance to addiction, then it might seem Bush's policies actually promise to exacerbate addiction rather than to reduce it.

Interestingly, one argument that Bush and his drug czar, William Bennett, frequently make is that they wish to discourage casual drug use as a way to combat addiction. In fact, during his speech, Bush noted that recreational drug use had decreased in the United States while regular, addicted drug use of cocaine had increased over the same period in the 1980s. One mechanism for this decrease in overall usage combined with increased adddiction may be that the incessant marketing of the idea that crack is addictive, and that no one can resist or free themselves from its power, is a self-fulfilling one that ensures that a greater percentage of the smaller numbers who try the drug are more likely to believe they will be addicted, and indeed become addicted.

More broadly, psychological theories have implications for our beliefs in the potential of humanity to influence its collective destiny and the best ways for doing so. Zajonc (1980a) described how both native American social psychologists and émigrés from Nazi Germany like Lewin and Heider were "ardently humanistic and liberal" and "believed that the perfectibility of man is not to be found in biological or genetic solutions, but in reason, in eduction, and in the self-imposed standards of conduct and morality."[1] At the same time, "they were impressed . . . with the powerful Nazi propaganda machine. . . . Germany was viewed as the product of a massive attitude change — a massive *cognitive* change —" indicating that "the role of cognitive processes in social life must be exceedingly important" (p. 189). Contrast this description with the analysis by Schachter in the same volume (a commemoration of Lewin's impact on American psychology):

> I suspect that the reductionist approach has the potential . . . of providing major insights into problems and areas that have seemed the exclusive province of social scientists and humanists — particularly, I anticipate, in . . . the understanding of aberrant mass phenomena. . . . Has there yet been a psychological, sociological, or historic analysis of Nazi Germany that made this period of human insanity comprehensible? . . . My opinion is based on the trusim that we all breathe the same air, drink the same water, eat similar food, smoke similar cigarettes, and so on. If something biological changes or goes wrong, it can affect all or most of a population. [Schachter proceeds to his analysis on the effects of smoking cessation efforts on a society, recorded above.] (p. 156)

---

[1]The Zajonc case is itself instructive. Labelled as a cognitive psychologist (the reason he was asked to write this review of the Lewin tradition), Zajonc's laboratory studies have become increasingly microscopic and have dissected human behavior into exceedingly small components. For example, his series of investigations on the "attitudinal effects of mere exposure" claimed to show that people liked best whatever they were exposed to most. Zajonc's scientific strategy has been that fundamental truths about human beings will be found in the most basic motivational/behavioral elements. Indeed, it is hard to see how his psychology of human beings differs from a psychology of animals, and Zajonc often draws parallels between human and animal behavior. In the logical extension of his views on the primacy of irrational motivations over the importance of reasoned thought (the opposite of the Lewinian anti-Nazi position he describes), Zajonc (1980b) argued that emotions drive thought and that cognition only enters a motivational-behavioral sequence after the fact, in order to explain a preordained reflexive reaction.

In 1962, Henry Murray delivered an audacious address entitled "The Personality and Career of Satan," in which he chided his audience for its "immaculate Scientism." He argued:

> The Devil's target . . . [is] the conception of a better world composed of better societies of better persons and . . . [the striving] to actualize it by self-transformations and social reconstructions. In other words, . . . the Satanic aim is to prevent all developments in this direction by shattering man's faith in the existence of the necessary potentialities within himself and reducing him to cynicism and despair. . . . And here is where our psychology comes in with the bulk of its theories, its prevailing views of human personality, its images of man, obviously in league with the objectives of the nihilistic Satanic spirit . . . [leaving] no ground at all for any hope that the human race can save itself from the fatality that now confronts it. (1981, pp. 533–534)

In prevailing views of obesity and smoking and in selected theories of human motivation and cognition, the image of human potential and the view of the sources of behavior are not the unambiguous results of empirical investigations – rather, they reflect and reinforce the perspectives from which the research was conducted. If not scientific in nature, where do these views originate? Murray provocatively evokes religious themes in his critique because the vision of human nature and human action that informs psychology is as open to a spiritual challenge as it is to an empirical one. And, from this vantage point, the Schachter group's work – and all of social psychology – is open to ethical criticism for its derogatory view of the human spirit as being ineluctably passive, fatalistic, and irrational.

References

Alexander, B.K., and Hadaway, P.F. (1982). Opiate addiction: The case for an adaptive orientation. *Psychological Bulletin, 92,* 367–381.

Bennett, W., and Gurin, J. (1982). *The dieter's dilemma.* New York: Basic Books.

Bernstein, D.A. (1969). Modification of smoking behavior: An evaluative review. *Psychological Bulletin, 71,* 418–440.

Biernacki, P. (1986). *Pathways from heroin addiction: Recovery without treatment.* Philadelphia: Temple University Press.

Cahalan, D. (1970). *Problem drinkers: A national survey.* San Francisco: Jossey-Bass.

Caplan, R.D., Cobb, S., and French, J.R.P., Jr. (1975). Relationships of cessation of smoking with job stress, personality, and social support. *Journal of Applied Psychology, 60,* 211–219.

Cartwright, D. (1978). Theory and practice. *Journal of Social Issues, 34,* 168–180.

Chein, I., Gerard, D.L., Lee, R.S., and Rosenfeld, E. (1964). *The road to H.* New York: Basic Books.

Christensen-Szalanski, J.J.J., and Beach, L.R. (1984). The citation bias: Fad and fashion in the judgment and decision literature. *American Psychologist, 39,* 75–78.

Festinger, L. (1953). Laboratory experiments. In L. Festinger and D. Katz (Eds.), *Research methods in the behavioral sciences* (pp. 136–172). New York: Dryden.

Festinger, L., Schachter, S., and Back, K. (1950). *Social pressures in informal groups.* New York: Harper.

Funder, D.C. (1987). Errors and mistakes: Evaluating the accuracy of social judgment. *Psychological Bulletin, 101,* 75–90.

Funder, D.C., and Dobroth, K.M. (1987). Differences between traits: Properties associated with interjudge agreement. *Journal of Personality and Social Psychology, 52,* 409–418.

Garn, S.M., Bailey, S.M., and Cole, P.E. (1980). Continuities and changes in fatness and obesity. In R. Schemmel (Ed.), *Nutrition, physiology and obesity* (pp. 51–78). Palm Beach, Florida: CRC.

Garn, S.M., Bailey, S.M., and Higgins, T.T. (1980). Effects of socioeconomic status, family line, and living together on fatness and obesity. In R.M. Lauer and R.B. Shekelle (Eds.), *Childhood prevention of atherosclerosis and hypertension* (pp. 187–204). New York: Raven Press.

Garn, S.M., Cole, P.E., and Bailey, S.M. (1979). Living together as a factor in family-line resemblances. *Human Biology, 51*, 565–587.

Garn, S.M., LaVelle, M., and Pilkington, J.J. (1984). Obesity and living together. *Marriage and Family Review, 7*, 33–47.

Garn, S.M., Pilkington, J.J., and LaVelle, M. (1984). Relationship between initial fatness level and long-term fatness change. *Ecology of Food and Nutrition, 14*, 85–92.

Gerin, W. (1982, August). (No) accounting for results. *Psychology Today*, p. 32.

Gilbert, D.G. (1979). Paradoxical tranquilizing and emotion-reducing effects of nicotine. *Psychological Bulletin, 86*, 643–661.

Goldblatt, P.B., Moore, M.E., and Stunkard, A.J. (1965). Social factors in obesity. *Journal of the American Medical Association, 192*, 1039–1044.

Gross, M.M. (1977). Psychobiological contributions to the alcohol dependence syndrome: A selective review of recent research. In G. Edwards, M.M. Gross, M. Keller, J. Moser, and R. Room (Eds.), *Alcohol-related disabilities* (WHO Offset Publication No. 32, pp. 107–131). Geneva: World Health Organization.

Herman, C.P., and Polivy, J. (1980) Restrained eating. In A.J. Stunkard (Ed.), *Obesity* (pp. 208–225). Philadelphia: Saunders.

Hughes, J.R., Gust, S.W., Keenan, R.M., Fenwick, J.W., and Healy, M.L. (1989). Nicotine vs. placebo gum in general medical practice. *Journal of the American Medical Association, 261*, 1300–1305.

Istvan, J., and Matarazzo, J.D. (1984). Tobacco, alcohol, and caffeine use: A review of their interrelationships. *Psychological Bulletin, 95*, 301–326.

Jarvick, M.E., Glick, S.D., and Nakamura, R.K. (1970). Inhibition of cigarette smoking by orally administered nicotine. *Clinical Pharmacology and Therapeutics, 11*, 574–576.

Katz, D. (1978). Social psychology in relation to the social sciences: The second social psychology. *American Behavioral Scientist, 5*, 779–792.

Kelley, H.H. (1980). The causes of behavior: Their perception and regulation. In L. Festinger (Ed.), *Retrospections on social psychology* (pp. 78–108). New York: Oxford.

Krasnegor, N.A. (Ed.). (1979). *Cigarette smoking as a dependence process* (Research Monograph Series No. 23). Rockville, Maryland: National Institute on Drug Abuse.

Leventhal, H., and Cleary, P.D. (1980). The smoking problem: A review of the research and theory in behavioral risk modification. *Psychological Bulletin, 88*, 370–405.

Maddux, J.F., and Desmond, D.P. (1981). *Careers of opioid users*. New York: Praeger.

Marlatt, G.A., and Gordon, J.R. (1980). Determinants of relapse: Implications for the maintenance of behavior change. In P.O. Davidson and S.M. Davidson (Eds.), *Behavioral medicine: Changing health lifestyles* (pp. 410–452). New York: Brunner/Mazel.

McClelland, D.C., Davis, W.N., Kalin, R., and Wanner, E. (1972). *The drinking man*. New York: Free Press.

McMorrow, M.J., and Foxx, R.M. (1983). Nicotine's role in smoking: An analysis of nicotine regulation. *Psychological Bulletin, 93*, 302–327.

Mechanic, D. (1979). The stability of health and illness behavior: Results from a 16-year follow-up. *Journal of Public Health, 69*, 1142–1145.

Mischel, W. (1984). Convergences and challenges in the search for consistency. *American Psychologist, 39*, 351–364.

Murray, H.A. (1981). The personality and career of Satan. In E.S. Schneidman (Ed.), *Endeavors in psychology* (pp. 518–534). New York: Harper & Row.

Nisbett, R.E. (1968). Taste, deprivation, and weight determinants of eating behavior. *Journal of Personality and Social Psychology, 10*, 107–116.

Nisbett, R.E. (1972). Hunger, obesity, and the ventromedial hypothalamus. *Psychological Review, 79*, 433–453.

Nisbett, R.E., and Ross, L. (1980). *Human inference: Strategies and shortcomings of social judgment*. Englewood Cliffs, New Jersey: Prentice-Hall.

Nisbett, R.E., and Wilson, T.D. (1977). Telling more than we can know: Verbal reports on mental processes. *Psychological Review, 84*, 231–259.

528 [282]   PEELE

Nurco, D.N., Cisin, I.H., and Balter, M.B. (1981). Addict careers III: Trends across time. *International Journal of the Addictions, 16*, 1353–1372.
Peele, S. (1981). Reductionism in the psychology of the eighties: Can biochemistry eliminate addiction, mental illness, and pain? *American Psychologist, 36*, 807–818.
Peele, S. (1983). *The science of experience: A direction for psychology.* Lexington, Massachusetts: Lexington.
Peele, S. (1984a). The cultural context of psychological approaches to alcoholism: Can we control the effects of alcohol? *American Psychologist, 39*, 1337–1351.
Peele, S. (1984b, December). The question of personality. *Psychology Today*, pp. 54–56.
Peele, S. (1985). *The meaning of addiction: Compulsive experience and its interpretation.* Lexington, Massachusetts: Lexington.
Pepitone, A. (1981). Lessons from the history of social psychology. *American Psychologist, 36*, 972–985.
Pierce, J.P., Fiore, M.C. Novotny, T.E., Hatziandrev, E.J., and Davis, R.M. (1989). Trends in cigarette smoking in the United States. *Journal of the American Medical Association, 261*, 49–65.
Polivy, J., and Herman, C.P. (1983). *Breaking the diet habit: The natural weight alternative.* New York: Basic Books.
Rodin, J. (1980). The externality theory today. In A.J. Stunkard (Ed.), *Obesity* (pp. 226–239). Philadelphia: Saunders.
Rodin, J. (1981). Current status of the internal-external hypothesis for obesity: What went wrong? *American Psychologist, 36*, 361–372.
Rodin, J., and Slochower, J. (1976). Externality in the nonobese: The effects of environmental responsiveness on weight. *Journal of Personality and Social Psychology, 33*, 338–334.
Rodin, J., Slochower, J., and Fleming, B. (1977). The effects of degree of obesity, age of onset, and energy deficit on external responsiveness. *Journal of Comparative and Physiological Psychology, 91*, 586–597.
Ross, L. (1977). The intuitive psychologist and his shortcomings: Distortions in the attribution process. In L. Berkowitz (Ed.), *Advances in experimental social psychology* (Volume 10, pp. 174–220). New York: Academic.
Sarason, S.B. (1981). An asocial psychology and a misdirected clinical psychology. *American Psychologist, 36*, 827–836.
Schachter, S. (1951). Deviation, rejection, and communication. *Journal of Abnormal and Social Psychology, 46*, 190–207.
Schachter, S. (1959). *The psychology of affiliation.* Stanford, California: Stanford University Press.
Schachter, S. (1964). The interaction of cognitive and physiological determinants of emotional state. In L. Berkowitz (Ed.), *Advances in experimental social psychology* (Volume 1, pp. 49–80). New York: Academic.
Schachter, S. (1968). Obesity and eating. *Science, 161*, 751–756.
Schachter, S. (1971a). *Emotion, obesity, and crime.* New York: Academic.
Schachter, S. (1971b). Some extraordinary facts about obese humans and rats. *American Psychologist, 26*, 129–144.
Schachter, S. (1977). Nicotine regulation in heavy and light smokers. *Journal of Experimental Psychology: General, 106*, 5–12.
Schachter, S. (1978). Pharmacological and psychological determinants of smoking. *Annals of Internal Medicine, 88*, 104–114.
Schachter, S. (1980). Non-psychological explanations of behavior. In L. Festinger (Ed.), *Retrospections on social psychology* (pp. 131–157). New York: Oxford University Press.
Schachter, S. (1982). Recidivism and self-cure of smoking and obesity. *American Psychologist, 37*, 436–444.
Schachter, S., Goldman, R., and Gordon, A. (1968). Effects of fear, food deprivation, and obesity on eating. *Journal of Personality and Social Psychology, 10*, 91–97.
Schachter, S., and Gross, L.P. (1968). Manipulated time and eating behavior. *Journal of Personality and Social Psychology, 10*, 98–106.
Schachter, S., and Rodin, J. (1974). *Obese humans and rats.* Washington, D.C.: Erlbaum.
Schachter, S., and Singer, J.E. (1962). Cognitive, social, and physiological determinants of emotional state. *Psychological Review, 69*, 379–399.

Shiffman, S. (1985). Coping with temptations to smoke. In S. Shiffman and T.A. Wills (Eds.), *Coping and substance use* (pp. 223–242). Orlando, Florida: Academic.

Stunkard, A.J. (1976). *The pain of obesity.* Palo Alto, California: Bull.

Stunkard, A.J. (Ed.). (1980). *Obesity.* Philadelphia: Saunders.

Stunkard, A.J., d'Aquili, E., Fox, S., and Filion, R.D. (1972). Influence of social class on obesity and thinness in children. *Journal of the American Medical Association, 221,* 579–584.

Tuchfeld, B.S. (1981). Spontaneous remission in alcoholics: Empirical observations and theoretical implications. *Journal of Studies on Alcohol, 42,* 626–641.

Vaillant, G. (1983). *The natural history of alcoholism.* Cambridge, Massachusetts: Harvard University Press.

Wing, R.R., and Jeffery, R.W. (1979). Outpatient treatment of obesity: A comparison of methodology and clinical results. *International Journal of Obesity, 3,* 261–279.

Zajonc, R.B. (1980a). Cognition and social cognition: A historical perspective. In L. Festinger (Ed.), *Retrospections on social psychology* (pp. 180–204). New York: Oxford University Press.

Zajonc, R.B. (1980b). Feeling and thinking: Preferences need no inferences. *American Psychologist, 35,* 151–175.

©1990 The Institute of Mind and Behavior, Inc.
The Journal of Mind and Behavior
Summer and Autumn 1990, Volume 11, Numbers 3 and 4
Pages 531 [285] – 544 [298]
ISSN 0271-0137
ISBN 0-930195-05-1

The Conceptual Bind in Defining the
Volitional Component of Alcoholism:
Consequences for Public Policy and Scientific Research

Richard E. Vatz

Towson State University

and

Lee S. Weinberg

University of Pittsburgh

An essential element in both lay and professional definitions of alcoholism is the a priori claim that afflicted individuals lack control over their drinking and/or over their behavior while drinking. The social, legal and scientific consequences of accepting this claim are examined. Based on specific evidence drawn from recent journal articles, we argue that alcohol researchers fail to adequately engage the issue of volition and that their research designs and findings are thereby flawed.

What does "alcoholism" mean? Contrary to the assumption of large numbers of Americans, there is no clear definition — not in medicine, not in law, and not in the community at large (Blakeslee, 1984). The conceptual confusion arises out of the implicit postulating of a necessary but untestable component of psychiatric and medical theoretical definitions of alcoholism: a lack of volition, or the inability to control one's drinking behavior.[1]

Requests for reprints should be sent to Richard E. Vatz, Ph.D., Department of Communication, Towson State University, Baltimore, Maryland 21204.

[1]The American Psychiatric Association (APA) speaks of "alcohol dependence" and "alcohol abuse" as two types of alcoholism, but the distinctions are not important for this paper, for both involve the criterion of alleged inability to cut down. Some sources delineate "species" of "alcoholism" relative to the pattern of drinking (American Psychiatric Association, 1987, p. 173), and in some there is a concession as well that there may be a type of "alcoholism" that does not include uncontrollability as a necessary component (Jellinek, 1960). The APA concedes only the possibil-

The definitional confusion surrounding the concept of "alcoholism" is of more than theoretical interest. The combined necessity and untestability of this alleged lack of control results in the dissemination of unreliable information in the popular press and in the generation of unreliable research in the professional sphere. Beliefs about the nature of excessive drinking have serious consequences for public policy dealing with heavy drinkers and the acts in which they engage while intoxicated. If we believe that physicians are able to medically identify what alcoholism is and who is an alcoholic, we can more easily justify: the expenditures made by thousands of firms and public agencies which have employee-assistance programs; the spending of millions of dollars by health insurance concerns for alcoholic services; and the extending to millions of Americans who drink heavily financial and legal protections accorded to handicapped individuals.

The costs of identifying and treating "alcoholics" plus the expense of paying for the damage done by excessive drinking in this country exceeds \$120 billion, according to the National Institute on Alcohol Abuse and Alcoholism (NIAAA) (Kolata, 1987b). Such estimates assume we are able to define alcoholism and identify which drinkers are "alcoholics," as opposed to just willful drinkers; moreover, the estimates of these costs are uniformly based on the assumption that alcohol is the *cause* of the actions of people who drink heavily, thereby combining cases wherein there is arguably such a connection (e.g., automobile accidents) with cases where there is arguably little if any causal connection (e.g., job absenteeism).

It is easy to understand why the public assumes such a causal connection. Statistically, alcohol consumption is highly correlated with a wide variety of anti-social and socially disvalued behaviors. There is near-ubiquitous quoting in both the popular and academic press of statistical estimates of alcohol-related social problems in America, statistics provided by alcohol interest groups, such as the NIAAA.[2] Significantly, when the NIAAA and other alcohol-interested parties present such statistics, they imply that the alcohol

ity of *unawareness* of "lack of control," and in only a minority of "people with alcoholism" (American Psychiatric Association, 1987, p. 173). More important, there is little or no reference in the popular or academic press to "alcoholism" that does not explicitly or implicitly involve the loss of control. One differentiation should be stressed, however. As we will refer to "alcoholism" as it is used in the popular press and academic research, we do not refer to either the pathoanatomical consequences of ingesting alcohol or what psychiatrists call "alcohol-induced organic mental disorders" (American Psychiatric Association, 1987). The latter notion does involve conceptual difficulties not dissimilar to those of the notion of "alcoholism," but that is beyond the scope of this paper.

[2]Here are some typical examples from typical lists: In about 90% of child abuse cases "alcohol is a significant factor" (Corbett, 1987, p. C5); almost one-half of all fatalities from driving accidents "involve alcohol" (Niven, 1984, p. 1913); "Alcohol is a factor in nearly half of America's murders, suicides and accidental deaths" (Lord, 1987, p. 56); and "Alcoholism and alcohol abuse . . . [creates] costs to the economy, which amount to about \$117 billion a year, most of it in lost productivity" (Holden, 1987, p. 1132).

consumption is the cause of the incidents, and "alcoholism," with all of its conceptual fuzziness, not "heavy drinking," is almost invariably the terminology used to characterize the excessive alcohol consumption.

Such consistent popular press and, to a lesser extent, academic press acceptance of alcoholism as a disease has been a major factor in convincing the public. Seventy-nine percent of respondents in a 1982 Gallup poll assented to the notion that alcoholism is a disease (Blume, 1983, p. 471), with the implications that alcoholism is well-defined, identifiable and renders its victims out of control.

The Issue of Control of One's Own Behavior

The issue of "control" of one's own behavior − the volitional question − has been historically and continues to be a central premise of the theory that alcoholism is a disease. This has been granted by both supporters (Blume, 1983) and skeptics (Fingarette, 1988) of that view, although not without exception (see footnote 5).

The question of volition is the critical question in the diagnosis of alcoholism, particularly with respect to the formation of legal and social policies concerning how we deal with the drinking and behavior of so-called alcoholics. Despite all of the confusion over the meaning of alcoholism, most medical experts see some loss of control over one's drinking to be a defining hallmark, although a few experts argue that there exists a minority of cases in which alcoholism can theoretically exist without implying loss of control or an inability to abstain (Blume, 1983).[3]

The component of volition is supremely important since the assumption that "alcoholics" cannot control their drinking or behavior-while-drinking on their own is the explicit or implicit justification for providing free help, as well as excusing some people for their actions. It is important to stress, however, that the argument over whether "alcoholism" is an "illness" is at the same time an argument over the volition question. While one might logically maintain that alcoholics cannot control their drinking but that this lack of control does not constitute an "illness," the conventional view rests on the implied assumptions that alcoholics lack control and that this lack of control itself constitutes an illness. Yet lack of control cannot be measured, since willfulness can only be assumed and not tested. Even the American Psychiatric Association (APA) takes the position that psychiatrists cannot measure volition, a position taken in response to attacks on the insanity plea

---

[3]The concept of volition, however, like the concept of alcoholism itself, is more complicated than generally acknowledged. In addition to the question of whether one can control whether he or she drinks is the crucial question of whether and to what extent the drinker can control his or her *behavior after* ingesting large quantities of alcohol.

several years ago (APA, 1982). Still, a thorough examination of reports in
the popular press before 1988 reveals not only an absence of *analysis* of the
confounding issue of volition, but also no mention of the problem of its
measurement.[4] Popular press articles from 1986–1987 (and certainly in years
prior to these) imply that alcoholism is a discrete phenomenon and can be
readily identified by professionals and even lay people who know the
"symptoms."

Although the public does not feel confused about "alcoholism," the medical
community is unable to provide a medically meaningful definition. The public
usually conceptualizes disease in a simple, straightforward way, meaning a
biologically unhealthy condition with a clear medical cause, such as infections. But the "disease" or "disorder," the term used by the APA's diagnostic
manual advisedly to avoid definitional specificity (APA, 1987, p. xxii) of
"alcoholism," is diagnosed by the psychiatric and medical communities mostly
by criteria of behavior and powerlessness to reduce drinking. Powerlessness,
or lack of volition, is typically assumed to exist if the drinker's family, legal
or financial problems are severe and seen as a consequence of the drinking.
Specifically, the APA's diagnostic manual posits uncontrollability of the heavy
drinking as a diagnostic criterion, but this loss of volition is not measured
directly, but inferred from the bad life experiences of the drinker and an
undefined "desire" to "cut down" the drinking (APA, 1987, p. 168).

The imprecision in psychiatric diagnosis of "alcoholism" is mirrored in the
medical community in general. There are no laboratory tests specific for
alcoholism, nor could there be in view of the inability to scientifically measure
a construct (Liskow and Goodwin, 1986, p. 196). Moreover, Liskow and Goodwin argue in a work well-received by the *Journal of the American Medical
Association* (Craig, 1987) that research on "alcoholism" is hopelessly confused
by conceptual inconsistency: "epidemiological studies of alcohol use and abuse
are bedeviled by the uncertainties of what to measure and how to measure
it. The terms alcoholism, alcohol dependence, alcohol abuse, problem drinking, and drinking problems continue to be used by different researchers in
different ways" (p. 191).

Partially due to these definitional difficulties, the search for genetic markers
for "alcoholism" has been unsuccessful (Nurnberger, Goldin, and Gershon,
1986). Researcher Donald Goodwin points out that "Almost without exception, whenever a report of an association between a marker and alcoholism
is followed by attempts to replicate the finding, the findings are contradictory" (Goodwin, 1979, pp. 57–58). In sum, as Goodwin points out, "we are
not certain that *anything* is inherited" (p. 60, emphasis in original). Most

---

[4]This includes a survey and content analysis of articles referenced under the title "alcoholism"
1985–1988 in *The National Newspaper Index*. The *Index* comprises *The New York Times, The
Washington Post, The Los Angeles Times, The Wall Street Journal,* and *The Christian Science Monitor.*

researchers agree that the behaviors we call "alcoholism" are a result of a complex combination of innate influences, simple learned behavior and freedom of choice. The suspicion that there is some genetic component to uncontrolled heavy drinking rests on the finding that alcoholism, however defined, tends to run in families, even though the vast majority of children of biological parents diagnosed as "alcoholics" do not become "alcoholics" (in fact, a disproportionate number become lifelong teetotalers) and most "alcoholics" have no such family history. Studies of twins, even when twins are separated at birth and adopted by nonalcoholic parents, show significantly higher rates of alcoholism (again, even with varying definitions) in children of alcoholic parents than in children of alcoholic parents whose biological parents were nonalcoholic (Goodwin, 1979).

Liskow and Goodwin (1986, p. 206) ask the key question that goes to the root of all the confusion: even if there is a hereditary factor, "What is inherited?" The speculations as to what may be inherited include most prominently (a) an increased euphoria from alcohol, and (b) the *lack* of intolerance to alcohol. The surest thing scientific studies can tell us is who is genetically *undisposed* to become "alcoholic" (Goodwin, 1979).

Legal Consequences

It is not surprising that the conceptual confusion and uncertainty evident in the medical community regarding alcoholism and volition is reflected in the law's posture as well, including the differentiating between volition concerning drinking and volition concerning behavior after heavy drinking (see footnote 3). In a 1962 case involving drugs, the Supreme Court (*Robinson versus California*, [1962]) held that California could not punish narcotics addicts merely for being addicts, i.e., to criminalize the "status or condition" of being an addict amounted to cruel and unusual punishment. But in 1968 the Court held that Texas could punish public drunkenness despite the offender's being a chronic alcoholic (*Powell versus Texas*, [1968]). The divided Court ruled that while punishing an alcoholic based on his or her status as an alcoholic is impermissible and that punishment of the mere act of drinking might be similarly impermissible, the further act of public drunkenness is punishable.

A 1988 Supreme Court decision (*Traynor versus Turnage* and *McKelvey versus Turnage*, [1988]) in combination with the publication of a book (Fingarette, 1988) on the issue earlier in that same year (and quoted by the Court in that decision), marked a new phase in the debate over whether alcoholism is a disease. These two highly-publicized events seem to have the potential to significantly change legal and public perceptions of the volitional issue as well as other issues and assumptions surrounding "alcoholism" and heavy drinking (see below). The actual Court ruling involved only a decision as to whether the refusal by the Veterans Administration (VA) to grant extensions of benefits to two "alcoholic" veterans on the ground that their "alcoholism" resulted from "willful misconduct" was inconsistent with Section 504 of the Rehabilitation Act.

Under the law governing veterans' benefits Congress has provided for extensions to "any eligible veteran who was prevented from initiating or completing such veteran's chosen program of education within such time period because of a physical or mental disability which was not the result of such veteran's willful misconduct" (38 U.S.C. Section 1662(a)(1) [1982]). The VA's refusal was based on its conclusion that alcoholism and the resulting inability of the claimants to complete their education during the allotted time resulted from their "willful misconduct." The VA took the view that some people simply choose to drink too much (primary alcoholism) while others drink too much as a secondary effect of an acquired psychiatric disorder (secondary alcoholism). The former are denied time extensions for benefits because their conditions presumably result from "willful misconduct," while the latter are granted extensions because it is believed that they do not willfully contract these psychiatric disorders.

The Supreme Court decision (April 20, 1988), however, did more than provide an interpretation of Section 504, which prohibits the denial of benefits to anyone "solely by reason of his handicap" (29 U.S.C. Section 794 [1982]). Protestations by the Court to the contrary notwithstanding, this decision amounted to official recognition that except for those suffering from an identifiable underlying mental illness, all other "alcoholics" may be conclusively presumed to have a willfully incurred disability. While noting the lack of agreement in the medical literature on the nature of "alcoholism," and explicitly refusing to address whether or not it is a disease, the logic of the majority opinion necessarily leads to the following conclusions: (a) "primary alcoholics" drink too much by choice, and (b) volitional conduct cannot logically constitute disease, although its *consequences*, of course, can — as in lung cancer resulting from smoking or cirrhosis resulting from drinking. Probably due to the highly publicized Supreme Court case and the Fingarette (1988) publication, many popular press articles in 1988, for the first time, make reference to the existence of an ongoing controversy regarding whether alcoholism is an illness (see footnote 4).

Research Consequences — Historical

More subtle but potentially more significant than the social and legal consequences of the confusing conceptualization of alcoholism concerns the effect on the very process by which our knowledge of "alcoholism" is acquired: scientific research on "alcoholism." If there is no scientifically meaningful concept of "alcoholism," the result must be the production of flawed scientific research. Fingarette (1988) examines the scientific evidence underlying the widely held public belief that excessive drinking may be meaningfully thought of as a disease, and he argues that most of the major assumptions of the alcoholism-as-disease ideology (e.g., the alcoholics' lack of control, the inexorable fall after an alcoholic takes one drink, the *medical* nature of alcoholic treatment, and the belief that the scientific community consensually recognizes alcoholism as a disease) are without scientific validity. He especially singles out assumptions concerning ability to control the consumption of alcohol. What makes Fingarette's contribution most noteworthy is his reliance on conventional medical sources and respected establishment "alcoholism" researchers (e.g., Donald Goodwin and George Vaillant) for proof of some of his contentions.[5]

For over two decades, psychiatrist and psychiatric critic Thomas Szasz has written on the myth of alcoholism as a disease (Vatz and Weinberg, 1983). For example, Szasz (1972) questioned the same myths addressed by Fingarette, including the argument that it is a *post hoc, ergo prompter hoc* fallacy by which the problems and failures of "alcoholics" — such as criminality, homelessness, job difficulties, and divorces — are assumed to be caused by drinking, and not vice-versa.

The new threat to the public's virtually unquestioned acceptance of the disease model of alcoholism made possible by changes in popular press reporting, rather than by new research discoveries, presages a new emphasis in research on alcoholism — genetic markers which can "prove" there is a "disease" of heavy drinking. For if "crises" generate the emergence of novel theories in science (Kuhn, 1970), then alcohol interests must soon find a mystifying escape from the new skepticism regarding alcoholism as a disease (Vatz and Weinberg, 1989). Thus, it is likely that there will be more frequent announcements of scientific "discoveries" to once again authenticate alcoholism as a disease (for a typical example, see Kolata, 1987a; "New Blood," 1988). These studies, as we will see below in our examination of current research, still plagued by the apparently inescapable conceptual problems in alcohol research, do not address the volitional question. In a recent issue of *The New England Journal of Medicine* (Vatz and Weinberg, 1988) the present authors have criticized one such typical and widely publicized study (published in that same journal) purporting to find a "genetic marker" for "alcoholism." In the study in question, "alcoholism" is never distinguished from any other kind

---

[5]George Vaillant, highly-respected among alcohol researchers, sees alcoholism as a "disease," but expresses skepticism as to whether "loss of control over the ingestion of alcohol [is either] a necessary or sufficient criterion for diagnosing alcoholism" (1983, p. 308), although he concedes, drinkers with "alcohol-related problems" perceive themselves as such (p. 308). Vaillant derides the notion of willpower as a method of controlling drinking (p. 196).

of heavy drinking, so the authors may be identifying at most a possible risk for heavy drinking, or, perhaps, as they themselves concede, a marker only for the *effects* of heavy drinking (Tabakoff et al., 1988). Yet, the lead author, scientific director of NIAAA, argues explicitly that his and other alcohol research demonstrates that "a biological predisposition to alcoholism exists in many individuals" (Tabakoff, 1987, p. A26).

Most of the private and public support, sympathy, and spending on alcohol-related problems are grounded in the alcoholism-as-disease assumption, an assumption which is historically characteristic of alcohol research in general. "Most alcoholism treatment programs," as Bower (1988) points out, "operate on the assumption that people seeking their help have a disease" (p. 88). Adoption of the view that heavy drinking is controllable behavior might result in the weakening of the support systems — medical, familial, business, and government — that lessen the penalties which society exacts from irresponsible drinkers.

Research Consequences — Current

Liskow and Goodwin (1986) acknowledge that "The clinical course of alcoholism is obscured by . . . a lack of agreement on the definition of the illness" (p. 197). But the increasing challenges to the illness model (for history and analysis of the "illness model" in psychiatry, see Conrad and Schneider, 1980) and attendant conceptual problems are only sporadically acknowledged in current alcohol research. For example, Klerman (1989) states the current view in *The New England Journal of Medicine*: "There has been gradual acceptance of the concept that alcoholism is a disease, as manifested in policy statements by the American Medical Association and the creation by Congress of the National Institute of Alcohol Abuse and Alcoholism as part of the Public Health Service" (p. 394).

Medical establishment publications have not yet reflected the logic that if control is necessarily central to the concept of alcoholism, then control should be addressed in all research designs. But if control cannot be measured, then valid research is not possible. Whether recognized or ignored, conceptual problems plague alcoholism research. And it is our contention that these problems therefore vitiate much of extant alcoholism research. To examine this contention we have reviewed major representative research on alcoholism published in 1988.

Based on our prior work (Vatz and Weinberg, 1988), our expectation was that the definitional debate, conceptual fuzziness, and frequent examples of illogic which have characterized the public and legal discussion of alcoholism and alcoholics would be evident in the current medical/scientific literature as well. Because of the centrality of the volition criterion for alcoholism, we sought to examine specifically the current handling of the issue of whether the concept of alcoholism entails the idea that afflicted individuals are impaired in their ability to choose not to drink. Our expectation on this issue, fueled by our general familiarity with research on alcoholism over the years, was that researchers would either acknowledge the importance of this issue but gloss over it because it cannot be measured, or, more likely, they would ignore volition, thus making it unnecessary to distinguish among different types of excessive drinkers and therefore beg the question of the need to establish the volitional component which is the critical and necessary factor for differentiating alcoholics from heavy drinkers. In the likely case of the latter situation, we expected to find either no effort to define "alcoholic" beyond the state of being a patient in an alcohol treatment program or, alternatively, where the effort is made, it would involve heavy reliance on the criteria for alcoholism in DSM-III-R, criteria which themselves do not address the volition issue except indirectly by inference from financial, legal or familial problems (APA, 1987, pp. 165–168). In order to more fully explore these expectations, we compiled a list of journals based upon a review of the journals cited most frequently by prominent defenders and attackers of the disease concept of alcoholism. These included: *Alcoholism: Clinical and Experimental Research, American Journal of Psychiatry, Archives of General Psychiatry, British Medical Journal, British Journal of Addiction, British Journal of Psychiatry, International Journal of the Addictions, Journal of Studies on Alcohol, Journal of the American Medical Association,* and *New England Journal of Medicine.*

We then reviewed the tables of contents of all of the issues of these journals for 1988 and identified all titles which specifically included the terms "alcoholism" or "alcoholic." From this list we chose for the most part major articles or original articles rather than commentaries, correspondence, or research notes. By focusing on articles which used the terminology "alcoholic" or "alcoholism," we eliminated the many pieces which address the impact of alcohol intake on various bodily functions and diseases. Our goal was not to examine all articles on alcohol, only articles expressly concerned with "alcoholism" or "alcoholics." We do not doubt the dangers of excessive drinking, nor do we criticize the research examining social or behavioral correlates of excessive drinking. However, we do argue that studies explicitly examining "alcoholism" or "alcoholics" should provide explicit definitions of these terms, and definitions that engage the volition issue. Yet, our review of the scientific literature in 1988 reveals disturbingly little discussion of the definition of "alcoholism" or "alcoholic." What follows are brief summaries and analyses of the manner in which the issue of volition and/or its measurement is dealt with or avoided in selected articles from 1988 alcohol research.

Hill, Steinhauer, Zubin, and Baughman (1988) attempt to explore whether a marker can be helpful in identifying those at risk "for developing alcoholism" (p. 545). In addition, however, Hill et al. report, "Those who agreed were sent a confirming letter asking them to refrain from using all alcohol and drugs . . . for 48 hours before coming into the laboratory" (p. 547), a request which concedes that the subjects of the study could, at least for 48 hours, choose not to drink. This dramatic point is made without argument or explanation as to its significant implications regarding volition and, therefore, the meaningfulness of the concepts "alcoholism" or "alcoholic."

In a companion article arising out of the same research (Hill, Aston, and Rabin, 1988), the same conceptual problems are evident. Hill et al. attempt here to show that "alcoholism is transmitted genetically" (p. 811) by looking for the "genetic linkage of an alcoholism susceptibility (AS) gene(s) to a well-defined polymorphic marker" (p. 811). Yet the subjects of the study were simply those who met the DSM-III-R criteria along with the Feighner criteria for alcoholism. Both the Feighner criteria (Feighner et al., 1972, pp. 60–61) and the DSM-III-R criteria, as indicated earlier, use the criterion of inability to control drinking, but neither provides a way to distinguish volitional heavy drinkers from non-volitional heavy drinkers. At best, therefore, Hill et al. might have demonstrated some evidence to show that heavy drinkers are more likely than the general population to have a particular blood marker which, in turn, might be linked to genetic make-up. However, like Tabakoff et al. (1988) and most other researchers, failing to compare volitional heavy drinkers with non-volitional heavy drinkers seriously weakens any claim to have found, as the title implies, "suggestive evidence of genetic linkage between alcoholism and the MNS blood group" (p. 811).

O'Sullivan, Rynne, Miller, O'Sullivan, Fitzpatrick et al.(1988) attempt to trace the drinking behavior of several types of alcoholics following discharge from the hospital. Such studies, of course, are contaminated at the outset in that they select for study those individuals who have been admitted for detoxification treatment at the hospital. No effort is made to measure volition among those in need of detoxification, and again there is no differentiation made between "alcoholics" and heavy drinkers.

Cyr and Wartman (1988) argue that many outpatients are alcoholics and that the asking of simple questions can identify them. Doctors should, according to Cyr and Wartman, routinely ask patients two questions which Cyr and Wartman's research purports to show to be effective measures of alcoholism. This is demonstrated by comparing answers to these questions to answers given on the Michigan Alcohol Screening Test (MAST) which is used to identify alcoholics. The two questions, which are not specifically asked on the MAST, are "Have you ever had a drinking problem?" and "When was your last drink?" Cyr and Wartman recommend "the routine incorporation of these . . . into the medical history" (p. 51). Again, however, the MAST standard by which Cyr and Wartman identify alcoholics may in fact only identify heavy drinkers and, at best, identifies heavy drinkers whose drinking poses problems for them and for their families. It, too, cannot distinguish volitional from non-volitional heavy drinkers.

The research reported by Schuckit, Risch, and Gold (1988) purports to show that currently non-alcoholic sons of alcoholic fathers have "less intense responses to ethanol" (p. 1391), a finding which suggests that the children of alcoholics may process alcohol differently than the children of non-alcoholics. This would lend support to the belief that inherited biochemical factors may play a role in drinking behavior. The methodology employed here to define "alcoholism," however, is flawed substantially beyond the lack of engagement of the criterion of volition. First, the very existence of an alcoholic father is determined only on the basis of questionnaire responses and follow-up interviews of students who claim that their biological fathers "met the DSM-III criteria for alcoholism" (p. 1392). Apparently, direct contact was not made with these fathers. Second, since sons who themselves "fulfilled the DSM-III criteria for alcoholism, drug abuse, or any major psychiatric disorders or who had any major medical disorders were excluded from the sample" (p. 1392), the finding that such individuals process ethanol differently from others ignores the necessary components for even a lay discussion of "alcoholism"; that is, the propensity to drink at all, let alone to drink to excess.

Ciraulo, Sands, and Shader (1988) review the literature concerning the abuse of benzodiazepine among "alcoholics" (p. 1501). The literature seems to indicate that while effective, this drug is more likely to create dependency problems among "alcoholics" than among recipients of the drug in general population. The authors raise three methodological concerns with the literature: inconsistent terminology variously purporting to study "abuse potential," "addictiveness," and several other conditions; inconsistent operational definitions of whatever terms are used; and a failure to distinguish among the types of benzodiazepines being prescribed to patients (p. 1502). Ironically, even to those expressing sophisticated sensitivity to aspects of the research method and design of the subject under examination, the issue of what is meant by the term "alcoholic," and what various operationalizations have been employed in the literature under review is not even mentioned. If the earlier studies claim that they have examined the effect of the drug on alcoholics, then it is accepted without question that all of these researchers meant the same thing by the term and that they all measured it in precisely the same manner.

Consistent with E. Fuller Torrey (1988) and others who argue that the homeless are overwhelmingly alcoholic and/or mentally ill, Koegel and Burnam (1988) examined "alcoholism" in a sample of homeless adults and compared them to a matched sample of Los Angeles residents. They found more alcoholism among the homeless and many more "mental illnesses" among the homeless alcoholics than among those alcoholics residing at home. Unlike the other studies reviewed, Koegel does address the definition of alcoholism and, interestingly, states that "our estimates of the prevalence of alcohol use disorder are based on the presence of either alcohol abuse or alcohol dependence. The term alcoholism, in this report, is likewise used to refer to people with either alcohol abuse or alcohol dependence" (p. 1013).

If Koegel and Burnam are using the term "alcoholism" to include all types of heavy drinkers, then they are tacitly admitting that volition is irrelevant to the diagnosis of alcoholism. The use of this broadened notion of the term "alcoholic" makes it indistinguishable from "heavy drinker" and contradicts even the much less rigorous popular conceptions of "alcoholism," as well as scientific or medical definitions. If their use of the term "alcoholism" is meant to convey a sense of uncontrollable drinking, the authors have failed to make any effort to measure it either in the homeless or resident populations under examination.

Ettorre (1988) presents data on Alcoholism Treatment Units in Britain and makes no attempt to explain the use of the term "alcoholism" or to suggest whether these units distinguish among relative levels of volitional drinking. We found that British journals and researchers appear in general even less cognizant of or concerned with the definitional conundrum than their American counterparts.

Our review demonstrates that the great preponderance of research articles published in the leading journals in the fields of medicine, psychiatry and alcohol studies continue to make two major errors. First, they study as "alcoholics" or those suffering from "alcoholism" patients receiving treatment for alcohol intoxication, while not examining the hospital admission criteria or diagnosis. Second, if they do attempt to classify subjects themselves rather than relying on hospitalized heavy drinkers, researchers employ DSM-III-R criteria which do not successfully address the question of volition, an element which constitutes the *sine qua non* for meaningfully and consistently conceptualizing "alcoholism" or "alcoholic."

The literature is uniform neither in its use nor its type of confusion over the concepts of "alcoholic" and "alcoholism." Indeed, many such articles make no reference to "alcoholism" or "alcoholic." For example, Shaper, Wannamethee, and Walker (1988) examined relationships between groups of drinkers ranging from none/occasional to heavy and the mortality rates in general and cardiovascular mortality rates in particular. Again, no methodological problem arises regarding the need to address volition in a study simply analyzing alcohol intake and its consequences. Studies such as this one have no bearing on our primary claim: those who do purport to be studying "alcoholism" and/or "alcoholics" make major and damaging conceptual and methodological errors.

Conclusion

That both sophisticated scientific researchers and journalists are consistently inattentive to the issues we have raised should once again alert us to the dangers of science being locked into extant paradigms. We do not intend by our efforts to minimize the human suffering experienced by heavy drinkers and their families, nor do we intend to denigrate the efforts made by medical and other professionals to alleviate that suffering. We do, however, seek to move both the scientific and public debates in the direction of rigorous engagement of important issues and away from passive acceptance of conventional assumptions.

In the end, decisions regarding the allocation of resources for research and/or for helping people should result from scientifically valid and honest debate on the relative merits of the claims of those seeking financial support from public sources. The evidence which we have presented in this paper of the low level of professional and public discourse about the problem of heavy drinking suggests that no such debate can be possible without clear, consistent and meaningful use of alcohol research concepts.

References

American Psychiatric Association. (1982). *American Psychiatric Association statement on the insanity plea*. Washington, D.C.: American Psychiatric Association.
American Psychiatric Association. (1987). *Diagnostic and statistical manual of mental disorders* (3rd edition, revised). Washington, D.C.: American Psychiatric Association.
Blakeslee, S. (1984, August 14). Scientists find key biological causes of alcoholism. *The New York Times*, pp. C1, C3.
Blume, S. (1983). The disease concept of alcoholism. *Journal of Psychiatric Treatment and Evaluation, 5*, 471–478.
Bower, B. (1988, August 6). Intoxicating habits: Some alcoholism researchers say they are studying a learned behavior, not a disease. *Science News, 134*, 88–89.
Ciraulo, D.A., Sands, B.F., and Shader, R.I. (1988). Critical review of liability for benzodiazepine abuse among alcoholics. *American Journal of Psychiatry, 145*, 1501–1506.
Conrad, P., and Schneider, J.W. (Eds.). (1980). *Deviance and medicalization: From badness to sickness*. St. Louis: C.V. Mosby Company.
Corbett, A. (1987, April 6). The alcoholics' legacy. *The Washington Post*, p. C5.
Craig, J.M. (1987). Psychiatry – Medicine [Review of *The Medical Basis of Psychiatry*]. *Journal of the American Medical Association, 258*, 1396–1397.
Cyr, M.G., and Wartman, S.A. (1988). The effectiveness of routine screening questions in the detection of alcoholism. *Journal of the American Medical Association, 259*, 51–54.
Ettorre, B. (1988). A follow-up study of alcoholism treatment units: Exploring consolidation and change. *British Journal of Addiction, 83*, 57–65.
Feighner, J.P., Robins, E., Guze, S.B., Woodruff, R.A., Winokur, G., and Munoz, R. (1972). Diagnostic criteria for use in psychiatric research. *Archives of General Psychiatry, 26*, 57–63.
Fingarette, H. (1988). *Heavy drinking: The myth of alcoholism as a disease*. Berkeley: University of California Press.
Goodwin, D.W. (1979). Alcoholism and heredity. *Archives of General Psychiatry, 36*, 47–61.
Hill, S.Y., Aston, C., and Rabin, B. (1988). Suggested evidence of genetic linkage between alcoholism and the MNS blood group. *Alcoholism: Clinical and Experimental Research, 12*, 811–814.

544 [298] VATZ/WEINBERG

Hill, S.Y., Steinhauer, S.R., Zubin, J., and Baughman, T. (1988). Event-related potentials as markers for alcoholism risk in high density families. *Alcoholism: Clinical and Experimental Research, 12,* 545–548.
Holden, C. (1987). Alcoholism and the medical cost crunch. *Science, 235,* 1132–1133.
Jellinek, E.M. (1960). *The disease concept of alcoholism.* New Haven: Hillhouse Press.
Klerman, G.L. (1989, February 9). Treatment of alcoholism. *The New England Journal of Medicine, 320,* 394–395.
Koegel, P., and Burnam, M.A. (1988). Alcoholism among homeless adults in the inner city of Los Angeles. *Archives of General Psychiatry, 45,* 1011–1018.
Kolata, G. (1987a, November 10). Alcoholism: Genetic links grow clearer. *The New York Times,* pp. C1–C2).
Kolata, G. (1987b, December 13). Alcoholism: The judgment of science is pending. *The New York Times,* p. 26E.
Kuhn, T.S. (1970). *Structure of scientific revolutions* (2nd edition). Chicago: University of Chicago Press.
Liskow, B.I., and Goodwin, D.W. (1986). Alcoholism: In G. Winokur and P. Clayton (Eds.), *The medical basis of psychiatry* (pp. 190–211). Philadelphia: W.B. Saunders Company.
Lord, L.J. (1987, November 30). Coming to grips with alcoholism. *U.S. News and World Report,* pp. 56–63.
New blood test can identify alcoholics. (1988, January 21). *The Washington Post,* p. A16.
Niven, R.G. (1984). Alcoholism – A problem in perspective [Editorial]. *Journal of the American Medical Association, 252,* 1912–1914.
Nurnberger, J.I., Jr., Goldin, L.R., and Gershon, E.S. (1986). Genetics of psychiatric disorders. In G. Winokur and P. Clayton (Eds.), *The medical basis of psychiatry* (pp. 486–521). Philadelphia: W.B. Saunders Company.
O'Sullivan, K., Rynne, C., Miller, J., O'Sullivan, S., Fitzpatrick, V., Hux, M., Cooney, J., and Clare, A. (1988). A follow-up study on alcoholics with and without co-existing affective disorder. *British Journal of Psychiatry, 152,* 813–819.
Powell v. Texas, 392 U.S. 514 (1968).
Robinson v. California, 370 U.S. 660 (1962).
Schuckit, M.A., Risch, S.C., and Gold, E.O. (1988). Alcohol consumption, ACTH level, and family history of alcoholism. *American Journal of Psychiatry, 145,* 1391–1395.
Shaper, A.G., Wannamethee, G., and Walker, M. (1988, December). Alcohol and mortality in British men: Explaining the U-shaped curve. *The Lancet,* pp. 1267–1273.
Szasz, T. (1972, July). Bad habits are not diseases: A refutation of the claim that alcoholism is a disease. *The Lancet,* pp. 83–84.
Tabakoff, B. (1987, December 17). Alcoholism: A treatable disorder [Letter to the editor]. *The Washington Post,* p. A26.
Tabakoff, B., Hoffman, P.L., Lee, J., Saito, T., Willard, B., and De Leon-Jones, F. (1988). Differences in platelet enzyme activity between alcoholics and nonalcoholics. *The New England Journal of Medicine, 318,* 134–139.
Torrey, E.F. (1988). *Nowhere to go: The tragic odyssey of the homeless mentally ill.* New York: Harper and Row.
Traynor versus Turnage and McKelvey versus Turnage, 108 S. Ct. 372 (1988).
Vaillant, G.E. (1983). *The natural history of alcoholism.* Cambridge: Harvard University Press.
Vatz, R.E., and Weinberg, L.S. (Eds.). (1983). *Thomas Szasz: Primary values and major contentions.* Buffalo: Prometheus Books
Vatz, R.E., and Weinberg, L.S. (1988). Correspondence. *The New England of Medicine, 319,* 179.
Vatz, R.E., and Weinberg, L.S. (1989, March 7). There's a new skepticism toward alcoholism as a disease. *The Washington Post,* p. WH6.

©1990 The Institute of Mind and Behavior, Inc.
The Journal of Mind and Behavior
Summer and Autumn 1990, Volume 11, Numbers 3 and 4
Pages 545 [299] – 556 [310]
ISSN 0271-0137
ISBN 0-930195-05-1

False Accusations of Sexual Abuse: Psychiatry's Latest Reign of Error

Lee Coleman

Berkeley, California

The problem of false accusations of child sexual abuse requires explanation. Investigators uncritically accepted theories and techniques from mental health authorities because of our society's traditional faith in such "experts." The history of this development is reviewed, illustrating the confusion resulting from a blending of investigative and therapeutic roles. Similarly hasty acceptance of unsupported medical interpretations are also reviewed. Recommendatons for reform stress a separation of investigators from mental health ideology, as well as more responsible investigative techniques.

Our society's belated recognition of child sexual abuse, in the late 1970s and early 1980s, seemed initially to promise greater protection to yet another oppressed segment of society. Prisoners, mental patients, rape victims (and abused women in general), the elderly, the handicapped – each group had in turn been the focus of greater awareness of and sensitivity to traditional abuses inflicted by persons or groups with unchecked power.

The much needed focus on physical abuse of children immediately preceded our recognition of sexual abuse. Spearheaded by pediatrician Henry Kempe and his colleagues at the University of Colorado, the "battered child syndrome" became a household word (Kempe and Helfer, 1968), and laws mandating that professionals report cases of suspected abuse were quickly passed by all the states.

As sexual abuse became the next target for efforts at greater protection of children, law enforcement and child protection agencies turned for guidance to mental health professionals and medical doctors, just as they had in the case of physical abuse. *This collaboration has led to a system of investigation which has gone terribly awry.* In the following discussion I will attempt to trace the

---

Requests for reprints should be sent to Lee Coleman, M.D., 1889 Yosemite Road, Berkeley, California 94707.

development of this partnership, illustrate what happens when a mental health model dictates the behavior of investigators, and I will propose alternative approaches which hold greater promise for protecting children from abuse while doing a better job of finding which allegations of abuse are true and which are false.

The Building Blocks

From the beginning, in the early 1970s, the distinction between investigator and therapist was missed. That this was a crucial oversight should become clear as we trace the development of certain key theories and practices which to this day are hindering responsible handling of sexual abuse accusations.

The Child Sexual Abuse Treatment Program (CSATP), started in San Jose, California in 1971, is the most important single precursor to our current methods of investigating alleged sexual abuse. It began as a project of the Santa Clara County Juvenile Probation Department, and was intended "to provide immediate humanistic treatment to the child and her family" (Giaretto, 1982, p. 3).

Perhaps because no responsible person could disagree with the idea of making prompt treatment services available for families caught in the web of sexual abuse, the crucial mistake which followed was lost on all concerned. CSATP joined forces with the San Jose Police Department and their respective roles became blurred. The police saw themselves as facilitators of treatment, while the therapists were thrust into the role of investigators. That neither side recognized what was happening only worsened the muddle.

Investigators as Therapists

If we consult CSATP's *Treatment and Training Manual* (Giaretto, 1982), which summarizes what has become a nationwide model for both sexual abuse therapists and investigators, we read that a major goal is to "learn how the police use CSATP as a resource to help obtain confessions and to convince the family to enter treatment. . ." (p. 109). This not only assumes that the accusation is true, but also that therapists should make the same assumption and do what they can to support the allegation.

This attitude — that allegations of sexual abuse should automatically be taken at face value — soon became an article of faith. To be both progressive and caring, professionals must "believe the child." Conversely, serious investigation which *tested* the validity of an allegation became virtually tantamount to non-support of the child. Because false allegations were not considered a serious possibility, it was assumed that those who raised doubts, as all investigators are mandated to do, were out of touch with what the experts were teaching — "children don't lie about sexual abuse."

Why were police and child protection investigators so ready to accept such reasoning, which runs counter to the very essence of the investigator's function? Because those who promoted these ideas were mental health professionals, and their expertise was taken for granted. The reliance by social agencies on mental health ideas and techniques had, of course, a long tradition to recommend it. As I have discussed elsewhere at greater length (Coleman, 1984), the language of psychiatry and psychology has done much to make the mental health professions appear more scientific, and therefore more reliable, than they are. If, for example, the new child protection movement uncritically accepted the false idea that sexual abuse was a "diagnosis," best made by mental health professionals, this was not too different from the idea that "dangerousness" or "criminal responsibility" were also issues best determined by experts from mental health.

In fairness to the reformers, we might recall that the need for protection from sexual abuse was (and is) real enough. Once confronted, child abuse in all its forms brings a sense of urgency to those now concerned about the problem and looking for tools to shake society out of its complacency. It may be that a medical/mental health model has been so attractive to reformers for the past 150 years, and was so again with the child abuse reformers, precisely because those with the power to make changes — especially legislators and polititians — are not likely to question advice from doctors.

History teaches, however, that the quickest response may not be the best. New ideas, uncritically adopted and molded into bureaucratic routine, are not easily undone. We have been living, for example, with the absurdities of the insanity defense for well over a century despite the widespread recognition that questions of criminal responsibility cannot be "examined" or "diagnosed" by mental health experts.

It has been argued by many (myself included) that the masquerading of a social problem as a medical/psychiatric problem often serves to disguise "hidden agendas" which are less palatable than surface appearances. I argued in *The Reign of Error* (Coleman, 1984), for example, that indeterminate sentencing of prisoners was never intended as a tool of rehabilitation as much as a tool of behavior control. Involuntary treatment of mental patients was more a matter of community and family convenience than individual treatment.

In the case of the child sexual abuse reformers, however, the problem was not a hidden agenda but the central role of uncritical assumptions about the nature of the problem and the nature of the solution. The whole problem, as reformers saw it, was getting the molested child to talk. And who would know better how to do this than the child therapists? Completely unrecognized was the baggage the therapists would bring with them. Thus, when police and social work investigators — but also legislators and judges — so easily adopted the ideas of the reformers, they may have had tradition on their side, but they nonetheless were unwittingly planting a mine field which was bound to blow up once the battle began.

Both the policy makers and the front line workers failed to realize that therapists are expected to be advocates for their clients and investigators are expected to be advocates for the truth. Put another way, the investigators failed to realize that therapists might be prone to assume victimization, that being good at "getting the child to talk" might create false information, and that in such cases child protection was furthered by finding the truth of a false accusation as much as finding the truth behind a true accusation.

Just how complete was the acceptance of the idea that investigators should act like therapists, and therapists should act like investigators, may be gleaned by returning to the program so successfully promoted by CSATP. Spokespersons for the San Jose Police Department's new Sexual Assault Investigation Unit became a standard part of CSATP's training program. Highlights of the approach include:

> We do what we have to do to get the father to admit and to protect the child.

> We . . . explain that there is help for the family from Parents United [CSATP].

> . . . [T]he mother must be supportive and agree to keep the father away.

> . . . [T]he officer interrogates the victim . . . we tell them we want them to know that they are victims and haven't done anything wrong . . . and that you did the right thing by telling. . . . [T]he children may deny it to us at first. Then we approach them with, "Daddy may have a sickness. . . . [I]f Daddy has something wrong with his head, with how he thinks, we would take him to a psychiatrist to get him help. You would want him to get help for any of these things that are wrong, wouldn't you?" The victim usually will concur by now. So we say, "Okay, I've been told that maybe Daddy has a little sickness in his head and we're here to try to help Daddy get better. . . ." So we finish the interview with the child, getting information about how the perpetrator approached her . . . where he touched her . . . whether he bribed her . . . etc.

> . . . [W]e want to get the family hooked into the CSATP as soon as possible. . . . [A]n intern or . . . volunteer will pick up the mother and victim and drive them back to the CSATP. . . . [T]here never is any question that they will make a connection one way or another with the CSATP. We let them know that this is part of the way they will cooperate with us. . . .

> . . . [S]ometimes a man won't come in. Then the department must use whatever means it has available to bring him in and get a confession. . . . *[T]here are generally two kinds of fathers, the ones who are so relieved to have the molestation exposed that they confess everything to the officer at once, and the others who deny or partially deny because they're too afraid to admit.* [italics added]

> . . . [T]he process of investigation and connecting the family to the CSATP is compressed into a few hours. We get a confession from the father, he is persuaded to stay out of the home and not have contact with this child, the connection to CSATP . . . is made, the

police go right to the district attorney with the evidence and a complaint is filed. . . . (Giaretto, 1982, pp. 113–120)

Such an "investigation" is obviously based on the assumption of guilt, from the outset. How else could there be only "two kinds of fathers" — those who are guilty and admit, and those who are guilty and deny? Why else would a referral to a sexual abuse treatment program be considered appropriate even before any real investigation had been done? How else can we explain not a single mention of false accusations in the CSATP manual?

Therapists as Investigators

If obtaining a confession from the accused became the natural goal for the investigator trained to think like a therapist, it was inevitable that therapists who functioned as investigators would adopt a similar style. At workshop after workshop on the sexual abuse of children, therapists had all their attention drawn to the fact that a molested child might conceal the information — even deny it when questioned — but no attention drawn to the possibility that a child could be influenced by adults to claim falsely to be the victim of abuse.

If we look, for example, at a highly influential article by Summit (1983), a leading proponent of such thinking, we read that "It has become a maxim among child sexual abuse intervention counselors and investigators that children never fabricate the kinds of explicit sexual manipulations they divulge in complaints or interrogations" (p. 190). Such a belief never had any data to support it, but it nonetheless became codified by phrases like "children don't lie about sexual abuse," or "believe the child."

In this same article which became standard fare for all who desired to be amongst the new wave in child protection, Summit outlined his "child sexual abuse accommodation syndrome." Situations where a child might be pressured to avoid disclosure were thoroughly discussed. Totally unmentioned was the possibility that such an "accommodation" to adult power and influence was not necessarily a one-way street, that a child might be pressured *into* an accusation, as well as *out of* one (Coleman, 1985).

In addition, therapists at sexual abuse workshops were taught to equate both their concern for children and their professional competence with the ability to bring a child to the point of "disclosure." If the leaders of this fledgling specialty were correct that children never fabricate tales of explicit sexual manipulations, then leading and suggestive questioning would do no harm. The non-molested child would not respond to such questioning with false statements, while the molested child might need just such techniques to overcome fear or embarrassment.

Having studied hundreds of video and audio tapes of children interviewed by therapists or investigators armed with such thinking, I have seen the results: the frequent training of a child to believe things which mirror the interviewers' questions and assumptions instead of the child's memories. The young child, especially, is soon unable to distinguish what is *remembered* from what is drawn out by the interviewer's insistent questioning. The child may not, therefore, be "lying" but still not telling the truth, because the child no longer *knows* the truth. This has been well documented not only in literature from mental health disciplines (Wakefield and Underwager, 1988) but also from official inquiries by the Attorneys General of Minnesota (Humphrey, 1985) and California (Van de Kamp, 1986).

Perhaps the most notorious example of this process is the way that the children from the McMartin preschool of Manhattan Beach, California were interviewed. In 1983, after the mother of a 2½-year-old boy became convinced that her son had been molested at the school, police investigators were unable to obtain corroboration from the boy or from other children attending the school. Convinced that the children were too frightened to reveal anything, the District Attorney decided that a mental health professional should have a try.

Social worker Kee MacFarlane had recently come from the Department of Health, Education and Welfare where she coordinated programs focusing on child sexual abuse. She was now at Los Angeles' Children's Institute International, and had a reputation as an expert at helping children disclose sexual abuse. Dolls and puppets were her forte. Especially because MacFarlane was (and in some circles still is) considered a model for others to emulate, let us take a closer look at the techniques said to be necessary to help children "disclose."

As we come to this excerpt from an interview with an eight-year-old boy who had attended the McMartin school four years earlier (Gorney, 1988), the child is holding a Pac-man puppet in his hand.

MacFarlane:	Here's a hard question I don't know if you know the answer to. We'll see how smart you are, Pac-man. Did you ever see anything come out of Mr. Ray's wiener? Do you remember that ?
Child:	(no response)
MacFarlane:	Can you remember back that far? We'll see how . . . how good your brain is working today, Pac-man. (Child moves puppet around)
MacFarlane:	Is that a yes?
Child:	(Nods puppet yes)

MacFarlane:	Well, you're smart. Now let's see if we can figure out what it was. I wonder if you can point to something of what color it was.
Child:	(Tries to pick up the pointer with the Pac-man's mouth.)
MacFarlane:	Let me get your pen here (puts a pointer in child's Pac-man puppet mouth.)
Child:	It was. . . .
MacFarlane:	Let's see what color is that.
Child:	(Uses Pac-man's hand to point to the Pac-man puppet.)
MacFarlane:	Oh, your pointing to yourself. That must be yellow.
Child:	(Nods puppet yes.)
MacFarlane:	You're smart to point to yourself. What did it feel like? Was it like water? Or something else?
Child:	Um, what?
MacFarlane:	The stuff that came out. Let me try. I'll try a different question on you. We'll try to figure out what the stuff tastes like. We're going to try and figure out if it tastes good.
Child:	He never did that to [me], I don't think.
MacFarlane:	Oh, well, Pac-man, would you know what it tastes like? Would you think it tastes like candy, sort of trying. . . .
Child:	I think it would taste like yucky ants.
MacFarlane:	Yucky ants. Whoa. That would be kind of yucky. I don't think it would taste like . . . you don't think it would taste like strawberries or anything good?
Child:	N o
MacFarlane:	Oh. Think it would sort . . . do you think that would be sticky, like sticky, yucky ants?
Child:	A little. (p. D1)

Tragically, those most responsible for developing interview techniques such as this, the mental health "experts," have thus far refused to acknowledge the terrible mistake inherent in the "believe the child" approach. They have also lacked the courage to admit that "believe the child" really meant a very select kind of belief. Denials from the child were *not* to be believed, as Mac-Farlane's behavior so clearly illustrates, but eventual disclosures (no matter how much they reflected adult pressures) were given blanket acceptance.

Summit (1986), for example, has tried to defend MacFarlane's interviews by writing, "there was both reason and precedent for the methods used. . . ." They represent the "state of the art . . . highly evolved, intensely specific and largely unknown outside the fledgling specialty of child abuse diagnosis" (p. 1). This new art form, Summit continues, is "an amalgam of several roles. . . . [T]he knowledge of a child development specialist to understand and translate toddler language, a therapist to guide and interpret interactive play, a police interrogator to develop evidentiary confirmation and a child abuse specialist to recognize the distinctive and pathetic patterns of sexual victimization." Police investigators need to copy such methods, Summit writes, because such techniques demonstrate "specialist understanding [that] is both unexpected and counterintuitive" (p. 2).

Using the format of workshops for police, child protection workers, district attorneys, and therapists, the style epitomized by MacFarlane's questioning of the boy from the McMartin school has become standard practice throughout the nation and even across the world. In my own experience studying tapes of children interviewed for alleged sexual abuse, I seldom encounter interview techniques which do not reflect the style started by CSATP and refined by specialists like MacFarlane. That such interviews are frequently done over and over with the same child, by therapists rather than investigators, with no tape recording to document what is happening, only adds to the impossibility in many cases of determining which statements of children are truly their own memories and which are the product of adult influence.

Politicized Medicine

The same motivation which spawned this blending of therapeutic and investigative roles — a sincere but badly muddled belief that concern for abused children was equal to assumption of guilt — has led a small group of medical doctors to overinterpret their findings on anal and genital examinations. Because victimized children may not voice a complaint immediately, if ever, and because non-violent forms of molestation may not leave any signs on examination, a few doctors have made claims to be able to interpret "subtle" evidence which "non-specialists" are unable to evaluate. To properly evaluate such "microtrauma," a "specialist" is needed.

Medical examinations for sexual abuse, done long after the alleged fact, are a new phenomenon. All but a handful of the articles on this subject are from the 1980s. An early but very influential discussion was that of Woodling and Kossoris (1981), a family physician and a district attorney from Ventura County, California. Their article describes variations of anal and genital anatomy, such as erythema (redness), anal muscles said to be too tight or too lax, fissures, or hymenal "irregularities." They claimed these findings were indicative of sexual abuse.

In support of such alleged indicators of prior sexual contact, Woodling offered only his "experience." This assumed, of course, that he had a way of knowing when his opinions were correct and when they were not. No discussion of this problem was included, and no studies comparing molested with non-molested children were cited. None had been done. Nonetheless, when a growing number of physicians and nurses began to take a special interest in forensic ano/genital examinations of possible abuse victims, these new specialists eagerly absorbed the "experience" of their trainers.

Frequently, these ideas were being transmitted in workshops sponsored by District Attorneys. No one seemed to see any problem with this blending of medical education and legal advocacy. The fervent desire to protect children from abuse simply overwhelmed scientific caution. As trainees went back to their communities, and in turn became trainers, these uncorroborated claims became the conventional wisdom of the experts. This second generation wrote more articles which passed along the same alleged "indicators" of molestation, but were conspicuous in their absence of any data showing that these indicators were limited to, or more frequently found in, molested children (Coleman, 1989). Most doctors refused to perform such examinations, deferring to those few who claimed to be "specialists." Law enforcement and child protection workers quickly learned which examiners were likely to make findings supportive of an allegation of molestation. Most often these examiners were members of a "sex abuse team."

What little research exists has failed to support the idea that molestation can be detected by such things as size of vaginal opening, shape of hymen, pattern of blood vessels, alleged "scars" of a few millimeters, or anal relaxation (Emans, Woods, Flagg, and Freeman, 1987; McCann, Voris, Simon, and Wells, 1989). Findings which are being described in courts across the land as clear indicators of sexual molestation are found with high frequency in normal, unmolested children (Coleman, 1989). A good many criminal convictions are currently being appealed on the grounds that medical testimony now discredited was an important part of the trial.

To illustrate another aspect of the human cost which such politicized medicine is capable of inflicting, led us take a brief look at what happened in Cleveland, England, where two pediatricians were sure that anal relaxation meant "buggery" (sodomy). Hobbs and Wynne (1986) had reported that "Dilatation and/or reflex dilatation of the anal canal" were not seen in normal children, and indicated sodomy. They added that, "In addition to reflex dilatation, we have also seen alternative contraction and relaxation of the anal sphincter or 'twitchiness' without dilatation. In our experience this also indicates abuse" (p. 794).

Despite a total absence of controlled data to support these notions, these claims were accepted as uncritically in Britain as similar ones here. This is how the *Report of the Inquiry into Child Abuse in Cleveland 1987* (Butler-Sloss, 1988) described what then started to unfold:

Dr. Higgs had, in the summer of 1986 . . . suspected sexual abuse and on examination saw for the first time the phenomenon of what has been termed "reflex relaxation and anal dilatation." She had recently learned from Dr. Wynne . . . that this sign is found in children subject to anal abuse. . . . (p. 14)

Higgs and a colleague (Wyatt) were soon diagnosing children right and left as victims of sodomy. So sure were they of their conclusions that when the finding disappeared and then returned — and the alleged perpetrator had no contact prior to the reappearance — they presumed a second sodomy by a different person. In one case, by the time of the fourth reappearance of anal relaxation, the grandfather, father, and finally two foster parents had all been accused of sodomizing the child! Before this farce played itself out, Higgs and Wyatt had, over a period of five months, "diagnosed" sexual abuse in 121 children from 57 families. Typically, the child was removed from the parents and then subjected to regular "disclosure work" interviews.

Eventually, outraged parents were able to arrange second examinations, and in almost all cases these second opinions differed drastically from the initial findings. And while most of the children were eventually returned home, there is no more indication in Britain than America that the medical community is ready to grapple with the problem.

What Is To Be Done?

While a few spectacular cases, such as the McMartin preschool case in Manhattan Beach, California or the multiple allegations in Jordan, Minnesota, have alerted many people to the fact that not all sexual abuse allegations are valid, few persons are aware of the magnitude of the problem. It is, of course, impossible to scientifically determine anything like a precise figure, since there is no scientific standard by which to determine the truth in individual cases. Statistics, therefore, will obviously reflect this uncertainty.

Most influential of those pointing to the frequent occurrence of false allegationstions is attorney Douglas Besharov. As a former prosecutor and former head of the National Center on Child Abuse and Neglect, his citations to data showing a national incidence of unfounded reports of abuse being near the sixty percent figure (Besharov, 1985) have added to the increasing awareness of this problem. In my own experience, cases labeled as "founded" or "validated" by police or child protection agencies are routinely full of improper invesigative methods and discrepancies which cast much doubt on where the truth lies.

I submit that we do not need to know the exact, or even approximate incidence of false allegations of sexual abuse. All we need to know is that false allegations are not at all rare and that they are occurring primarily because of ill-conceived assumptions and methods on the part of police, caseworkers, therapists, and doctors. I propose the following changes.

Investigators from police and child protection agencies will require a systematic re-training, focusing on neutral investigative techniques. The intimate alliance with mental health theory and practice will need to be examined and removed, freeing investigators to see themselves as seekers of truth rather than advocates for any particular person.

State legislatures should mandate tape-recording of all child interviews by professionals from law enforcement, child protection, mental health, and medicine, in which the subject of possible sexual abuse is discussed. Such tapes would, of course, be available to all parties involved in civil or criminal accusations of molestation, but otherwise protected as confidential material.

The medical community should review the current state of the art of sexual abuse examinations, widely publicize its findings, and censure those doctors who persist in offering reports and testimony which go beyond what is known.

Written records of child protection agencies and therapists interviewing children for molestation must be available to persons accused of molestation and their attorneys. This is especially important prior to the day when taping becomes mandatory. Secret interrogations of children, by adults trained to believe that false allegations are seldom if ever a problem, and trained to encourage "disclosure," are a sure recipe for injustice toward accused adults and victimization of children by a form of abuse unintended but nonetheless real.

References

Besharov, D.J. (1985). Right versus rights: The dilemma of child protection. *Public Welfare, 43 (2),* 19–27.
Butler-Sloss, D.B.E. (1988). *Report of the inquiry into child abuse in Cleveland, 1987.* Presented to Parliament by the Secretary of State for Health and Social Services by Command of Her Majesty. London, England: Her Majesty's Stationery Office.
Coleman, L. (1984). *The reign of error.* Boston: Beacon.
Coleman, L. (1985, January/February). False allegations of sexual abuse: Have the experts been caught with their pants down? *Forum* [Journal of the California Attorneys for Criminal Justice], pp. 12–22.
Coleman, L. (1989). Medical examination for sexual abuse: Have we been misled? *Issues in Child Abuse Accusations, 1,* 1–9.
Emans, S.J., Woods, E.R., Flagg, N.T., and Freeman, A. (1987). Genital findings in sexually abused, symptomatic and asymptomatic girls. *Pediatrics, 79,* 778–785.
Giaretto, H. (1982). *Integrated treatment of child sexual abuse: A treatment and training manual.* Palo Alto, California: Science and Behavior Books.
Gorney, C. (1988, May 18). The community of fear. *Washington Post,* p. D1.
Hobbs, C.J., and Wynne, J.M. (1986, October, 4). Buggery in childhood – a common syndrome of child abuse. *Lancet,* pp. 792–796.
Humphrey, H.H. III (1985). *Report on Scott County investigations.* Minneapolis, Minnesota: Attorney General's Office.
Kempe, C.H., and Helfer, R.E. (1968). *The battered child.* Chicago: University of Chicago Press.

McCann, J., Voris, M., Simon, M., and Wells, R. (1989). Perianal findings in prepubertal children selected for nonabuse: A descriptive study. *Child Abuse and Neglect, 13,* 179–193.

Summit, R. (1983). The child sexual abuse accommodation syndrome. *Child Abuse and Neglect, 7,* 177–183.

Summit, R. (1986, February 5). No one invented McMartin "secret." *Los Angeles Times,* Part II, pp. 1, 2.

Van de Kamp, J. (1986). *Report on Kern County Investigations.* Sacramento, California: Attorney General's Office.

Wakefield, H., and Underwager, R. (1988). *Accusations of child sexual abuse.* Springfield, Illinois: C.C. Thomas.

Woodling, B., and Kossoris, P.D. (1981). Sexual misuse: Rape, molestation and incest. *Pediatric Clinics of North America, 28,* 481–499.

©1990 The Institute of Mind and Behavior, Inc.
The Journal of Mind and Behavior
Summer and Autumn 1990, Volume 11, Numbers 3 and 4
Pages 557 [311] – 564 [318]
ISSN 0271-0137
ISBN 0-930195-05-1

Law and Psychiatry: The Problems That Will Not Go Away

Thomas Szasz

State University of New York

The practice of psychiatry rests on two pillars: mental illness and involuntary mental hospitalization. Each of these elements justifies and reinforces the other. Traditionally, psychiatric coercion was unidirectional, consisting of the forcible incarceration of the individual in an insane asylum. Today, it is bidirectional, the forcible eviction of the individual from the mental hospital (which became the home) supplementing his or her prior forcible incarceration in it. So intimate are the connections between psychiatry and coercion that noncoercive psychiatry, like noncoercive slavery, is an oxymoron.

Ever since I first reflected on matters such as madness and madhouses and especially the incarceration of insane persons in insane asylums — long before I went to college, much less medical school — it has seemed to me that the entire edifice of psychiatry rests on two false premises, namely: that persons called "mental patients" have something others do not have — mental illness; and that they lack something others do have — free will and responsibility. In short, psychiatry is a house of cards, held up by nothing more, or less, than mass belief in the truth of its principles and the goodness of its practices. If this is so, then psychiatry is a religion, not a science, a system of social controls, not a system of treating illness.

But if I knew this long ago, why — I am often asked — did I enter psychiatric and psychoanalytic training? I did so for two reasons: because I wanted to practice psychotherapy, and because I wanted to see if I could mount a successful critique of the fundamental principles and practices of psychiatry.

After floating a few cautiously phrased articles in professional journals, in 1961 I published *The Myth of Mental Illness*, and all hell broke loose.

This article is adapted from the Preface to the Syracuse University Press edition of *Law, Liberty, and Psychiatry* (1989). Requests for reprints should be sent to Thomas Szasz, M.D., Department of Psychiatry, State University of New York, Health Science Center, 750 East Adams Street, Syracuse, New York 13210.

Psychiatrists greeted my assertion that there is no mental illness with as much enthusiasm as priests might greet a fellow clergy's assertion that there is no God; not, mind you, because the assertion is clearly false, or because they are sure that it is false, but because the person making it is not supposed to say such a thing — especially if it is true.

The controversy about mental illness still rages, and the nature of the controversy is often still stubbornly misunderstood: mental health professionals and lay persons alike seem to believe that the demonstration of a genetic defect or neurological lesion in some so-called mental patients proves that mental illness exists — "like any other illness." But this is silly: if mental illness is a metabolic or neurological disease, then it is a disease of the body, not of the mind; and if mental illness is behavior, then it is behavior, not disease. A screwdriver may be a tool or a drink; no amount of empirical research on orange juice–and–vodka can establish that it is, in reality, an unrecognized manifestation of a carpenter's tool.

With the simple but uncompromising idea that mental illness is a metaphor I hoped to inflict a fatal blow, philosophically speaking, on the conceptual foundations of psychiatry. Perhaps I succeeded. But then, given what the greatest scientist of the mind who ever lived considered to be a typical instance of mental illness, this may not have been so difficult. In 1937, Freud wrote,

> The moment a man questions the meaning and value of life, he is sick, since objectively neither has any existence; by asking this question one is merely admitting to a store of unsatisfied libido to which something else must have happened, a kind of fermentation leading to sadness and depression. (cited in E. Freud, 1960, p. 36)

Recognizing a metaphor — as well as a dangerous deception and self-deception — when I saw one, I next turned my energies to constructing a critique of psychiatric practices, especially those taking place outside the privacy of the consulting room.

Once again, my basic idea could not have been simpler. In *The Myth of Mental Illness* I tried to clarify why mental illness is not, and cannot be, a bona fide illness — because the mind is not a bodily organ, and because, as everyone knows but few acknowledge, the term "mental illness" is typically affixed to misbehavior, not brain disease. In *Law, Liberty, and Psychiatry* (1963) I set out to document two equally obvious observations: first that mental hospitalization is not, and cannot be, the same as medical hospitalization — because the mental patient is not free to leave the building in which he or she is housed, whereas the medical patient is. Second, that the two paradigmatic practices of psychiatry — involuntary mental hospitalization or civil commitment and the insanity defense or the exculpation of persons guilty of crimes as not guilty by reason of insanity — rests on a philosophically indefensible and morally odious proposition, namely, that unlike the behavior of the sane person, which is governed by free will, the behavior of the insane person is governed by impulses which the subject finds irresistible and for which he or she is, therefore, not responsible. With the rejection of these fundamental propositions as well, my excommunication from psychiatry became complete and irreversible.

Why should such ideas cast one out of an ostensibly scientific, professional discipline? Because of their consequence: if mental illness is like any other illness, and if psychiatrists are like any other medical practitioners, then psychiatrists ought to act like physicians. The individual suffering from diabetes or multiple sclerosis is not hospitalized involuntarily, nor is the individual excused from punishment if he or she commits an crime. Why, then, commit the mentally ill person innocent of lawbreaking, and why acquit that person as not guilty by reason of insanity when he or she is, in fact, guilty of a premeditated crime?

After all, it is self-evident that the so-called mentally ill criminal has committed a crime. What psychiatrists contend, and what most people now accept, is not that such a person does not commit crimes, but only that he or she does so from psychotic motives, exemplified by the phrase "I heard God's voice and he told me to kill my child." But "Crimes," asserted Sir Hartley Shawcross (1946) at the Nuremberg trials of the Nazi war criminals, "do not cease to be criminal because they have a political motive" (p. 467). Obviously so. By the same token, I maintain that crimes do not cease to be criminal because they have a psychotic motive.

Thus it was not just liberty that I sought for the mental patient unjustly deprived of it. More important, I sought to impose on the mental patient, if guilty of misbehavior or crime, the same responsibility and punishment we impose on the mentally healthy person. With respect to psychiatry–and–law, my whole argument can thus be condensed into a few paragraphs, exposing two phony psychiatric claims and their consequences. The claims are: "I can't/couldn't help it . . ." and "He/she can't/couldn't help it. . . ."

In the first phrase, "it" may refer to eating too much or too little, drinking, smoking, gambling, having adulterous affairs, killing one's baby or someone else, and so forth. If such a claim about one's non-responsibility is legally and socially accepted, then the claimant is not only excused of his or her immoral or illegal behavior, but may even be accredited as a person with special expertise in diagnosing and treating eating disorders, alcoholism, tobacco dependence, sexual addiction, and countless other (alleged) mental maladies.

In the second phrase – "He/she can't/couldn't help it . . ." – "it" may refer to hearing voices no one else can hear, seeing things no one else can see, expressing a desire to kill oneself or someone else, or virtually any other socially disturbing or illegal behavior. If such a claim about another person's non-responsibility is legally and socially accepted, then the person so identified becomes a fit subject for imprisonment without trial (involuntary psychiatric hospitalization) and punishment without having been sentenced (psychiatric treatment). But this is heresy: psychiatrists have correctly perceived that if involuntary psychiatric interventions of all sorts along with the insanity defense were abolished, as I proposed, psychiatry as we know it would cease to exist.

My sustained critique of the conceptual foundations and legal-social uses of psychiatry has proved to be very influential, though not, at least not yet, in the ways I had hoped. My aim was, and still is, to usher in a new way of seeing and treating individuals who are called, or call themselves, mentally ill: accord them the same rights, and impose on them the same responsibilities we accord and impose on other adults in our society. We have abandoned the tradition-sanctioned coercive-paternalistic control of blacks and women; we should similarly abandon the legally and psychiatrically sanctioned coercive-paternalistic control of mental patients.

I did not expect this to happen overnight, and it did not. Maybe it will never happen. What did happen is that psychiatrists, and many others too, began to feel guilty about the mistreatment of the mentally ill and embarked on yet another cycle of so-called reforms. Mental patients, it became clear, were deprived of their rights. Okay, said the reformers, we will give them some rights. Thus did it come about that since the publication of *Law, Liberty, and Psychiatry* in 1963, mental patients have become the involuntary recipients of rights they never dreamed of — such as the right to a lawyer, to treatment, to refuse treatment, to be incarcerated in the least restrictive setting, and so forth. This time the Potemkin's Village called Psychiatry was spruced up in earnest. Before the 1960s, the abuse of the psychiatric patient was undisguised: the mental hospital was a "snake-pit." Clearly, the snakes had to go. American psychiatry and the society it serves replaced the reptiles with lawyers and therapists:

> The right to refuse antipsychotic medication is now more than a decade old. . . . Refusal is not uncommon, but refusing patients appear almost always to receive treatment in the end. These findings point up the essential illogic of allowing committed persons to refuse treatment that would permit their freedom to be restored. The future evolution of the right [to treatment] . . . will restore the equivalence between the power to commit and the power to treat. (Appelbaum, 1988, p. 413)

Exhilarated by the prospect of possessing not just one but two different powers over his patient, Appelbaum adds "That such a right to refuse treatment might exist was unimaginable before the 1970s" (p. 414). But the practice of rulers giving meaningless rights to their subjects can hardly be called unimaginable in our century saturated with slogans of phony freedoms. Sadly, but not surprisingly, if the pillars of society go through enough trouble to conceal their dark deeds, they are likely to succeed. That the concealments practiced by legal and psychiatric reformers have, this time around, been more successful than heretofore is suggested by the fact that they now fool even seasoned, critical observers. How else are we to explain the views of Roger Scruton, Professor of Aesthetics at Birkbeck College in London and editor of the *Salisbury Review?* In an editorial note appended to an essay entitled "Do Liberals Love Liberty?", Scruton states:

> It is worth pointing out that the thinking represented by Szasz has been so successful that US law has been revised so as to forbid compulsory hospitalization of the insane. The chaotic and disturbing result of this change can be witnessed in every major American city. (1988, p. 30)

The assertion that "US law has been revised so as to forbid compulsory hospitalization of the insane" is news, indeed. Does Scruton actually believe that John Hinckley, Jr. is staying at St. Elizabeth's Hospital, the nation's premier madhouse, because he likes it there, and because the government likes him so much that it houses and feeds him at taxpayer's expense? I go through the trouble of refuting Scruton's absurd misstatement because it reflects the widespread perception, carefully cultivated by psychiatric propagandists, that involuntary mental hospitalization has become so rare in America as to be irrelevant. This is not so. As I write these lines there comes to my hand the February 1989 issue of *The American Journal of Psychiatry* featuring a "Special Section" containing four articles collectively entitled "Dangerousness and the Civil Commitment Process" (Special Section, 1989). An Editorial introducing these studies states:

> The most recent national data (1980) show that of 1,176,558 inpatient admissions, 26% were involuntary noncriminal commitments. More than 51% of admissions to state and county mental hospitals are, however, involuntary (noncriminal). (Roth, 1989, p. 135)

Moreover, these figures do not even begin to reflect the escalating ugliness of the American psychiatry scene, noted in an essay in *The Sunday Times Magazine* (London):

> Thousands of [New York] homeless are former inmates of mental hospitals which [Mayor] Koch emptied, largely on economic grounds; on the other hand, he has decreed that a "sidewalk dweller" should be carted off to a mental hospital, on the grounds that anyone sleeping rough and pestering passers-by must be mentally disturbed. New Yorkers see no method in what some of them call the mayor's madness. (McCrystal, 1989, p. 32)

In the past, thousands of individuals were forcibly incarcerated in mental hospitals, often for life; that was bad enough, but at least many of these unfortunate persons could make the asylum their home. Now the situation is even worse, thousands of persons being not only forcibly incarcerated in mental hospitals, but also forcibly evicted from them as soon as they show any sign of adapting to their new environment. Then the cycle of forcible hospitalization and dehospitalization is repeated over and over again, depriving the "mental patient" of a predictable and stable environment both within and without the insane asylum.

Thus, what Scruton observed "in every major American city" is not the triumph of my ideas as social policy but only a singularly unattractive feature of the American national character (if one can so generalize), otherwise often good and generous. Perhaps precisely because Americans strive so hard to be good and generous, they do not like to be told that they have done wrong. Charles Dickens' observation on just this point is unerring:

> I believe [he wrote in 1842] there is no country, on the face of the earth, where there is less freedom of opinion on any subject in reference to which there is a broad difference of opinion than in this [the United States]. . . . I write the words with reluctance, disappointment, and sorrow; but I believe it from the bottom of my soul. . . . The wonder is that a breathing man can be found with temerity enough to suggest to the Americans the possibility of their having done wrong. (cited in Forster, 1966, vol. 1, p. 194)

Dickens was right. Instead of simply acknowledging their wrongdoing, Americans prefer to deny it with a dramatic gesture of undoing. Indians on reservations, blacks on plantations, epileptics in colonies, the mentally ill in snake pits — all these embarrassing wrongs must be quickly righted and forgotten: the Indians are treated like citizens of fictitious independent nations; the blacks get reverse discrimination; epileptic colonies are written out of medical and psychiatric history; the men and women imprisoned in mental hospitals for decades are suddenly and forcibly evicted.

The result, pretentiously called deinstitutionalization, "proves" not only how very respectful psychiatrists really are of the civil rights of mental patients, but also how very right psychiatrists have been all along in stigmatizing and segregating mental patients as dangerous deviants. The failure of the quick cure then justifies the re-repression of the mad: mental illness exists and the mentally ill are dangerous; ergo, mental patients, lacking free will and responsibility, have a right to be hospitalized against their will, treated against their will, lawyered against their will, even acquitted of crimes against their will; and if they commit mayhem and murder, then, suffering as they do from mental illness, they cannot be held responsible for their actions, need to be hospitalized against their will, treated against their will, and so on.

In short, I interpret Scruton's howler (and its inclusion into the pages of so prestigious a publication) as evidence that psychiatry is a religion and that Voltaire was right: if mental illness did not exist, it would be necessary to invent it. Clearly, people now passionately believe in psychiatric explanations, excuses, and coercions – the educated perhaps even more than the uneducated, the latter stubbornly clinging to Jesus and the televangelists, refusing to embrace Freud and the soul-doctors. "Analyzing humor," remarked E.B. White, "is like dissecting a frog. Few people are interested and the frog dies of it." The same goes for dissecting a popular delusion, such as psychiatry today: few people are interested and the delusion dies of it – except people do not let it die. Indeed, why should they, if they want it to live? Freedom of belief lies at the heart of individual liberty and dignity. That is why I maintain that the "deluded" patient is as entitled to his or her belief as the "enlightened" psychiatrist is to his or her belief. Like clergy of different faiths, or believers and unbelievers, each should be protected from being coerced by the other. To insure our protection from unwanted saviors – whether clerical or clinical – is a fundamental duty of the American government.

In the United States, the pursuit of happiness is an opportunity and an obligation that belongs to each and every individual. We are supposed to chase and catch that elusive quarry ourselves. We can delegate the task to experts, but no one – no pope, no prince, no politician, not even a psychiatrist – should be able to take it away from us. For – after all is said and done – is justifying the armed hunt for the happiness of the Other not the most dangerous delusion to which we can succumb?

References

Appelbaum, P.S. (1988). The right to refuse treatment with antipsychotic medications: Retrospect and prospect. *American Journal of Psychiatry, 145,* 413–419.

Forster, J. (1966). *The life of Charles Dickens.* London: Dent/Everyman's Library.

Freud, E.L. (Ed.). (1960). *Letters of Sigmund Freud* [T. and J. Stern, Trans.]. New York: Basic Books.

McCrystal, C. (1989). The Big Apple turns sour. *The Sunday Times Magazine* (London). February 12, pp. 24–37.

Roth, L.H. (1989). Editorial: Four studies of mental health commitments. *American Journal of Psychiatry, 146,* 135–137.

Scruton, R. (1988, September). Editorial note. *The Salisbury Review,* p. 30.

Special Section: Dangerousness and the civil commitment process. (1989). *American Journal of Psychiatry, 146,* 170–193.

Shawcross, H. (1946). *Trial of the major war criminals before the International Military Tribunal.* Proceedings 19 July - 29 July, Vol. XIX. July 26. Nuremberg, Germany.

Szasz, T.S. (1961). *The myth of mental illness: Foundations of a theory of personal conduct.* New York: Hoeber-Harper.

Szasz, T.S. (1963). *Law, liberty, and psychiatry: An inquiry into the social uses of mental health practices.* New York: Macmillan.

BOOKS RECEIVED FOR REVIEW

Abnormal Psychology: Its Experience and Behavior. Peter McKellar. Routledge, Chapman & Hall, 1990. $49.95 hard, $14.95 paper, 378 pages.

The Adventure of Self-Discovery. Stanislav Grof. State University of New York Press, New York, 1988. $12.95 paper, 321 pages.

Altered States of Consciousness and Mental Health: A Cross-Cultural Perspective (Volume 12, Cross Cultural Research and Methodology Series). Colleen A. Ward (Editor). Sage Publications, Newbury Park, California, 1989. $35.00 hard, 316 pages.

American Psychiatric Press Review of Psychiatry Volume 9. Allan Tasman, M.D., Stephen M. Goldfinger, M.D., and Charles A. Kaufman, M.D. (Editors). American Psychiatric Press, Washington, D.C., 1990. $54.95 hard, 699 pages.

Annual Progress in Child Psychiatry and Child Development 1989. Stella Chess, M.D. and Margaret E. Hertzig (Editors). Brunner/Mazel, New York, 1990. $50.00 hard, 576 pages.

Archetypal Process: Self and Divine in Whitehead, Jung, and Hillman. David Griffin. Northwestern University Press, Evanston, Illinois, 1990. $39.95 hard, $14.95 paper, 300 pages.

Artificial Intelligence in Psychology: Interdisciplinary Essays. Margaret A. Boden. The MIT Press, Cambridge, Massachusetts, 1989. $9.95 paper, 188 pages.

Attachment in the Preschool Years: Theory, Research, and Intervention. Mark T. Greenberg, Dante Cicchetti, and E. Mark Cummings (Editors). The University of Chicago Press, Chicago, 1990. $39.95 hard, 507 pages.

Auditory Scene Analysis: The Perceptual Organization of Sound. Albert S. Bregman. The MIT Press, Cambridge, Massachusetts, 1990. $55.00 hard, 773 pages.

Beginning to Read: Thinking and Learning About Print. Marilyn Jager Adams. The MIT Press, Cambridge, Massachusetts, 1990. $29.95 hard, 494 pages.

Behavior Settings: A Revision and Extension of Roger G. Barker's Ecological Psychology. Phil Schoggen. Stanford University Press, Stanford, 1989. $39.50 hard, 419 pages.

Best Friends and Marriage: Exchange Among Women. Stacey J. Oliker. University of California Press, Berkeley, 1989. $20.00 hard, 253 pages.

Beyond Self-Interest. Jane J. Mansbridge (Editor). The University of Chicago Press, Chicago, 1990. $53.00 hard, $14.95 paper, 402 pages.

Biological Assessment and Treatment of Posttraumatic Stress Disorder. Earl L. Giller, Jr., M.D. (Editor). American Psychiatric Press, Washington, D.C., 1990. $28.50 hard, 208 pages.

The Birth of the Family: An Empirical Inquiry. Jerry M. Lewis, M.D. Brunner/Mazel, New York, 1989. $26.95 hard, 224 pages.

Brief Therapy Approaches to Treating Anxiety and Depression. Michael D. Yapko. Brunner/Mazel, New York, 1989. $39.95 hard, 384 pages.

Carl Jung and Christian Spirituality. Robert L. Moore (Editor). Paulist Press, New York, 1988. $12.95, 252 pages.

A Casebook in Psychiatric Ethics (GAP Report No. 129). Group for the Advancement of Psychiatry, Committee on Medical Education. Brunner/Mazel, New York, 1990. $21.95 hard, $14.95 paper, 113 pages.

Century's End: A Cultural History of the Fin De Siecle From the 990s Through the 1990s. Hillel Schwartz. Doubleday, New York, 1990. $19.95 hard, 368 pages.

The Challenge of Art to Psychology. Seymour B. Sarason. Yale University Press, New Haven, Connecticut, 1990. $25.00 hard, 188 pages.

The Child in Our Times: Studies in the Development of Resiliency. Timothy F. Dugan, M.D. and Robert Coles, M.D. (Editors). Brunner/Mazel, New York, 1989. $25.00 hard, 224 pages.

Child Prodigies and Exceptional Early Achievers. John Radford. The Free Press, New York, 1990. $22.95 hard, 255 pages.

Childhood and Human Nature. Sula Wolf. Routledge, Chapman & Hall, New York, 1990. $52.50 hard, $16.95 paper, 242 pages.

Cognitive Foundations of Natural History. Scott Atran. Cambridge University Press, New York, 1990. $49.50, 360 pages.

Cognitive-Behavioral Marriage Therapy. Donald H. Baucom and Norman Epstein. Brunner/Mazel, New York, 1990. $47.95 hard, 496 pages.

Computational Neuroscience. Eric L. Schwartz (Editor). The MIT Press, Cambridge, Massachusetts, 1990. $45.00 hard, 441 pages.

Computer Applications in Psychiatry and Psychology (Clinical and Experimental Psychiatry Series, Monograph #2). David Baskin (Editor). Brunner/Mazel, New York, 1990. $23.95 hard, 192 pages.

Computers and Thought: A Practical Introduction to Artificial Intelligence. Mike Sharples, David Hogg, Chris Hutchinson, Steve Torrence, and David Young. The MIT Press, Cambridge, Massachusetts, 1990. $25.00 hard, 401 pages.

Concepts, Kinds, and Cognitive Development. Frank C. Keil. The MIT Press, Cambridge, Massachusetts, 1989. $29.95 hard, 328 pages.

Concern For Others: A New Psychology of Conscience and Morality. Tom Kitwood (Concepts in Developmental Psychology, Edited by David Cohen). Routledge, London and New York, 1990. $52.50 hard, 256 pages.

Concise Guide to the Evaluation and Management of Sleep Disorders. Martin Reite, Kim Nagel, and John Ruddy. American Psychiatric Press, Washington, D.C., 1990. $18.50 paper, 185 pages.

Connectionist Modeling and Brain Function: The Developing Interface. Stephen Jose Hanson and Carl R. Olson (Editors). The MIT Press, Cambridge, Massachusetts, 1990. $37.50 hard, 423 pages.

Consciousness in Contemporary Science. A.J. Marcel and E. Bislach (Editors). Oxford University Press, New York, 1988. $75.00 hard, 407 pages.

Contemporary Approaches to Psychological Assessment. Scott Weltzer and Martin M. Katz (Editors). Brunner/Mazel, New York, 1989. $40.00 hard, 366 pages.

The Crisis of Competence: Transitional Stress and the Displaced Worker (Brunner/Mazel Psychosocial Stress Series, No. 16). Carl Maida, Norma S. Gordon, and Norman L. Faberow. Brunner/Mazel, New York, 1990. $27.50 hard, 226 pages.

Critical Terms for Literary Study. Frank Lentricchia and Thomas McLaughlin. The University of Chicago Press, Chicago, 1990. $45.00 hard, $16.95 paper.

Critical Theories of Psychological Development. John M. Broughton. Plenum Press, New York, 1987. $39.50 hard, 313 pages.

Current and Historical Perspectives on the Borderline Patient (Current Issues in Psychoanalytic Practice: Monographs of the Society for Psychoanalytic Training, Number 1). Rueben Fine (Editor). Brunner/Mazel, New York, 1989. $40.00 hard, 448 pages.

Darwin and the Emergence of Theories of Mind and Behavior. Robert J. Richards. The University of Chicago Press, Chicago, 1989 (paperback edition). $17.95 paper, 700 pages.

A Day Hospital Group Treatment Program for Anorexia Nervosa and Bulima Nervosa (Brunner/Mazel Eating Disorders Monograph Series). Niva Prian and Allan S. Kaplan (Editors). Brunner/Mazel, New York, 1990. $25.00 hard, 168 pages.

Defining American Psychology: The Correspondence between Adolf Meyer and Edward Bradford Titchener. Ruth Leys and Rand B. Evans (Editors). Johns Hopkins University Press, Baltimore, 1990, $42.50 hard, 292 pages.

Depression and Families: Impact and Treatment. Gabor I. Keitner, M.D. American Psychiatric Press, Inc., Washington, D.C., 1990. $25.00 hard, 192 pages.

Depression in Schizophrenia. Lynn E. Delisi, M.D. American Psychiatric Press, Washington, D.C., 1990. $22.50 hard, 162 pages.

Descriptions. Stephen Neale. MIT Press, Cambridge, Massachusetts, 1990. $29.95 hard, 286 pages.

Developing Theories of Mind. Janet W. Astington, Paul L. Harris, and David R. Olson (Editors). Cambridge University Press, New York, 1990. $17.95 paper, 447 pages.

DSM-III-R Training Guide for Diagnosis of Childhood Disorders. Judith L. Rapoport, M.D. and Deborah R. Ismond. Brunner/Mazel, New York, 1990. $27.50 hard, $17.95 soft, 224 pages.

The Dynamics of the Social. Isabel Menzies Lyth. Free Association Books, London, England, 1990. $19.50 paper, 274 pages.

Economics and Power: The Inquiry into Human Relations and Markets. Randall Bartlett. Cambridge University Press, New York, 1990. $32.50 paper, 210 pages.

The 11th Annual Conference of the Cognitive Science Society (August 18–19, 1990, University of Michigan). Lawrence Erlbaum Associates, Englewood Cliffs, New Jersey. $79.95 paper, 1000 pages.

The Emperor's New Mind. Roger Penrose. Oxford University Press, Oxford, England, 1989. $24.95 hard, 466 pages.

The Encyclopedia of Alternative Health Care. Kristin Gottschalk Olsen. Pocket Books, New York, 1990. $8.95 paper.

Envisioning Information. Edward R. Tufte. Graphics Press, Cheshire, Connecticut, 1990. $48.00 hard, 126 pages.

Epistemology. Stephen Eversen (Editor). Cambridge University Press, New York, 1990. $54.50 hard, $16.95 paper, 286 pages.

Evolution of the Brain: Creation of the Self. John C. Eccles. Routledge, Chapman & Hall, New York, 1990. $25.00 hard, 282 pages.

Extending Psychological Frontiers: Selected Works of Leon Festinger. Stanley Schachter and Michael S. Gazzaniga (Editors). Russell Sage Foundation, New York, 1990. $45.00 hard, 613 pages.

Extrapolations: Demonstrations of Ericksonian Therapy (Ericksonian Monographs, No. 6). Stephen R. Lankton and Jeffrey K. Zeig. Brunner/Mazel, New York, 1989. $25.00 hard, 138 pages.

Fear and Courage (Second Edition). S.J. Rachman. W.H. Freeman and Company, New York, 1989. $17.95 paper, 405 pages.

Foundations of Cognitive Science. Michael I. Posner (Editor). The MIT Press, Cambridge, Massachusetts, 1990. $45.00 hard, 888 pages.

The Fragmentation of Reason. Stephen Stich. The MIT Press, Cambridge, Massachusetts, 1990. $22.50 hard, 181 pages.

Fragments of Genius: The Strange Feats of Idiots Savants. Michael J.A. Howe. Routledge, Chapman & Hall, New York, 1990. $29.95.

From Fear to Fury. H.D. Johns. Vantage Press, New York, 1990. $14.95 hard, 155 pages.

From Reading to Neurons. Albert M. Galaburda (Editor). The MIT Press, Cambridge, Massachusetts, 1990. $45.00 hard, 545 pages.

Fundamentals of Human Psychology (Third Edition). Bryan Kolb and Ian O. Whishaw. W.H. Freeman and Company, New York, 1990. 910 pages.

The Grace of Great Things: Creativity and Innovation. Robert Grudin. Ticknor & Fields,

New York, 1990. $20.95 hard, 257 pages.
A Guide to Journals in Psychology and Education. Wing Hong Loke. Scarecrow Press, Metuchan, New Jersey, 1990. $39.50 hard, 415 pages.
Hamlet's Enemy: Madness and Myth in Hamlet. Theodore Lidz. International Universities Press, Madison, Connecticut, 1990. $19.95 paper, 258 pages.
Historical Fictions: Essays by Hugh Kenner. North Point Press, Berkeley, California, 1990. $24.95 hard, 338 pages.
How to Build a Person: A Prolegomenon. John Pollock. The MIT Press, Cambridge, Massachusetts, 1990. $22.50 hard, 189 pages.
Hypnotherapy Scripts: A Neo-Ericksonian Approach to Persuasive Healing. Ronald A. Havens and Catherine Walters. Brunner/Mazel, New York, 1989. $27.95 hard, 196 pages.
I Hear Voices. Paul Abelman. McPherson and Company, Kingston, New York, 1990. $10.00 paper, 168 pages.
Imagery: Current Developments. Peter J. Hampson, David E. Marks, and John T.E. Richardson (Editors). Routledge, New York, 1990. $57.50 hard, 386 pages.
Information and the Origin of Life. Bernd-Olaf Kuppers. The MIT Press, Cambridge, Massachusetts, 1990. $22.50, 215 pages.
Insights in Decision-Making: A Tribute to Hillel J. Einhorn. Robin M. Hogarth (Editor). The University of Chicago Press, Chicago, 1990. $24.50 paper, 356 pages.
Intention, Plans, and Practical Reason. Michael E. Bratman. Harvard University Press, Cambridge, Massachusetts, 1987. $25.00 hard, $12.95 paper, 200 pages.
Intentions in Communication (System Development Foundation Benchmark Series). Philip R. Cohen, Jerry Morgan, and Martha E. Pollack (Editors). The MIT Press, Cambridge, Massachusetts, 1990. $45.00 hard, 508 pages.
Interpretation and Explanation in the Study of Animal Behavior, Volume I: Interpretation, Intentionality, and Communication. Marc Bekoff and Dale Jamieson (Editors). Westview Press, Boulder, Colorado, 1990. $45.00 (paper), 465 pages.
Interpretation and Explanation in the Study of Animal Behavior, Volume II: Explanation, Evolution, and Adaptation. Marc Bekoff and Dale Jamieson (Editors). Westview Press, Boulder, Colorado, 1990. $45.00 (paper), 505 pages.
Intuition in Organizations: Leading and Managing Productively. Weston H. Agor (Editor). Sage Publications, Newbury Park, California, 1989. $35.00 hard, $18.95 paper, 285 pages.
Intuitive Judgments of Change. Linda Silka. Springer-Verlag, New York, 1989. $49.00 hard, 214 pages.
An Invitation to Cognitive Science (Three Volumes: Volume 1, *Language*; Volume 2, *Visual Cognition*; Volume 3, *Thinking*). Daniel N. Oherson (Editor). The MIT Press, Cambridge, Massachusetts, 1990. $55.00 hard, 273, 356, and 308 pages.
Issues in Psychobiology. Charles R. Legg. Routledge, Chapman & Hall, New York, 1990. $47.50 hard, $17.95 paper, 224 pages.
Jung's Three Theories of Religious Experience (Studies in the Psychology of Religion, Volume 3). J. Harley and M. Chapman. The Edwin Mellen Press, Lewiston, New York, 1988. 178 pages.
Language and Species. Derek Bickerton. The University of Chicago Press, Chicago, 1990. $24.95 hard, 297 pages.
The Last Intellectuals. Russell Jacoby. The Noonday Press, New York, 1987. $9.95 paper, 274 pages.
Leading Edges in Social and Behavioral Science. R. Duncan Luce, Neil J. Smelser, and Dean R. Gerstein (Editors). Russell Sage Foundation, 1990. $59.95 hard, 713 pages.
Learnability and Cognition: The Acquisition of Argument Structure. Steven Pinker. The

MIT Press, Cambridge, Massachusetts, 1990. $29.95 hard, 411 pages.
Lexical Representation and Process. William Marslen-Wilson (Editor). The MIT Press, Cambridge, Massachusetts, 1989. $49.95 hard, 576 pages.
Life Changes: Growing Through Personal Transitions. Sabina Spencer and John D. Adams. Impact Publishers, San Luis Obispo, California, 1990. $8.95, 192 pages.
The Logic of Architecture: Design, Computation, and Cognition. William J. Mitchell. The MIT Press, Cambridge, Massachusetts, 1990. $35.00 hard, $19.95 paper, 292 pages.
The Lourdes of Arizona. Carlos Amantea. Who & Who Works, San Diego, California, 1989. $17.95 hard, $10.95 paper, 175 pages.
Machine Learning: Paradigm and Methods. Jaime Carbonell (Editor). The MIT Press, Cambridge, Massachusetts, 1990. $27.50 paper, 394 pages.
Making a Difference: Psychology and the Construction of Gender. Rachel T. Hare-Mustin and Jeanne Marecek (Editors). Yale University Press, New Haven, Connecticut, 1990. $18.95 hard, 212 pages.
Manhood in the Making: Cultural Concepts of Masculinity. David D. Gilmore. Yale University Press, New Haven, Connecticut, 1990. $22.50 hard, 258 pages.
Marginalism and Discontinuity: Tools for the Crafts of Knowledge and Decision. Martin H. Krieger. Russell Sage Foundation, New York, 1989. $25.00 hard, 206 pages.
Mazes. Hugh Kenner. North Point Press, Berkeley, 1989. $22.95, 336 pages.
Meaning and Grammar: An Introduction to Semantics. Gennaro Chierchia and Sally McConnell-Ginet. The MIT Press, Cambridge, Massachusetts, 1990. $29.95 hard, 476 pages.
Microcognition: Philosophy, Cognitive Science, and Parallel Distributed Processing. Andy Clark. The MIT Press, Cambridge, Massachusetts, 1989. $19.95 hard, 226 pages.
The Middle Years: New Psychoanalytic Perspectives. John M. Oldham, M.D. and Robert S. Liebert, M.D. Yale University Press, New Haven, Connecticut, 1990. $30.00 hard, 300 pages.
Mind, Body and Culture: Anthropology and the Biological Interface. Geoffrey Samuel. Cambridge University Press, Cambridge, England, 1990. 192 pages.
Mind Bugs: The Origins of Procedural Misconceptions. Kurt Vanlehn. The MIT Press, Cambridge, Massachusetts, 1990. $27.50 hard, 253 pages.
The Mind: Its Origin, Evolution, Structure and Functioning. Malcolm I. Hale. Hale-van Rutz, Pittsburgh, Pennsylvania, 1989. $7.95 paper, 300 pages.
Mind Sights: Original Visual Illusions, Ambiguities, and Other Anomalies, with a Commentary on the Play of the Mind in Perception and Art. Roger N. Shephard. W.H. Freeman and Company, New York, 1990. $24.95 hard, $14.95 paper, 228 pages.
The Miracle Within: Secrets of Self-Healing and Self-Improvement. Joseph Moccia, M.D. Vantage Press, New York, 1990. $13.95 hard, 192 pages.
Modern Perspectives in the Psychiatry of the Affective Disorders. John G. Howells, M.D. (Editor). Brunner/Mazel, New York, 1989. $60.00 hard, 440 pages.
Motivation and Explanation: An Essay on Freud's Philosophy of Science (Psychological Issues, Monograph 56). Nigel Mackay. International Universities Press, Inc., Madison, Connecticut, 1989. $27.50 hard, 254 pages.
The Mundane Matter of the Mental Language. J. Christopher Maloney. Yale University Press, 1989. $39.50 hard, 274 pages.
Naturally Intelligent Systems. Maureen Caudill and Charles Butler. The MIT Press, Cambridge, Massachusetts, 1990. $19.95 hard, 304 pages.
The Need for Reassurance. Nicholas Hariton, M.D. Vantage Press, New York, 1990. $14.95 hard, 249 pages.
Neural Network Design and the Complexity of Learning. J. Stephen Judd. The MIT Press, Cambridge, Massachusetts, 1990. $24.95 hard, 150 pages.

A Neurocomputational Perspective: The Nature of Mind and the Structure of Science. Paul M. Churchland. The MIT Press, Cambridge, Massachusetts, 1990. $25.00 hard, 321 pages.

New Horizons: Explorations in Science. P.D. Ouspensky. Globe Press, Yorktown, New York, 1990. $4.95.

New Perspectives on Narcissism. Eric M. Plakun, M.D. (Editor). American Psychiatric Press, Washington, D.C., 1990. $28.50 hard, 240 pages.

Noradrenergic Neurons. Marianne Fillenz. Cambridge University Press, New York, 1990. $44.50 hard, $19.95 paper, 240 pages.

Office Treatment of Schizophrenia. Mary V. Seeman and Stanley E. Greben (Editors). American Psychiatric Press, Washington, D.C., 1990. $28.50 hard, 208 pages.

The Organization of Learning. Charles R. Gallistel. The MIT Press, Cambridge, Massachusetts, 1990. $45.00 hard, 648 pages.

An Orientation to the Trance Experience (Audiocassette). Ronald A. Havens and Catherine Walters. Brunner/Mazel, New York, 1989. $10.00, Running Time: 31:39.

Paradigms in Behavior Therapy: Present and Promise. Daniel B. Fishman, Frederick Rotgers, and Cyril M. Franks (Editors). Springer Publishing Company, New York, 1988. $42.95, 376 pages.

Perils of the Night: A Feminist Study of Nineteenth-Century Gothic. Eugenia C. DeLamotte. Oxford University Press, New York, 1990. $34.50 hard, 352 pages.

Personology: Method and Content in Personality Assessment and Psychobiography. Irving E. Alexander. Duke University Press, Durham, North Carolina, 1990. $42.50 hard, $18.95 paper, 280 pages.

The Power of Unconditional Love. Ken Keyes, Jr. Love Line Books, Coos Bay, Oregon, 1990. $7.95 paper, 214 pages.

The Practical Application of Medical and Dental Hypnosis. Milton H. Erickson, M.D., Seymour Hershman, M.D., and Irving I. Secter, D.D.S. Brunner/Mazel, New York, 1989. $18.95 soft, 480 pages.

Preventing Mental Health Disturbances in Childhood. Stephen E. Goldston, Joel Yager, Christoph M. Heinicke, Robert S. Pynoos (Editors). American Psychiatric Press, Inc., Washington, D.C., 1990. $36.00 hard, 254 pages.

Principles of Mental Imagery. Ronald A. Finke. The MIT Press, Cambridge, Massachusetts, 1990. $19.95 hard, 179 pages.

Propositional Attitudes: An Essay on Thoughts and How We Ascribe Them. Mark Richard. Cambridge University Press, New York, 1990. $44.50 hard, $16.95 paper, 276 pages.

Psychoanalysis: Toward the Second Century. Arnold M. Cooper, M.D., Otto F. Kernberg, M.D., and Ethel Spector Person, M.D. Yale University Press, New Haven, Connecticut, 1990. $27.50 hard, 228 pages.

Psychoanalytic Terms and Concepts. Burness E. Moore, M.D. and Bernard D. Fine, M.D. (Editors). Yale University Press, New Haven, Connecticut, 1990. $35.00 hard, 210 pages.

Psychological Consulting to Management: A Clinician's Perspective. Lester L. Tobias. Brunner/Mazel, New York, 1990. $25.00 hard, 208 pages.

The Psychotherapist's Guide to Psychopharmacology. Michael J. Gitlin, M.D., The Free Press, New York, 1990. $35.00, 410 pages.

Racism. Robert Miles. Routledge, Chapman & Hall, New York, 1989. $11.95 paper, 158 pages.

Rat Man. Stuart Schneiderman. New York University Press, New York and London, 1987. $25.00 hard, $15.00 paper, 115 pages.

Realms of Strife: The Memoirs of Juan Goytisolo, 1957–1982. North Point Press, Berkeley, California, 1990. $19.95 hard, 261 pages.

Recognizing Child Abuse: A Guide to the Concerned. Douglas J. Besharov. The Free Press, New York, 1990. 270 pages.

Reconstructing Schizophrenia. Richard P. Bentall (Editor). Routledge, New York, 1990. $49.95 hard, 308 pages.

Recovering the Soul: A Scientific and Spiritual Search. Larry Dossey, M.D. Bantam Books, New York, 1989. $9.95 paper, 321 pages.

Relativized Minimality (Linguistic Inquiry Monograph Sixteen). Luigi Rizzi. The MIT Press, Cambridge, Massachusetts, 1990. $14.95 paper, 147 pages.

Schizophrenia: Treatment of Acute Psychotic Episodes. Steven T. Levy, M.D. and Philip T. Ninan (Editors). American Psychiatric Press, Inc., Washington, D.C., 1990. $34.50 hard, 223 pages.

Schooling: The Developing Child. Sylvia Farnham-Diggory. Harvard University Press, Cambridge, Massachusetts, 1990. $17.95 hard, $8.95 paper, 236 pages.

The Science of Mind. Kenneth Klivington. The MIT Press, Cambridge, Massachusetts, 1990. $39.95 hard, 239 pages.

Seeing Voices. Oliver Sacks. University of California Press, Berkeley, 1989. $15.95 hard, 180 pages.

Selecting Effective Treatments. Linda Seligman. Jossey-Bass, San Francisco, 1990. $29.95 hard, 408 pages.

Separation and the Very Young. James and Joyce Robertson. Columbia University Press, New York, 1989. $40.00 hard, 242 pages.

Sex Differences in Depression. Susan Nolen-Hoeksema. Stanford University Press, Stanford, 1990. $25.00 hard, 258 pages.

Sexual Personae: Art and Decadence from Nefertiti to Emily Dickinson. Camille Paglia. Yale University Press, New Haven, Connecticut, 1990. $35.00 hard, 718 pages.

Sexuality and the Devil: Symbols of Love, Power, and Fear in Male Psychology. Edward J. Tejirian. Routledge, New York, 1990. $29.95 hard, 254 pages.

Single Session Therapy: Maximizing the Effect of the First (and Often Only) Therapeutic Encounter. Moshe Talmon. Jossey-Bass, Inc., San Francisco, California, 1990. $29.95 hard, 146 pages.

Solving the Puzzle of Your Hard-To-Raise Child. William G. Crook, M.D. and Lura Stevens. Professional Books, Jackson, Tennessee.

Staying the Course: The Emotional and Social Lives of Men Who Do Well at Work. Robert S. Weiss. The Free Press, New York, 1990. $24.95 hard, 314 pages.

Step Workbook for Adolescent Chemical Dependency Recovery: A Guide to the First Five Steps. Steven L. Jaffe. American Psychiatric Press, Inc., Washington, D.C., 1990. $45.00 paper, 60 pages.

The Structure of Love. Alan Soble. Yale University Press, New Haven, Connecticut, 1990. $32.50 hard, 374 pages.

Suicide and Ethnicity in the United States (GAP Report No. 128). Group for the Advancement of Psychiatry Committee on Cultural Psychiatry. Brunner/Mazel, New York, 1990. $21.95 hard, $15.95 paper, 148 pages.

Superpersonalities: The People Inside Us. John Rowan. Routledge, Chapman & Hall, 1990. $14.95 paper, 242 pages.

Symbol and Image in Celtic Religious Art. Miranda Green. Routledge, Chapman & Hall, New York, 1990. $45.00 hard, 279 pages.

Sympathy. Jean Ambrosi. Vantage Press, New York, 1990. $13.95 hard, 117 pages.

Systemic Treatment of Incest: A Therapeutic Handbook (Brunner/Mazel Psychological Stress Series, No. 13). Mary S. Trepper and Mary Jo Barrett. Brunner/Mazel, New York, 1989. $30.00 hard, 288 pages.

Theoretical Perspectives on Language Deficits. Yosef Grodzinsky. The MIT Press, Cambridge, Massachusetts, 1990. $25.00 hard, 192 pages.

Theories of Creativity. Mark A. Runco and Robert S. Albert (Editors). Sage Publications, Newbury Park, California, 1990. $36.00 hard, $17.95 soft, 276 pages.

A Theory of Content and Other Essays. Jerry A. Fodor. The MIT Press, Cambridge, Massachusetts, 1990. $29.95 hard, 270 pages.

These Tools. Francis Diaz Hernandez. Vantage Press, New York, 1990. $7.95 hard, 40 pages.

Thoughtful Foragers: A Study of Prehistoric Decision Making. Steven J. Mithen. Cambridge University Press, New York, 1990. $59.50 hard, 290 pages.

Time and Mind: The Study of Time VI. J.T. Fraser (Editor). International Universities Press, Madison, Connecticut, 1990. $37.50 hard, 314 pages.

Trancework: An Introduction to the Practice of Clinical Hypnosis. Michael D. Yapko. Brunner/Mazel, New York, 1990. $42.50 hard, 480 pages.

Transitions 2: Music to Help Baby Sleep (Compact Disk Womb Sound Musical Recording). Placenta Music, Inc., Atlanta, Georgia, 1990. $14.98 CD, $10.98 Cassette.

Trauma, Transformation and Healing: An Integrative Approach to Theory, Research, and Post-Traumatic Therapy (Brunner/Mazel Psychological Stress Series No. 14). John P. Wilson. Brunner/Mazel, New York, 1989. $40.00 hard, 368 pages.

Unintended Thought. James S. Uleman and John A. Bargh (Editors). The Guilford Press, New York, 1989. $45.00 hard, 469 pages.

Virginia Woolf: The Impact of Childhood Sexual Abuse on Her Life and Work. Louise DeSalvo. Beacon Press, Boston, 1989. $22.95 hard, 372 pages.

Where the Spirits Ride the Wind: Trance Journeys and Other Ecstatic Experiences. Felicitas D. Goodman. Indiana University Press, Bloomington, Indiana, 1990. $35.00 hard, $12.95 paper, 256 pages.

Wittgenstein's Philosophy of Psychology. Malcolm Budd. Routledge, Chapman & Hall, New York, 1990. $39.95 hard, 186 pages.

The Workings of the Brain: Development, Memory, and Perception (Readings from *Scientific American Magazine*). Rodolfo R. Llinas (Editor). W.H. Freeman and Company, New York, 1990. $11.95 paper, 173 pages.

A World of Propensities. Karl R. Popper. Thoemmes Antiquarian Books, Bristol, England, 1990. £5.00 paper, 64 pages.

AUTHOR INDEX VOLUME 11

NETWORK AGAINST COERCIVE PSYCHIATRY
172 West 79th Street, #2E
New York, NY 10024

The Network Against Coercive Psychiatry is an organization comprised of psychotherapists (including psychiatrists), survivors of psychiatric incarceration (commonly known as "mental patients"), scholars and other concerned citizens. Our position is uncompromising. We believe the "mental health" Establishment has conned the American people. The idea of "mental illness" is a misleading and degrading metaphor. "Psychiatric treatments" in mental hospitals are for the most part forms of physical and emotional abuse. Psychiatric "diagnoses" are demeaning labels without any scientific validity. The psychiatric Establishment is pushing dangerous drugs which they euphemistically term "medication." Treatments in this century have ranged from revolving chairs to lobotomies to electrical assaults on the human brain to neurologically damaging drugs. There has been no revolution in the treatment of individuals who are psychiatrically labeled: it is an unbroken history of barbaric practices, justified by professionals as medical procedures designed to control patients' ostensible mental diseases.

The Network is emerging at an historical juncture that constitutes a time of potential danger as well as opportunity. The danger lies in the continued expansion of psychiatric power and of the merger of the "mental health" system with the American government. This forebodes a social control apparatus as totalitarian as that foreseen by George Orwell in *1984*. In this case conformity to social norms would be enforced by mental health professionals playing the role of Big Brother.

For well over thirty years a number of theorists and therapists have been writing devastating critiques of the medical model of human behavior. Thomas Szasz was the first to argue that to describe individuals who are having "problems in life" as "mentally ill" is to use a metaphor that is misleading and demeaning. It obscures the individual's real problems and it serves to justify psychiatric coercion and the gratuitous deprivation of individual liberty. R.D. Laing, the British psychiatrist, argued that "psychiatric treatment" of "schizophrenia" typically aborts what is essentially a natural process tending toward the reconstitution of the self on a more mature level. Theodore Sarbin and James Mancuso conclude in their exhaustive study that despite over 80 years of popularity the "disease model" has failed to establish its value as either an explanatory theory or a practical tool. Family therapists like Jay Haley, Salvador Minuchin and the Mental Research Institute have demonstrated the extraordinary success of an approach that is not based on the metaphor of mental illness. These theorists/practitioners have had virtually no effect on public policy.

The American public is aware through exposure to a variety of documentary materials — including such realistic works of the imagination as *One Flew Over the Cuckoo's Nest* by Ken Kesey — that "mental health" professionals in the public sector in another era abused the authority vested in them. The public has not confronted the fact — and the media has not exposed the fact — that the same kind of monstrous abuse of power is occurring right now. If the radical humanitarian changes advocated by the critics of the mental health system are to be implemented, it will be because the American people will begin to realize that they have been abused and mystified by the mental health professions and because they will seize the opportunity to assert their rights and to demand accountability from those who claim to serve them.

Psychiatric survivors have been organizing for human rights and against psychiatric oppression since the mid-1970s. George Ebert, a psychiatric survivor, recently described the reason for his twelve year involvement in the movement against psychiatric oppression. "As long as the psychiatric state remains, as long as people are being tortured, oppressed, dehumanized, and denied ownership of their lives, we who have survived are obligated to struggle to break the silence." The Network Against Coercive Psychiatry calls upon all socially conscious persons to join the movement.

For more information: Manhattan (212) 799-9026

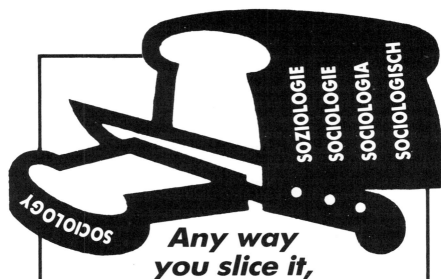

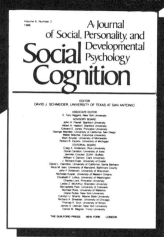

Volume 8, Number 4 – 1988-89

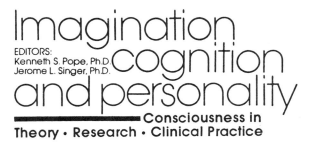

EDITORS:
Kenneth S. Pope, Ph.D.
Jerome L. Singer, Ph.D.

Consciousness in
Theory • Research • Clinical Practice

Assessing the Phenomenological Effects of Several Stress Management Strategies
Ronald J. Pekala, Elizabeth J. Forbes, and Patricia A. Contrisciani

The Relationship between Planned and Actual Responses to
Hypnotic Suggestions
Donald R. Gorassini

Sampling Conscious Thought: Influences of Repression—Sensitization and
Reporting Conditions
George A. Bonanno

A Circadian Rhythm in the Frequency of Spontaneous Task-Unrelated Images
and Thoughts
*Leonard M. Giambra, Edwin H Rosenberg, Siegfried Kasper, William Yee, and
David A. Sack*

Cognitive Complexity and Creativity
Steve Charlton and Paul Bakan

Understanding William James's Conception of Consciousness with the Help of
Gerald E. Myers
Thomas Natsoulas

This *Journal* presents thoughtful explorations of the flow of images, fantasies, memory
fragments and anticipations, which constitute our moment-to-moment experience of
awareness. It presents original scientific research examining the relationship of consciousness
to brain structure and function, to sensory process, to human development, to aesthetic
experience, and to the flow of life events.

ISSN 0276-2366
INSTITUTIONAL PRICE: $87.00
INDIVIDUAL PRICE: $36.00 (Paid by personal check or credit card.) Add $4.50
for postage in the U.S.A. and Canada and $9.35 elsewhere. Subscription per
volume only (4 issues), must be prepaid in U.S. dollars on a U.S. bank. Prices
subject to change without notice.

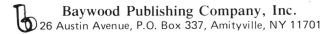
Baywood Publishing Company, Inc.
26 Austin Avenue, P.O. Box 337, Amityville, NY 11701   IC8T

British Journal of Social Psychology
Special Issue on Social processes in small groups

Call for Papers

Empirical, theoretical, or review papers are invited for a special issue of the journal dedicated to social processes in small groups. Papers may deal with any aspect of small group behaviour, but we particularly welcome contributions that reflect new theoretical perspectives on small groups, illustrate innovative methods for investigating such groups, or focus on types of groups that are not often studied. Further information about this special issue can be obtained from the Guest Editors.

Closing date for submissions: 30 June 1991

Papers should be prepared in accordance with APA guidelines, and submitted in quadruplicate to the relevant Guest Editor. Any papers that cannot be included in the special issue will automatically be considered for publication in regular issues of the journal, unless authors expressly decline this option.

Submissions should be addressed to: Michael A. Hogg, Department of Psychology, University of Queensland, Brisbane, QLD 4067, AUSTRALIA.

Submissions from North America should be addressed to: Richard L. Moreland, Department of Psychology, University of Pittsburgh, 432 Langley Hall, Pittsburgh, PA 15260, USA.

The **British Journal of Social Psychology** is published quarterly. Volume 30 (1991) is available price £73 (US$142) from **The British Psychological Society**, The Distribution Centre, Blackhorse Road, Letchworth, Herts. SG6 1HN, UK. Special prices are available for individual members of related societies.

British Journal of Developmental Psychology
Special Edition, 1992: Developmental Psychology in Europe:
An agenda for the 1990s

Call for Papers

The Journal is producing a Special Edition in 1992, edited by Robert Grieve, University of Edinburgh, devoted to: Developmental psychology in Europe: An agenda for the 1990s. Papers are now invited. Authors are encouraged to adopt a broad perspective, and write papers which address research topics thought likely to feature notably during the 1990s, for theoretical, methodological, applied and/or policy reasons.

Papers in any area of research in developmental psychology will be considered. Papers (single or joint authored) from any one country in Europe, or collaborative papers by several authors from more than one country, will be welcomed, as will papers concerned with collaborative research between Europe and other continents. Papers on interdisciplinary approaches to aspects of developmental psychology in Europe in the 1990s will be particularly welcomed.

Papers should be submitted to the **British Journal of Developmental Psychology**, Editorial Office, 13A Church Lane, London N2 8DX, England, and marked 'Special Edition, Europe, 1992'.

The deadline for submissions is 30 September 1991.

The **British Journal of Developmental Psychology** is published quarterly. Volume 9 (1991) price £70 (US$137) is available from The British Psychological Society, The Distribution Centre, Blackhorse Road, Letchworth, Herts. SG6 1HN, UK. Special prices are available for individual members of related societies.